Experimental
Hepatocarcinogenesis

Experimental Hepatocarcinogenesis

Edited by

M. B. Roberfroid

and

V. Préat

Université Catholique de Louvain
Brussels, Belgium

Plenum Press • New York and London

Library of Congress Cataloging in Publication Data

European Meeting on Experimental Hepatocarcinogenesis (2nd: 1987: Spa, Belgium)
   Experimental hepatocarcinogenesis.

   "Proceedings of a European Meeting on Experimental Hepatocarcinogenesis, held
May 27–30, 1987, in Spa, Belgium" – T. p. verso.
   Includes bibliographies and index.
   1. Liver – Cancer – Congresses. 2. Carcinogenesis – Congresses. 3. Liver – Cancer –
Animal models – Congresses. 4. Oncology, Experimental – Congresses. I. Roberfroid,
M. B. II. Préat, V. III. Title. [DNLM: Liver Neoplasms, Experimental – Congresses. W3
EU886F 2nd 1987e 1 WI 735 E887 1987e]
RC280.L5E97 1987   616.99′436   87-35725
ISBN-13: 978-1-4612-8264-8   e-ISBN-13: 978-1-4613-0957-4
DOI: 10.1007/978-1-4613-0957-4

Proceedings of a European Meeting on Experimental Hepatocarcinogenesis,
held May 27–30, 1987, in Spa, Belgium

© 1988 Plenum Press, New York
A Division of Plenum Publishing Corporation
233 Spring Street, New York, N.Y. 10013
Softcover reprint of the hardcover 1st edition 1988

PREFACE

        The meeting on experimental hepatocarcinogenesis
which took place in Spa, Belgium at the end of May 1987 was
the Second European Meeting. About 100 scientists, mostly
from Europe but also from the United States, met there for
three days in a very friendly atmosphere to exchange knowledge
and ideas on experimental and human liver carcinogenesis. The
main topics discussed during the meeting included general
reviews on hepatocarcinogenesis, experimental models of hepatocarcinogenesis, biology of hepatocarcinogenesis, and in
vitro studies in hepatocarcinogenesis. They are all covered by
the various chapters of this proceedings volume, which
reflects the present state of knowledge in this important
field of cancer research.

        The final aim of that research is to understand the
basic mechanisms of carcinogenesis. The liver offers a particularly interesting tool to reach such a goal. Indeed, its
biochemistry, its morphology, and its physiology are very
diverse, but relatively well known. Various protocols have
been developed to produce hepatocellular carcinomas or other
malignant tumors. Their appearance is most often preceded by
phenotypically altered foci and nodules which have been
isolated and characterized. The major cell populations of
normal, neoplastic, and malignant livers have been cultivated.

        Once again the major conclusion of the meeting was the
complexity of the carcinogenic process. More than ever, it has
become clear that understanding the carcinogenic process will
require collecting and integrating information and discoveries
from different disciplines. Even though we each have to speci-
alize in order to obtain the most detailed and complete information possible, at the same time, we have to be very
open-minded and try to understand each other's results. No one
single discipline alone will give the explanation we are
looking for. The cancer problem is at the heart of the major
biological problems, it involves all the complexity of life.

        Keeping that in mind, all the participants helped
create during the meeting, an atmosphere of modesty and since-
rity, which made all discussion very fruitful and highly

constructive. Various projects of mutual exchanges and collaboration were discussed, which are the best guarantees for
further progress. We hope that greater advances will be
presented at the next meeting, which is expected to take place
in the near future. Thanks to our Hungarian colleagues, who
have made a very attractive offer to organize the Third
European Meeting on Hepatocarcinogenesis in their country. On
behalf of the international organizing committee, I invite you
to join us in 1990.

Prof. M. Roberfroid

CONTENTS

Preface 1

EXPERIMENTAL AND HUMAN LIVER CARCINOGENESIS :
CAUSE AND MODULATION

Hepatocarcinogens 5
   H. Neuman

The Induction of Localized Tumors by Carcinogens
   Implanted into the Liver 15
   K. Aterman

Two Stage Theory of Carcinogenesis : a critical review
   Introducing the Concept of Modulation   29
   M. Roberfroid

Modulating Factors of Hepatocarcinogenesis 41
   V. Préat and N. Delzenne

Sex Hormones as Modulators of Liver Tumor Development . 51
   S.D. Vesselinovitch, N. Mihailovich and S. Negri

Liver Cancer and Viruses 63
   Z. Schaff and K. Lapis

MORPHOLOGICAL ALTERATIONS DURING LIVER CARCINOGENESIS

Metabolic Zonation of the Liver 79
   K. Jungermann

Cellular Differentiation during Neoplastic Develop-
   ment in the Liver 89
   P. Bannasch, H. Enzmann, Y. Ruan, E. Weber and
   H. Zerban

Histochemical Analysis of Hepatocarcinogenesis 105
   H.J. Hacker, G. Seelman-Eggebert, F. Klimek,
   P. Peschke and R. Kletzien

CELL PROLIFERATION, CELL DEATH AND LIVER CARCINOGENESIS

Cell Proliferation and Hepatocarcinogenesis 121
   H.M. Rabes

Initiation of Chemical Hepatocarcinogenesis : Compen-
    satory Cell Proliferation versus Mitogen Induced
    Hyperplasia 133
    A. Columbano, G.M. Ledda-Columbano, P. Coni, D.S.R.
    ' Sarma and P. Pani

Cell Death (Apoptosis) in Normal and Preneoplastic Liver
    Tissue 143
    W. Bursch and R. Schulte-Hermann

        BIOCHEMICAL ALTERATIONS DURING LIVER CARCINOGENESIS

A Study of the Activities of Carbohydrate Metabo-
    lizing. Enzymes and the Levels of Carbohydrate
    Metabolites and Amino Acids in Normal Liver
    and in Hepatocellular Carcinoma 163
    V. Gerbracht, E. Roth, K. Becker, M. Reinacher and
    E. Eigenbrodt

The Expression of Cell Surface Receptors in Regene-
    rating and Neoplastic Liver Tissue 175
    L. Eriksson, P. Rissler, N. Andersson, Ch. Möller,
    G. Norstedt and G. Andersson

Cholesterol Metabolism during Cell Proliferation 185
    P. Pani, S. Dessi, B. Batetta

Mechanism of the Inhibition of Liver Carcinogenesis
    Promotion by S-adenosyl-L-methionine 195
    F. Feo, R. Garcea, L. Daino and R. Pascale

    NUCLEAR AND GENETIC ALTERATIONS DURING LIVER CARCINOGENESIS

Long Term Effect of Diethylnitrosamine (DEN) on the
    Production of Micronuclei in Precancerous Rat
    Liver 211
    H. Barbason, B. Bouzahzah, S. Massart, D. Brumioul,
    B. Robaye and Ch. Herens

Nuclear Alterations during Hepatocarcinogenesis :
    Promotion by 2-acetylaminofluorene 221
    P. Seglen, G. Saeter and P. Schwarze

Cytogenetic and Genetic Alterations during Hepato-
    carcinogenesis 231
    M. Kirsch-Volders, S. Haesen, A. Deleener, Ph. Cas-
    telain, M. Alexandre and V. Préat

Role of Oncogenes in Hepatocarcinogenesis 245
    C. Guguen-Guillouzo, G. Baffet, P.L. Etienne, D.
    Glaise, N. Defer, M. Corral, D. Corcos and J. Kruh

            IN VITRO STUDIES IN LIVER CARCINOGENESIS

Separation and Biochemical Characterization of Rat
    Liver Parenchymal Cell Subpopulations 257
    P. Steinberg, B. Seibert and F. Oesch

Growth Control of Hepatocytes, their Immortalization
    and Transformation by Transforming Genes of
    Polyoma Virus and of SV40 Virus 267
    D. Paul

Changes in Hepatocyte TGFβ Receptors and Gene Expres-
    sion during Normal and Neoplastic Liver Growth ... 275
    B.L. Carr, R.H. Whitson and K. Itakura

Regulation of Carbohydrate Metabolism in a Glycogen-
    storing Liver Cell Line 283
    D. Mayer

Techniques in Measuring DNA Synthesis and Mitosis Induced
    by Tumor Promoters in Hepatocytes Primary Cultu-
    res 297
    W. Parzefall and F.A. Puhringer

CONCLUSIONS

Concluding Remarks 309
    R. Schulte Hermann

Contributors 313

Index 317

INTRODUCTION

EXPERIMENTAL AND HUMAN LIVER CARCINOGENESIS : CAUSE AND MODULATION

HEPATOCARCINOGENS

Hans-Günther Neuman

Institute of Pharmacology and Toxicology,

University of Würzburg, Fed.Rep.Germany

INTRODUCTION

According to a recent worldwide survey, liver cancer ranks seventh among tumors in males and ninth in females.[1] Only a few agents have so far been associated more directly with the development of these tumors in man. Among them are: aflatoxins, cycasin, vinyl chloride, and estrogens, agents of quite different chemical nature. In experimental animals, mostly the rat and the mouse, quite a number of diverse chemicals have been demonstrated to produce liver tumors. Accordingly, such chemicals are called hepatocarcinogens.

In order to demonstrate carcinogenic potential, the compounds are usually administered over an extended period of time either mixed into the feed or the drinking water or, occasionally they are given by gavage if the compound is unstable or exact dosing is intended. It is, however, also possible to produce rat liver tumors with a single or a few doses of a potent hepatocarcinogen.[2,3] This would indicate that the whole process of carcinogenesis, which may include a long latency period until finally a malignant tumor develops, is triggered by the primary lesion. Although different phases can be morphologically distinguished, some feel that this does not necessarily mean that different stages exist which depend on separate actions of the chemical. According to this supposition, all the necessary lesions are produced at or shortly after the administration of the compound. Thereafter, transformed cells are only subject to endogenous growth control (or factors modulating that control). Within this framework a single lesion, presumably of genotoxic nature, could suffice to explain the effects of a hepatocarcinogen.

However, experimental data are accumulating which suggest that tumors develop in a multi-stage process and chemicals exist which affect predominantly only one or another of these stages. This concept was originally derived from the initiation-promotion type of experiments on mouse skin, which was later extended to rat liver as well.[4] This concept implies that chemicals with initiating properties produce effects in the target cells which are different from those exerted by chemicals with promoting

properties. Typically, the latter effect their action on initiated cells and therefore after initiation. This raises the
question as to whether complete hepatocarcinogens have multiple
properties and how these could become effective in single or
oligo dose experiments. Serious objections have been raised
against the multi-stage concept, one of the arguments being that
there are no pure initiators or pure promoters, there are only
strong and weak carcinogens.[5]

A classical model hepatocarcinogen is 2-acetylaminofluorene
(AAF). When AAF was fed at a level of 0.02% in the diet to
weanling male Sprague-Dawley rats for a short period of time (18
d), 20-30% of the animals developed liver tumors.[6] This demonstrates that AAF is a complete liver carcinogen. When this
treatment was followed by feeding DDT, tumor incidence increased
to almost 100% within the same time. DDT alone did not produce
any tumors and was therefore designated a promoter in these
experiments.[6] What is the basis for the tumor promoting effect -
a weak genotoxic effect, an unspecific cytotoxic effect or a
specific effect related neither to direct DNA-damage nor to cell
killing?

We became interested in these questions when we compared
the properties of different aromatic amines, all of which yield
genotoxic metabolites which bind to DNA in rat liver and yet
are not all hepatocarcinogens. Among AAF, trans-4-acetylamino-
stilbene (AAS) and 2-acetylaminophenanthrene (AAP) only AAF is a
complete rat liver carcinogen. AAS and AAP are strong initiators
in this system, which makes it difficult to call them weak liver
carcinogens, but seem to lack some properties necessary to make
them liver tumor promoters. The results which will be discussed
in this brief overview suggest that complete aromatic amine
hepatocarcinogens in addition to their direct genotoxic potential have promoting activity which is unrelated to metabolic
activation and is possibly receptor mediated.

DNA-DAMAGE IS NOT CORRELATED WITH HEPATOCARCINOGENESIS

A major argument against the notion that a single early
effect, genotoxic in nature, is sufficient to trigger the whole
process of hepatocarcinogenesis is the lack of correlation between DNA-damage and tumor formation. The metabolic activation of
aromatic amines has been thoroughly studied and many of the
primary reaction products with nucleic acids held to be responsible for genotoxic effects such as gene mutations and chromosomal defects are known.[7,8] After oral administration to rats AAF,
AAS and AAP yield similar amounts of DNA adducts. Actually,
higher doses of AAF are required to obtain the same number of
adducts than with AAS.[9] However, the structures of the adducts
are not the same, and their genotoxic effects may vary. We have
recently identified a number of AAS-adducts, among them cyclic
adducts hitherto unknown for aromatic amines.[10,11] In addition,
we have collected data which indicate that AAS, but not AAF,
produces DNA-DNA cross links. These results could explain the
generally higher mutagenicity of AAS in in vitro test systems if
compared to other aromatic amines, and it would be highly unexpected if these DNA modifications were not relevant for the
generation of rat liver tumors.

In order to clarify this point, AAS was tested as an initiator in an initiation-promotion experiment in female Wistar rats.[12] When initiating doses of AAS were followed by partial hepatectomy and/or liver promoters such as phenobarbital, DDT or diethylstilbestrol, preneoplastic lesions and liver tumors developed. This proves that AAS is able to initiate rat liver cells. Does it also prove that AAS is a pure initiator in this tissue?

A positive answer to this question is supported by the results of another initiation-promotion experiment in which we tried to demonstrate that AAS also initiates cells in rat kidneys. Initiating doses of AAS were followed by unilateral nephrectomy and/or nephrotoxic antibiotics. With unilateral nephrectomy alone, three tumors were observed in the remaining kidneys of two out of ten animals. With ß-cyclodextrin five kidney tumors in 3/10 animals were observed. Unilateral nephrectomy plus gentamycin produced a total of nine tumors in 3/10 animals. Some animals developed ear duct tumors which are typical for AAS, but in none of the animals could we find preneoplastic foci, neoplastic nodules or tumors in the liver. The initiating dose (4 x 20µmol/kg) of AAS given was sufficient to produce ear duct tumors but clearly did not produce any morphologically recognizable liver lesions within the 88 weeks of this experiment (Hoffmann et al., unpublished results).

AAS was not hepatocarcinogenic in the two initiation-promotion experiments described, but initiated cells in liver and kidney, and most likely in other tissues as well. With regard to liver and kidney, AAS may be called a pure initiator.

Similarly, AAF and AAP have been compared. The amount of compound acutely und persistently bound to rat liver DNA is comparable for the two compounds following single injections into adult Fischer rats[13] or weanling Sprague-Dawley rats[14]. Administration of AAP to weanling Sprague-Dawley rats, however, failed to initiate liver tumors.[14] More recently, liver tumors were obtained in male Fischer rats when the initiating treatment with AAP was followed by partial hepatectomy and DDT feeding (N.K.Scribner, personal communication).

The initiating potency of various acetamides was directly compared in another initiation-promotion experiment.[15] Weanling male Fischer rats were given the compound at different dose levels as a single oral dose. Two weeks later all animals were treated with a single dose of AAF (30 mg/100g) in order to raise the background of GGT-positive foci to an observable level. Another week later a partial hepatectomy was performed followed after 2 weeks by feeding DDT for 6 weeks. With GGT-positive foci as an endpoint, the initiating potencies were ranked in the order AAS ≫ AAP > AAF > AABP.

The DNA adduct pattern and the time course of adduct elimination was compared in male Sprague-Dawley rats after single injections of the N-hydroxy derivatives (40 mg/kg) of the last three amides mentioned above.[16] Total binding to DNA was highest for the hepatocarcinogen N-hydroxy-AAF only at 1.5 h (159 fmol/µg); at 24 h it was 51, 62, and 5 fmol/µg, respectively, for N-hydroxy-AAF, N-hydroxy-AAP, and N-hydroxy-AABP; at 9 days it was highest for the non-hepatocarcinogen N-hydroxy-AAP (36 fmol/µg).

Another example is 2-methyl-4-dimethylaminoazobenzene (2-

Me-DAB). Metabolites bind to rat liver DNA and the level of persistent adducts is comparable to those of hepatocarcinogenic azo dyes. Yet, 2-Me-DAB is not carcinogenic even after prolonged periods of feeding. It can, however, produce liver tumors when proliferation is stimulated by partial hepatectomy or when phenobarbital is applied as a promoter.[17,18] The compound has been called a weak carcinogen, or a good initiator with only weak promoting properties[18], and has been proposed for use in initiation-promotion studies as a "pure initiator".[19]

The ever increasing accumulation of information appears to indicate that DNA-damage as we measure it in the form of (persistent) base adducts does correlate with an early genotoxic effect related to initiation, but not with hepatocarcinogenesis.

WHAT IS THE DIFFERENCE BETWEEN INITIATORS AND COMPLETE HEPATOCARCINOGENS?

The answer most frequently given to this question is: a complete hepatocarcinogen has to be cytotoxic. However, there is a complete lack of understanding as to how toxicity is brought about, and there are conceptual differences behind this general term. On the one hand, toxicity is considered to produce a proliferative stimulus which, like partial hepatectomy, is necessary to complete the process of initiation in a tissue such as liver with a low rate of cell replication. On the other hand toxicity is considered to produce selective pressure under which initiated cells grow more favourably than normal cells.

Agents with liver tumor promoting properties are often assigned to two different classes:[20] (1) Those which normally do not produce acute signs of toxicity in liver but are able to induce liver growth by hyperplasia and/or hypertrophy (hormones and compounds with hormon-like effects belong to this class) and (2) hepatocarcinogens ("complete" carcinogens) or diets which cause massive necrosis or shorten the life-span of hepatocytes if toxic damage develops more slowly. Phenobarbital belongs to the first category and is thought to promote by increase in cell proliferation, inhibition of cell death and enhanced expression or stabilization of the altered phenotype. AAF is considered to be hepatotoxic, thereby creating a cell deficit and subsequently a growth stimulus for the remaining liver cells. Most advanced is the resistant cell hypothesis which is based on the observation that hepatocytes in foci or nodules exhibit a remarkable resistance to cytotoxic effects of AAF and other hepatotoxins.[21] It appears important therefore to look more closely into the role and mechanism of cytotoxicity.

THE ACUTE TOXICITY OF AROMATIC AMINES

Some early observations were published by Laird and Barton.[22] They noted that in the first 4 - 8 weeks during continuous feeding of 0.045 - 0.06% AAF no significant change in the total number of liver cells occurs, and necrosis cannot be found. Thereafter, cell proliferation sets in and the number of liver cells increases at a constant rate. In the initial lag period of cell multiplication liver weight actually decreases. This decrease in liver weight was later interpreted as a clear indication of liver damage and necrosis.[23] Studying the fine structure of rat hepatocytes during the early phases of chronic AAF intoxication, Flaks[24] did not observe necrosis but rather what now is considered typical for enzyme inducing liver tumor promoters. Others noted a replacement of the functional hepatocytes by oval cells.[25] The cirrhotic reactions coincide with an increase of DNA synthesis, which, however, starts only some 42 d after the beginning of AAF feeding. Histological and biochemical evidence for early cell death was not obtained. Although AAF generally is said to be acutely hepatotoxic, the early effects appear not to be well documented.

Although AAS is acutely toxic and kills the animals by damaging the glandular stomach, thereby inducing severe bleeding, we were not able to detect acute toxic effects in rat liver with lethal doses.[26,27] This is the more surprising since metabolites react to a greater extent with nucleic acids and proteins in liver than in the glandular stomach[27] and also more so than those of AAF[9]. We therefore looked for differences in "nonbinding" reactions which could explain the different hepatotoxicity of AAF and AAS. One possibility would be the generation of radicals or reactive oxygen species by redox cycling[28]. To test this hypothesis, the efflux of oxidized glutathione from liver into the bile of animals with cannulated bile ducts was measured after i.p. injection of the test compounds (Hillesheim and Neumann, unpublished results). A single injection of AAS, AAF, 2-aminofluorene (AF), trans-4-aminostilbene (AS) or paracetamol into adult female Wistar rats did not increase the efflux of oxidized glutathione. The doses of AAF and AAS (1 mmol/kg) were higher than those usually administered for tumor induction but no signs of acute liver toxicity were evident from blood analysis. The same doses of the amines, AF and AS, were toxic for the animals and the experiment could not be continued for 4 h under comparable conditions, but this could not be attributed to effects in the liver. With lower doses (0.1 mmol/kg) the efflux of oxidized glutathione was not increased, nor was it elevated with massive doses of paracetamol (2.65 mmol/kg). A negative result with toxic doses of paracetamol was also obtained by Smith and Mitchell.[29] Menadione is a classical redox-cycler and was used as a positive control in our experiments. Much to our surprise doses above 0.4 mmol/kg were necessary to raise the efflux of oxidized glutathione. This demonstrates the high capacity of rat liver to cope with oxidative stress, and we conclude from these results that it is highly unlikely that reactive oxygen causes cytotoxic effects in liver with aromatic amines under almost any conditions relevant in vivo. The causes for acute AAF liver toxicity, if it exists, thus remain to be specified.

SPECIFIC EFFECTS OF AROMATIC AMINES

The last two decades have been dominated by the paradigm that reactive metabolites are responsible for acute toxic and carcinogenic effects caused by aromatic amines and many other xenobiotics. The time now seems ripe to look with less prejudice at the primary reactions and to consider the possibility that chemically unreactive compounds may also interact with cellular constituents.

We have recently observed that the function of the glandular stomach in rats may be impaired by the systemic action of

AAS. With acutely toxic doses metabolic elimination in liver is saturated, more of the parent compound reaches the circulation and accumulates for unknown reasons in this tissue. Stomach functions seem to be impaired for up to 24 h.[27]

More relevant for tumor induction may be the observation made in an initiation-promotion experiment in which we tested the synergistic effects of AAS and AAF as initiators in rat liver.[30] The compounds were administered either alone or sequentially combined. The promotion phase was started by partial hepatectomy followed by phenobarbital added to the drinking water. Enzyme altered foci and hyperplastic nodules were used as biological endpoints. First of all, the biological effects were more than additive in the combination groups. This clearly demonstrates a synergism of the genotoxic effects of the two different chemicals. But secondly, the biological effects depended on the sequence in which the initiators were given. Enzyme altered foci developed much faster when AAF was given after AAS than before AAS. This suggested that the complete hepatocarcinogen AAF in addition to its initiating properties has some other activity acting on AAS-initiated cells. However, it could not be excluded that interactions with metabolism or repair of DNA-damage modified the extent of DNA-lesions on which the applied promoting measures acted. The pattern of DNA-adducts and their total amount at the time when partial hepatectomy was performed was, however, virtually indistinguishable in the combination groups and in those groups in which only one of the compounds was administered during the appropriate time interval.[9] These results indicate that AAF and AAS generate DNA-damage independently of each other under these conditions and that AAF affects the overall biological outcome by effects unrelated to adduct formation.

In a first attempt to demonstrate compound-specific interactions Cikryt and his coworkers studied the affinity of several aromatic amides to the rat hepatic aromatic hydrocarbon (Ah) receptor.[31] AAF and AAP decrease the binding of 2,3,7,8-tetra-chlorodibenzo-p-dioxin (TCDD) to the Ah-receptor in a concentration dependent manner. The 50% inhibition concentration of AAF is 5 μM, that of AAP 13 μM, the apparent inhibition constants, respectively, are 1 and 2.6 μM. AAS and the non-carcinogenic 4-acetylaminofluorene do not compete with TCDD. It is interesting to note that AAF reaches inhibiting concentrations in rat liver cytosol in vivo after a 100 μmol/kg dose.

These authors also studied the inducibility of the Ah-receptor.[32] AAS, although without notable affinity to the receptor, is able to double the receptor concentration in vivo, whereas AAF is inactive in this respect. On the other hand the induction of Ah-receptor related enzymes was determined. AAS was inactive and did not change cytochrome P-450 activities in rat liver. This is in accordance with previous findings showing that the metabolism of aminostilbene derivatives is not altered upon repeated administration.[33] AAF (100 μmol/kg for 5 d) induced ethoxyresorufin-O-deethylase activity 1.3-fold and aryl hydrocarbon hydroxylase activity 1.9-fold in female Wistar rats. Changes of AAF metabolism upon repeated administration have previously been attributed to enzyme induction.[34]

Ornithine decarboxylase (ODC) is another enzyme whose induction is mediated by the Ah-receptor. This has been shown in

mouse liver[35] and has now been studied in rat liver.[36]
AAF, AAS, methylcholanthrene as a positive control and the non-
carcinogen 4-AAF increased ODC activity between 3.6- (MC) and
5.7-fold (AAS). The different time course of induction paralleled, by and large, the cytosolic concentrations of the inducer. ODC induction, therefore, does not correlate with the
apparent promoting properties or the affinity for the Ah receptor of the tested compounds in rat liver.

Although a role of the Ah-receptor in liver tumor promotion
has been suggested, it has not been firmly established. At this
time, however, it should be emphasized that a differential
interaction of the amides with a cellular constituent has been
demonstrated, and that the complete hepatocarcinogen AAF was
most active. The results encourage further work in this direction.

Finally, the results provide a possible explanation for the
above experiments demonstrating the synergistic effects of AAF
and AAS. The combination AAS first and AAF second could be more
efficient than the reverse combination because AAS induces the
Ah receptor to which AAF has the affinity. The promoting effects
of AAF could be enhanced in this way and act upon AAS initiated
cells.

ACKNOWLEDGEMENTS

Work in our laboratory was supported by the Deutsche Forschungsgemeinschaft, SFB 172. The more recent results were generated predominantly by Dr. Roland Franz, Wolfgang Hillesheim
Andre Hoffmann and Mannfred Ruthsatz with the expert help of
Elisabeth Rüb-Spiegel and Ingrid Trnka. Their cooperation is
gratefully acknowledged.

REFERENCES

1. D. M. Parkin, J. Stjernward, and C. S. Muirs, Estimates of
       cancer occurrance throughout the world, International
       Agency for Research on Cancer, Lyon, France (1986).
2. P. Bannasch and H. A. Müller, Lichtmikroskopische Untersu-
       chungen über die Wirkung von N-Nitrosomorpholin auf die
       Leber von Ratte und Maus, Arzneim. Forsch., 14:805
       (1964).
3. P. Bannasch, U. Brenner., H. Enzmann, and H. J. Hacker,
       Tigroid cell foci and neoplastic nodules in the liver of
       rats treated with a single dose of aflatoxin B_1,
       Carcinogenesis 6:1641 (1985).
4. H. C. Pitot and A. E. Sirica, The stages of initiation and
       promotion in hepatocarcinogenesis, Biochim. Biophys. Acta
       605:191 (1980).
5. O. H. Iversen and E. G. Astrup, The paradigm of two-stage
       carcinogenesis: a critical attitude, Cancer Investig.
       2:51 (1984).
6. C. Peraino, R. J. M. Fry, E. Staffeldt, and J. P.
       Christopher, Comparative enhancing effects of phenobarbi-
       tal, amobarbital, diphenylhydantoin, and dichlorodiphenyl-
       trichloroethane on 2-acetylaminofluorene-induced hepatic
       tumorigenesis in the rat, Cancer Res. 35:2884 (1975).

7. H.-G. Neumann, the role of DNA damage in chemical carcinogenesis of aromatic amines, <u>J. Cancer Res. Clin. Oncol.</u> 112:100 (1986).

8. F. F. Kadlubar and F. A. Beland, Chemical properties of ultimate carcinogenic metabolites of arylamines and arylamides, in: R. G. Harvey, ed., Polycyclic Hydrocarbons and Carcinogenesis, ACS Symposium Series, No. 283, American Chemical Society, Washington (1985), pp 341.

9. M. Ruthsatz, R. Franz, and H.-G. Neumann, DNA-damage, initiation and promotion by aromatic amines, in: Primary changes and control factors in carcinogenesis, T. Friedberg and F. Oesch, ed., Deutscher Fachschriften-Verlag, Wiesbaden (1986).

10. R. Franz, H.-R. Schulten, and H.-G. Neumann, Identification of nucleic acid adducts from trans-4-acetylaminostilbene, <u>Chem.-Biol. Interactions</u> 59:281 (1986).

11. R. Franz and H.-G. Neumann, Reaction of trans-4-N-acetoxy-N-acetylaminostilbene with guanosine, deoxyguanosine, RNA and DNA in vitro: predominant product is a cyclic N^2,N3-guanine adduct, <u>Chem.-Biol. Interactions</u> in press.

12. D. Hilpert, W. Romen, and H.-G. Neumann, The role of partial hepatectomy and of promoters in the formation of tumors in non-target tissues of trans-4-acetylaminostilbene in rats, <u>Carcinogenesis</u> 4:1519 (1983).

13. J. D. Scribner and G. Koponen, Binding of the carcinogen 2-acetamidophenanthrene to rat liver nucleic acids: lack of correlation with carcinogenic activity, and failure of the hydroxamic acid ester model for in vivo activation, <u>Chem.-Biol. Interactions</u> 28:201 (1979).

14. J. D. Scribner and N. K. Mottet, DDT acceleration of mammary gland tumors induced in the male Sprague-Dawley rat by 2-acetamidophenanthrene, <u>Carcinogenesis</u> 2:1235 (1981).

15. N. K. Scribner, K. S. Rector, and B. A. Woodworth, Relative orders of initiating potencies of four aromatic amides may be similar in target and in non-target tissues, Proc. Third Intern. Conference on Carcinogenic and Mutagenic N-Substituted Aryl Compounds, Detroit (1987).

16. R. C. Gupta and N. R. Dighe, Formation and removal of DNA adducts in rat liver treated with N-hydroxy derivatives of 2-acetylaminofluorene, 4-acetylaminobiphenyl, and 2-acetylaminophenanthrene, <u>Carcinogenesis</u> 5:343 (1984).

17. G. P. Warwick, The covalent binding of metabolites of tritiated 2-methyl-4-dimethylaminoazobenzene to rat liver nucleic acids and proteins, and the carcinogenicity of the unlabeled compound in partially hepatectomized rats, <u>Eur. J. Cancer</u> 3:227 (1967).

18. T. Kitagawa, H. C. Pitot, E. C. Miller, and J. A. Miller, Promotion by dietary phenobarbital of hepatocarcinogenesis by 2-methyl-N,N-dimethyl-4-aminoazobenzene in the rat, <u>Cancer Res.</u> 39:112 (1979).

19. R. Daoust, Toxic effects of 2-methyl-4-dimethylaminoazobenzene in normal and partially hepatectomized rats, <u>Chem.-Biol. Interactions</u> 48:221 (1984).

20. R. Schulte-Hermann, Tumor promotion in the liver, <u>Arch. Toxicol.</u> 57:147 (1985).

21. E. Farber and R. Cameron, The sequential analysis of cancer development, <u>Adv. Cancer Res.</u> 31:125 (1980).

22. A. K. Laird and A. D. Barton, Cell growth and the development of tumours, <u>Nature</u> (London) 183:1655 (1959).

23. J. C. Arcos and M. F. Argus, Chemical Induction of Cancer, Vol. II B, Academic Press, London (1974), pp 49.

24. B. Flaks, Changes in the fine structure of rat hepatocytes during the early phases of chronic 2-acetylaminofluorene intoxication, Chem.-Biol. Interactions 2:129 (1970).
25. R. E. Albert, F. J. Burns, L. Bilger, D. Gardner, and W. Troll, Cell loss and proliferation induced by N-2-fluorenylacetamide in the rat liver in relation to hepatoma induction, Cancer Res. 32:2172 (1972).
26. P. Marquardt, W. Romen, and H.-G. Neumann, Tissue specific acute toxic effects of the carcinogen trans-4-dimethylaminostilbene, Arch. Toxicol. 56:151 (1985).
27. A. Pfeifer and H.-G. Neumann, Organ specific acute toxicity of the carcinogen trans-4-acetylaminostilbene is not correlated with macromolecular binding, Chem.-Biol. Interactions 59:185 (1986).
28. A. Stier, R. Clauss, A. Lücke, and I. Reitz, Radicals in carcinogenesis by aromatic amines, in: D. C. H. McBrien and T. F. Slater, eds., Free radicals, lipid peroxidation and cancer, Academic Press, London, New York (1982).
29. C. V. Smith and J. R. Mitchell, Acetaminophen hepatotoxicity invivo is not accompanied by oxidant stress, Biochim. Biophys. Res. Commun. 133:329 (1985).
30. J. Kuchlbauer, W. Romen, and H.-G. Neumann, Syncarcinogenic effects on the initiation of rat liver tumors by trans-4-acetylaminostilbene and 2-acetylaminofluorene, Carcinogenesis 6:1337 (1985).
31. P. Cikryt, Cytosolic binding proteins for aromatic hydrocarbons and their affinity for aromatic amines, in: T. Friedberg and F. Oesch, eds., Primary changes and control factors in carcinogenesis, Deutscher Fachschriften-Verlag, Wiesbaden (1986).
32. M. Göttlicher and P. Cikryt, Induction of the aromatic hydrocarbon receptor and of drug metabolizing enzymes by various aromatic amines in rat liver, Naunyn Schmiedeberg's Arch. Pharmacol. 335:R8 Suppl. (1987).
33. H.-G. Neumann, The metabolism of repeatedly administered trans-4-dimethylaminostilbene and 4-dimethylaminobibenzyl, Z. Krebsforsch. 79:60 (1973).
34. A. Aström and J. W. DePierre, Characterization of the induction of drug metabolizing enzymes by 2-acetylaminofluorene, Biochim. Biophys. Acta 673:225 (1981).
35. D. W. Nebert, N. M. Jensen, J. W. Perry, and T. Oka, Association between ornithine decarboxylase induction and the Ah locus in mice treated with polycyclic aromatic compounds, J. Biol. Chem. 255:6836 (1980).
36. M. Göttlicher and P. Cikryt, Induction of ornithine decarboxylase by aromatic amines in rat liver, Cancer Letters 35:65 (1987).

THE INDUCTION OF LOCALIZED TUMOURS BY CARCINOGENS IMPLANTED INTO THE LIVER

Kurt Aterman

Dept. of Biology, University of Brunswick
and
Regional Laboratory, Dr. Everett Chalmers Hospital
Fredericton, N.B., Canada.

The experiment presented here is the third in a series started some 20 years ago (Aterman 1965, 1967), originally with the intention of separating the process of fibrogenesis and scarring in the liver - the result of toxic injury caused by the rather large doses of hepatocarcinogens then used - from the phenomenon of hepatocarcinogenesis proper. It was assumed that the implantation of known hepatocarcinogens into the liver would lead only to a gradual release and metabolisation of the water - insoluble material deposited which, in the low concentrations thus produced, would not cause serious acute liver cell damage and necrosis and therefore would minimize or obviate the subsequent connective tissue proliferation. With luck, it was reasoned, the presence of a persisting depot of carcinogenic material would in time also lead to the development of tumours, as had been shown to be the case in other organs. A few early studies applying that approach to the liver had, however, yielded negative results (Jones et al. 1935, Woglom 1938, Esmarch 1940, Rusch et al. 1940, Shear et al. 1940) and only scanty positive findings (Ilfeld 1936, Oberling et al. 1939, Eisen 1946) in the induction of liver tumours by the application of substances such as 3-methylcholanthrene or benzopyrene had been reported. The tumours, however, were all fibrosarcomas, and no hepatocellular neoplasms had apparently been produced by the local application of hepatocarcinogens - with the doubtful exception of such a tumour in a mouse (Ilfeld 1936 which was questioned already then (Esmarch 1940) as being probably a "spontaneous" tumour in genetically predisposed species.
Kinosita's (1936, 1937, 1940, 1955) classical experiments may well have prejudged the issue when he reported that he had produced hepatocellular tumours in rats by feeding or injecting them with 4-dimethylaminoazobenzene ("butter yellow"), but had failed to do so when this "strongly carcinogenic" substance was introduced directly into the liver. This "negligible response of the liver" (Shear et al. 1940) led in due course to the view that this organ was "surprisingly insensitive" (Berenblum 1974) to the local application of hepatocarcinogens - indeed a surprising

conclusion seeing that the liver is known to be highly
susceptible to hepatocarcinogenesis by diverse carcinogens
given in the food or by injection. No explanation of this
glaring discrepancy had been advanced. It was, moreover,
realized that most of the older experiments could also be
questioned on technical grounds (Aterman 1967) such as the
choice and number of experimental animals, or the use of
solvent substances with possible modifiying effects (Arcos
1968). These considerations contributed to the decision to
reinvestigate the question of hepatocarcinogenesis by local
application. Only the most recent of 3 separate long-term
experiments will be described here. It should, however, be
pointed out that the last two - identical - experiments had
yielded surprisingly congruent results, although they had
been performed almost 10 years apart and in different
locations.

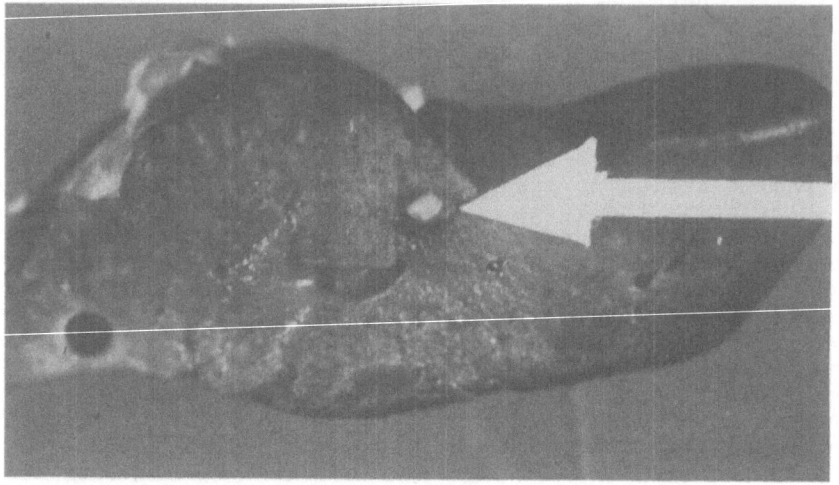

Fig. 1 A pellet of DAB is shown 624 days after implantation.
       There was no gross or micrococoscopic change in the
       liver parenchyma.

This fact tends to support the view that the induction of
localized hepacarcinogenesis should now be considered a
reproducible phenomenon. A more detailed description and
discussion can be found in a recent paper on "Localized
hepatocarcinogenesis" (Aterman 1987).

METHODS

     Pure carcinogens (3-methylcholanthrene (3-M.C.); 4-
dimethylamino-azobenzene (DAB)) and their non-carcinogenic
controls (cholesterol (CHOL); anthracene (ANT); ∝ -naphthy-
lisothiocyanate (ANIT)) were compressed in a pellet press to
yield fairly comparable pellets. No solvent or binding
material whatever was used. A slightly curved incision was
made into one lobe of the exposed rat's liver and the pellet
was inserted underneath the flap of liver tissue thus
created. No anchoring sutures were needed, since the pellet
was retained by the flap and the clotted blood. All the
animals used were recently weaned male Holtzman rats. 11

groups of 5 littermates in each group were chosen for the
main part of the experiment. A pellet of CHOL. was placed
into the liver of the first animal, the second brother
received a pellet of ANT, the third one of ANNIT, the fourth
one of DAB, and the fifth one of 3-M.C. These rats were kept
in individual cages to the end of their lives, so that the
incidence of tumours could be assessed. In the second part
of this experiment, designed to study the evolution of
lesions, groups of rats carrying pellets of 3-M.C. or of DAB
were killed at arbitrary intervals over a period of 44 to 668
days after implantation. At necropsy the presence and
appearance of the pellets was verified in each case, (Fig.
1); multiple sections, placed into formalin, were taken from
the implantation site and the adjacent parenchyma, as well as
from more distant areas of the implanted lobe and the other,
non-involved lobes. The same procedure was followed in the
case of the tumours.

RESULTS

The immediate and the long-term response of the liver to
the implantation of the carcinogenic and the control pellets
(Aterman 1967) did not differ from the response to any other
foreign body (Aterman et al. 1971): Granulation tissue
replaced the initial necrosis and inflammation and was in due
course transformed into a firm connective tissue capsule that
enveloped the entire pellet (Fig. 2).

The carcinogenic pellets also tended to provoke a variable,
lymphocytic infiltrate that was not noticed in the control
implants. This observation needs to be confirmed. A most
unusual response was obtained with implants of ANIT which
provoked an intense outpouring of a largely acellular exudate
around the pellet, and calcification to such a degree that
the pellet came to be surrounded by a distinct shell that
could easily be separated from the surrounding liver. In
none of the control animals, however, did a tumour develop
that could be attributed to the implants.

The situation was radically different when carcinogens
had been implanted. In 10 out of 11 (90.9%) rats that had
received a pellet of 3-M.C. there developed after 202-644
days a large, solitary, fleshy, bosselated tumour with, in
some cases, numerous implantations metastases in the
abdominal cavity. Of the rats with pellets of DAB in the
liver 3 out of 11 (27.2%) animals developed after 484 to 732
days a tumour of a grossly similar appearance. It should be
noted that

    a) all the tumours had formed around the pellet which
    could always be found embedded in the tumour mass,

    b) the tumours involved only the implanted lobe, al-
    though they could invade locally an adjacent lobe.
    The rest of the liver appeared grossly normal. On
    microscopic examination too only occasional foci of
    altered hepatocytes of the types described in ageing
    rats (van Bezooijen 1984, Ward and Obshima 1985) could
    be found, but these changes were also seen to the same
    extent in the control livers. There were not found any

17

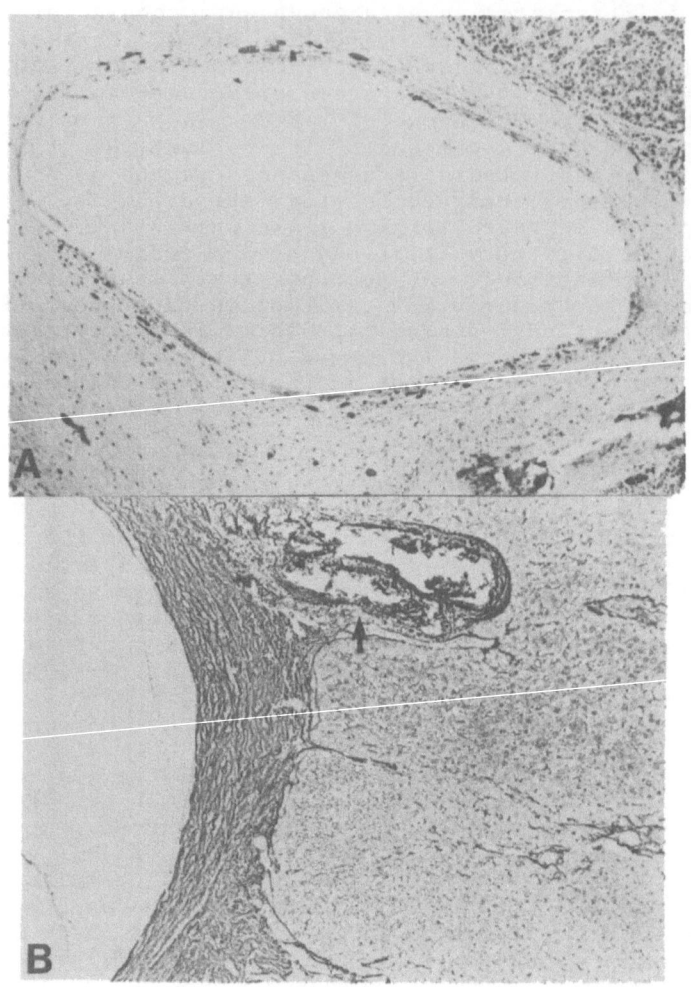

Fig. 2 Showing the firm fibrous tissue capsule around a
pellet of DAB. The arrow (fig. B) points to a
focal deposit of calcium, a common occurence
(A = H.E; B = reticulin stain).

of the other changes frequently described as a feature
accompanying or preceding the development of tumours -
to be more precise, hepatocellular tumours.
Specifically, no cirrhosis (eg. Bannasch, 1969; Orr,
1940), glycogen accumulations (eg. Bannasch, 1967;
Bannasch et al., 1980), "oval cell" proliferations (eg.
Farber, 1956a; Rubin, 1964; Ogawa et al., 1974; Sell et
al., 1981; Ohshima et al., 1984) or "nodule formation"
(eg. Kinosita, 1955; Farber, 1956b, 1973, 1984;
Bannasch, 1976; Hirota and Williams, 1979; Farber and
Cameron, 1980) were seen in any area of the pellet- or
tumour-carrying livers. This applied also to those rats
whose livers were removed at varying time intervals to
observe the evolution of the lesions.

The tumours induced by 3-M.C. had in the past (Aterman 1967) been largely classified as pleomorphic fibrosarcomas, although they would now probably be viewed as "malignant fibrous histiocytomas". They frequently, but not always, showed a characteristic "swirling" arrangement with pleomorphic, active fibroblasts, bizarre giant cells, numerous mitoses, and reticulin and collagen fibres embedded in a variably dense matrix. A striking feature was (Fig. 3) the remarkable variability of their histologic appearance. Beside classical fibrosarcomatous areas with spindle-shaped cells there were distinctly haemangiomatous or even haemangiosarcomatous regions which could alternate with aggregates of distinctly epithelial-like -? histiocytic - cells (Fig. 4), which on occasions strongly resembled the appearance found in hepatomas. In other specimens a cystic dilatation and proliferation of bile ducts could be found (Fig. 5), a phenomenon that in an earlier experiment (Aterman, 1967) had also been accompanied by squamous metaplasia, even metastasizing squamous cell carcinoma formation (ExpII., Aterman, 1987), of the biliary epithelium.

Of even greater interest from our point of view was the development of hepatocellular carcinomas after the implantation of DAB - the first time that this phenomenon had been produced. The tumours closely resembled in their appearance those induced by injecting or feeding this "hepatospecific" carcinogen. The only difference was, as has already been stated, the absence of "precursor" lesions that could be demonstrated by routine-histiological procedures. It must, however, be stressed here that so far no enzyme-histochemical reactions had been used to study the presence of "altered cell" foci, which one would expect in the light of present views of hepatocarcinogenesis. In standard sections the tumours presented a greater inter-than intra-tumorous variability, with ranging in appearance from almost spindle-shaped to "oncocytic", with occasional giant cells (Fig. 6, Fig. 7), PAS-positive globules and inclusions, a variable number of mitotic figures, and little connective tissue. The one feature they all had in common, including their intra-abdominal implants, was the presence of glandular spaces with a lining that varied from flat to distinctly cylindrical, thereby producing the appearance of bile ducts of a variable degree of differentiation (Fig. 8). In contrast to an earlier experiment (Aterman, 1987) no metastases could be found in extrahepatic organs.

DISCUSSION

The development of a firm connective tissue capsule around pellets of carcinogens contradicts earlier reports in which such a development - in other tissues - had been denied. (See Aterman, 1967, 1987). It does, however, raise the question which cell type is predominantly involved in this development. This question is of interest not only because it touches on the still debated nature of "fibroblastic" cells in the liver (Aterman, 1986), but because it may also help to understand the relation of the pellet capsule to the origin of the mesenchymal tumours induced. Nothing is known about the cell type that gives rise to the sarcomas seen with such frequency after the

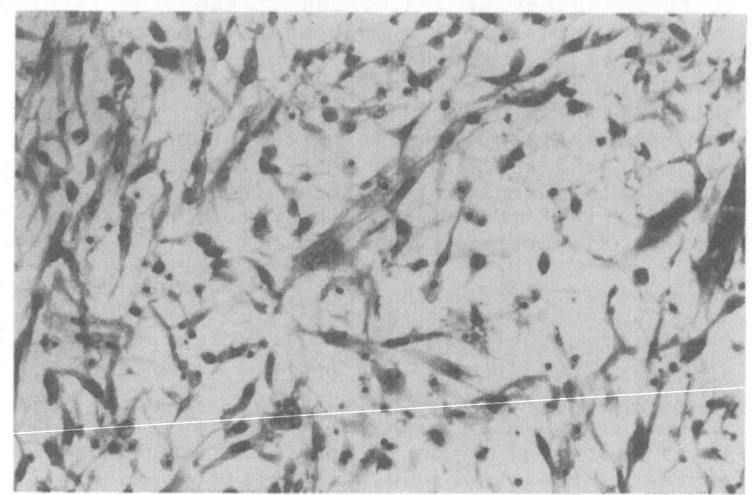

Fig. 3 517 days after implantation of a pellet of 3-M.C.
this rat died with an almost myxoid "malignant
fibrous histiocytoma".

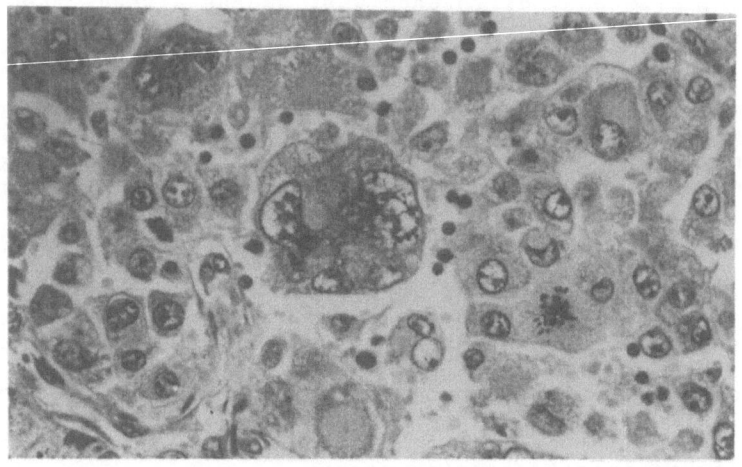

Fig. 4 Epithelial-like (? histiocytic cells) in another
"malignant fibrous histiocytoma" of the liver (641
days. Please note the bizarre giant cell.

implantation of 3-M.C. The presence also of other elements -
the histiocytic, haemangiosarcomatous of biliary component -
in these tumours suggests that 3-M.C. is a rather indiscrimi-
nate carcinogen involving also the other cell types in the
rodent liver, not only the "fibroblasts". This in turn
raises the question whether the hepatoma-like areas seen
in the 3-M.C.-induced tumours were perhaps derived from
hepatocytes. 3-M.C. has not been viewed as a hepatocarcinogen under ordinary conditions (Farber et al., 1979),
although there exist some, unconfirmed, publications

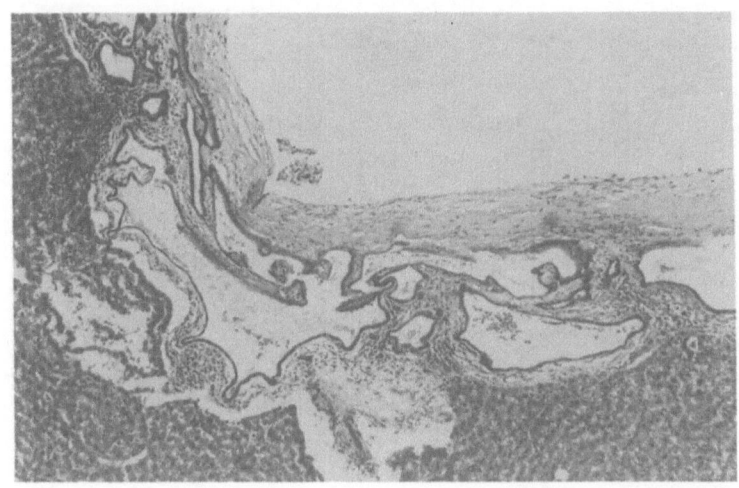

Fig. 5 Biliary changes induced by a pellet of 3-M.C.
right upper corner) 330 days after implantation.
Please note the absence of changes in the capsule.

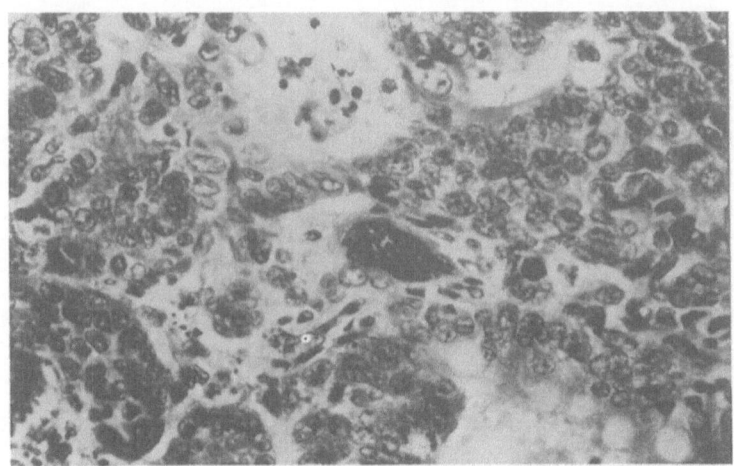

Fig. 6 A hepatocellular carcinoma 484 days after the
implantation of a pellet of DAB, showing a giant
cell (center) and the formation of ill-defined
glandular spaces. Please compare with Fig. 7.

pointing in this direction (Aterman, 1987). It has not been
possible to confirm or refute the hepatocellular nature of
the areas in question found in the sarcomatous tumours of the
present series, and this is a problem that requires clarification.

Little has so far been said about the state of the
implanted pellets towards the end of the experiments. Some
older reports had indicated that pellets of cholesterol
implanted into the liver were in time reduced in size, indicating absorption (Aterman, 1987). The histological findings of giant cells and intracellular crystals in macropha-
ges would agree with this observation. In the present

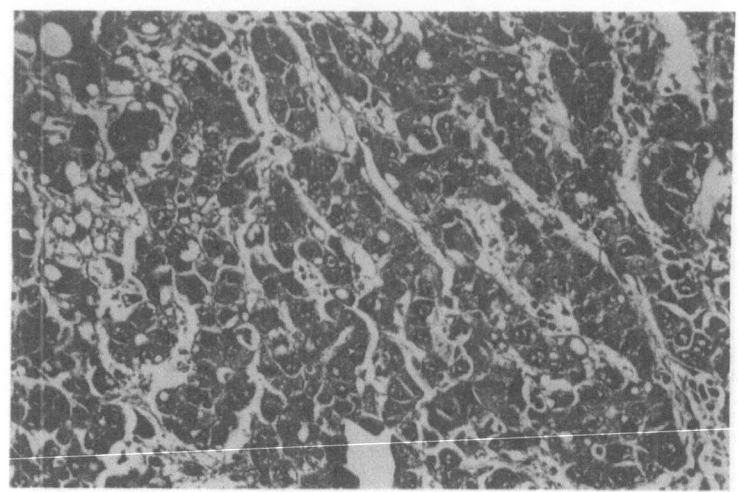

Fig. 7   Another DAB-induced hepatocellular cancer (732 days)
to show the classical trabecular arrangement not seen
in Fig. 6.

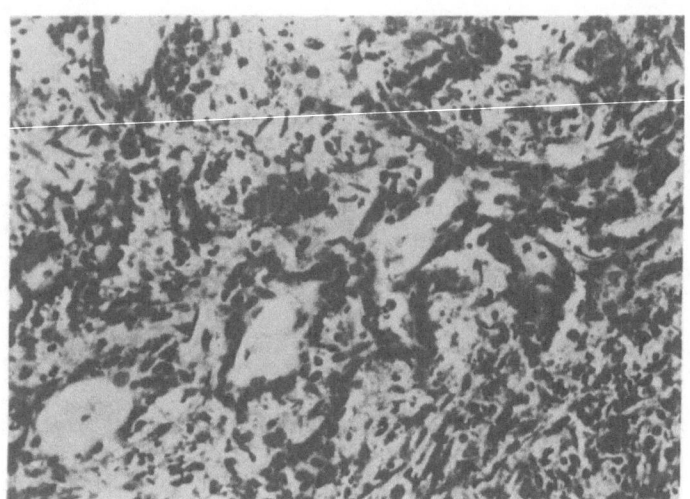

Fig. 8   The occurence of numerous duct-like spaces lined
by rather flat cells is a prominent feature of this
hepatocellular, DAB-induced, tumour.

experiments too there could be little doubt that, in the case
of DAB, the implanted pellets had become distinctly smaller -
despite the presence of a complete connective tissue envelope.
This gradual degradation of the carcinogenic depot has to be
viewed in the context of:

a) the absence of significant degenerative or of
demonstrable "preneoplastic" hepatocellular changes such
as the formation of "nodules", and

b) the development of hepatocellular tumours in some

animals in the absence of such changes.

It must, however, be stated here that these findings
should still be viewed as somewhat tentative, since some of
the observations and interpretations should still be
verified by further experiments. They should, on the other
hand, also be viewed in the light of the repeatedly made
statement by Farber and Sarma (1986, 1987) that "so far no
model has been described in which hepatocellular cancers
occur without a prior appearance of hepatocyte nodules." The
emphasis on "nodules" is to be noted. If the absence of such
"nodules", which were not seen here - as opposed to "foci"
which were not specifically searched for - can be confirmed,
we may have here the model that so far has been missing, and
that may experimentally confirm the intuitive views of those
few workers (Foulds, 1975; Bannasch, 1976; Weisburger et al.,
1972; Williams, 1980; Peraino et al., 1983) who have questioned the significance of nodules as an unavoidable pre-
condition of hepatocellular cancer.

The model discussed here raises a number of other
interesting questions which await answers. It has already
shown the myth of the insensitivity of the liver to the local
application of carcinogens to be one of those pseudotruth
which are only too common. Perhaps it is not too much to
hope that it will also help to illuminate some of the other
facets of the complex problem of hepatocarcinogenesis.

SUMMARY

Contrary to the previously held view that the liver -
which readily responds to carcinogens given by mouth or by
injection - is resistant to carcinogens applied locally, it
is shown here that the implantation of pellets of carcinogens
into the rat's liver can induce hepatic tumours. Whereas
control pellets of cholesterol, anthracene or α-naphthyliso-
thiocyanate only provoked, like other foreign bodies, a
connective tissue response encapsulating the implants, a
significant number of rats that had received a pellet of
3-methylcholanthrene developed pleomorphic fibrosarcomas of
the liver presenting features of the currently so-called
"malignant fibrous histiocytomas". Areas of a haemangiomatous to haemangiosarcomatous appearance, fields of an epithelial-like, possibly hepatomatous nature and foci of
cystic biliary dilatation and proliferation were also seen
in these tumours. Implants of 4-dimethylaminoazobenzene,
on the other hand, provoked in about 27% of the experimental
rats the development of a hepatocellular carcinoma that morphologically resembled the tumours induced by feeding or
injecting carcinogens. The tumours induced here, however,
were always solitary and arose only in the lobe that had
received the implant. The other liver lobes appeared
grossly and microscopically always normal, except for
changes known to occur in old animals; these were seen
to the same degree also in the control animals. The
points to be stressed here are:

a) the fact that the pellets were always found embedded
in the tumour mass, and

b) the absence of demonstrable "pre-neoplastic" changes
such as glycogen-containing areas, oval cell
proliferations, or hepatocellular nodules.

This applied to the non-involved lobes of tumour-bearing animals as much as to the liver parenchyma in the vicinity of the carcinogenic implants in those animals that did not develop tumours. The development of hepatocellular carcinomas in the absence of preceding hepatocellular "nodules" is an interesting phenomenon that should be studied further.

ACKNOWLEDGEMENTS

Parts of the experiments were supported by the generous assistance of Prof. M.D.B. Burt, Department of Biology, University of New Brunswick, Fredericton, N.B., Canada (N.S.E.R.C. Operating Grant No. A2358). The excellent technical assistance of Mr. J. Keillor and the skilled photographic work of Mr. E. Gouchie are gratefully acknowledged.

REFERENCES

Arcos, J.C., Argus, M.F. and Wolf, G., 1968, Chemical induction of cancer. Structural bases and biological mechanisms, 1:391, Academic Press, New York.

Aterman, K., 1965, The response of the rat liver to implanted carcinogens, Fed. Proc., 24:685.

Aterman, K., 1967, The response of the rat liver to implanted carcinogens, in: Liver Research, Tijdschrift Gastroenterol, 10B, Suppl., 341.

Aterman, K., Lau, H., and Gillis, D.A., 1971, The response of the liver to the implantation of artificial bile ducts, J. Pediatric Surg., 6:413-420.

Aterman, K., 1986, The parasinusoidal cells of the liver. A historical survey, Histochem J., 18:279-305.

Aterman, K., 1987, Localized hepatocarcinogenesis: The response of the liver and of the kidney to implanted carcinogens, J. Cancer Res. Clin. Onc., In Press.

Bannasch, P., 1967, Glykogen und endoplasmatisches Retikulum der Leberzelle während der Carcinogenese, Ber. Physik-Med. Ges., Würzburg, N.S., 73:83-86.

Bannasch, P., 1969, Grundsätzliche cytopathologische Unterschiede in der Genese von Lebercirrhose und Leberzellcarcinom, Ver. Dtsch. Ges. Path., 53:335-344.

Bannasch, P., 1976, Cytology and cytogenesis of neoplastic (hyperplastic) hepatic nodules, Cancer Res., 36:2555-2562.

Bannasch, P., Mayer, D. and Hacker, H.J., 1980, Hepatocellular glycogenesis and hepatocarcinogenesis, Biochim. Biophys. Acta, 605:217-245.

Berenblum, I., 1974, Carcinogenesis as a biological problem. in: "Frontiers of Biology", Vol. 34, p. 12, Neuberger, A. and Tatum, E.L., ed., American Elsevier Publishing Co., New York.

Eisen, M.J., 1946, Induction of sarcoma of the liver in the
    rat with methylcholanthrene and benzpyrene,
    Cancer Res., 6:421-425.

Esmarch, O., 1940, Dépot de méthylcholanthrene dans quelques-
    uns des organes de la souris, Acta. Pathol. Microbiol.
    Scand., 17:9-21.

Farber, E., 1956a, Carcinoma of the liver in rats fed ethio-
    nine, Arch. Path., 62:445-453.

Farber, E., 1956b, Similarities in the sequence of clearly
    histological changes induced in the liver of the rat
    by ethionine, 2-actylaminofluorene, and 3'-methyl-
    4-dimethylaminoazobenzene, Cancer Res., 16:142-148.

Farber, E., Cameron, R.G. Laishes, B., Lin, J.C., Medline,
    A., Ogawa, K., and Solt, D.B., 1979, Physiological and
    molecular markers during carcinogenesis, pp. 319-335.
    In: Carcinogens: Identification and mechanisms of
    action. (eds.: A.C. Griffin & C.R. Shaw). Raven
    Press, New York.

Farber, E., and Cameron, R., 1980, The sequential analysis
    of cancer development, Adv. Cancer Res., 31:125-226.

Farber, E., and Sarma, D.R. 1986, Chemical carcinogenesis:
    the liver as a model, Pathol. Immunopathol. Res., 5:1.

Farber, E., and Sarma, D.R., 1987, Hepatocarcinogenesis:
    A dynamic cellular perspective, Lab. Invest., 56:4.

Foulds, L., 1975, Neoplasia in the liver, pp. 205-237.
    In: Neoplastic development, Vol. 2, Academic
    Press, New York.

Hirota, N. and Williams, G.M., 1979, Persistence and growth
    of rat liver neoplastic nodules following cessation of
    carcinogen exposure, J. Natl. Cancer Inst., 63:(5)
    1257-1265.

Ilfeld, F.S., 1936, The experimental production of visce-
    ral tumors with hydrocarbons, Am. J. Cancer,
    26:743-753.

Jones, B.F., Rothman, A.J., and Shear, M.J., 1935, Unpu-
    blished Experiments, (Quoted by: Shear et al., 1940).

Kinosita, R., 1936, Researches on the cancerogenesis of the
    various chemical substances, Gann, 30:423-426.

Kinosita, R., 1937, Special report: "Studies on the
    cancerogenic chemical substances", Trans. Jap.
    Path. Soc., 27:665-727.

Kinosita, R., 1940, Studies on the cancerogenic azo and
    related compounds, Yale J. Biol. Med., 12:287-300.

Kinosita, R., 1955, Some recent findings concerning

hepatomas induced with p-dimethylaminoazobenzene,
J. Natl. Cancer Inst., 15:1443-1445.

Oberling, Ch., Guerin, P. and Guerin, M., 1939, La
production de tumeur hépatique par le 3-4 benzopyrene
chez le rat blanc, Compt. Rend. Soc. Biol.,
130:417-419.

Ogawa, K., Minase, T., and Onoe, T., 1974, Demonstration
of glucose-6-phosphatase activity in the oval cells
in azo-dye carcinogenesis, Cancer Res., 34:3379-3386.

Ohshima, M., Ward, J.M., Brennan, L.M., and Creasia, D.A.,
1984, A sequential study of metapyrilene hydrocho-
loride-induced liver carcinogenesis in male F344
rats, J. Natl. Cancer Inst., 72:(3), 759-768.

Orr, J.W., 1940, The histology of the rat's liver during
the course of carcinogenesis by butter-yellow
(p-dimethylaminoazobenzene), J. Pathol.
Bacteriol., 50:393-408.

Peraino, C., Richards, W.L., and Stevens, F.J., 1983,
Multistage hepatocarcinogenesis, pp. 1-53. In:
mechanisms of tumor promotion, v.1. Tumor promotion
in internal organs. (ed.: T.J. Slaga). CRC Press
Inc., Boca Raton, Florida.

Rubin, E., 1964, The origin and fate of proliferated bile
ductular cells, Exp. Molec. Path., 3:279-286.

Rusch, H.P., Baumann, C.A., and Maison, G.L., 1940, Production of internal tumors with chemical carcinogens,
Arch. Path., 29:8-19.

Sell, S., Leffert, H.L., Shinozuka, H., Lombardi, B., and
Gochman, N., 1981, Rapid development of large numbers
of α-fetoprotein-containing "oval" cells in the
liver of rats fed N-2-fluorenylacetamide in a choline-
devoid diet, Gann, 72:479-487.

Shear, M.J., Stewart, H.L., and Seligman, A.M., 1940,
Studies in carcinogenesis XIII. Tumors of the spleen
and liver in mice following the introduction of hydrocarbons into these organs, J. Natl. Cancer Inst.,
1:291-302.

van Bezooijen, C.F.A., 1984, Influence of age-related changes
in rodent liver morphology and physiology on drug
metabolism - a review. Mechanisms of Ageing and
Devolpm., 25:1-22.

Ward, J.M., and Ohshima, M., 1985, Evidence for lack of promotion of the growth of the common naturally
occurring basophilic focal hepatocellular proliferative lesions in aged F344/NCr rats by phenobarbital, Carcinogenesis, 6:1255-1259.

Weisburger, J.H. Yamamoto, R.S., Williams, G.M., Grantham,
P.H., Matsushima, T., and Weisburger, E.K., 1972, On
the sulfate ester of N-hydroxy-N-2-fluorenylacetamide

as a key ultimate hepatocarcinogen in the rat, Cancer Res., 32:491-500.

Williams, G.M., 1980 The pathogenesis of rat liver cancer caused by chemical carcinogens, Biochim. Biophys. Acta. 605:167-189.

Woglom, W.H., 1938, Agent and soil in experimental carcinogenesis, Am. J. Cancer, 32:447.

TWO STAGE THEORY OF CARCINOGENESIS: A CRITICAL REVIEW

INTRODUCING THE CONCEPT OF MODULATION

Marcel Roberfroid

Unite de Biochimie Toxicologique et Cancerologique
Universite Catholique de Louvain
U.C.L., Av. Mounier 73.69, B-1200
Brussels, Belgium

INTRODUCTION

Carcinogenesis is a long lasting process which, progressively, transforms part of a differentiated tissue to a malignant tumor. Initiation is the first event which introduces the tissue or some of its cells into that process. That event may be a physical (radiation) or a chemical mostly mutagenic treatment but also a viral infection or even a transfection of a piece of viral DNA (Lacey et al.1986). In most experimental protocols reported so far for viral and physical induction of cancer, only the initiation step seems to be required so that after a single or a few infections by the virus or a single or a few doses of irradiation is (are) sufficient to induce the appearance of malignant tumors in a majority of the animals. Eventhough such single step protocols do exist for the chemical induction of cancer using large doses of carcinogen, most of the protocols which are classically used for that purpose are multisteps in that sense that they involve a sequence of different treatments. Since, during the last two decades, chemically induced carcinogenesis has been the most studied process, it has become selfevident that carcinogenesis is a multistep process. The pathologists who have made extensive description of the history of a neoplastic development in human have clearly reported that, very often, preneoplastic and neoplastic lesions preceed the appearance of malignancy. Since many experimental protocols used to chemically induce cancer similarily produce preneoplastic or benign neoplastic lesions before cancer, it has also become selfevident that the various steps required for the carcinogenesis process induce stages or phases which sequence the events inherent to carcinogenesis.

Thus, since experimental, mainly chemical carcinogenesis has developed with the aim to give "scientific bases to the experimental dissection of the history of neoplastic development" (Pitot, 1983), carcinogenesis is, as a conclusion of such studies, regarded as a long lasting multistep, multistage or multiphase process.

However, the concept of cancer arissing as the end point of a long lasting process during which stages/phases do appear which imply steps to take place or to be completed relies most exclusively on operational rather than on biological evidences. It means that each "stage or phase" had been identified as resulting from the effect(s) of specific chemical, nutritional or surgical treatments considered as step(s). None has been clearly defined by its biological nature. "The concept that carcinogenesis is a two or multistage process has developed mainly by indirect ways from experiments in which certain operational steps were used (Bannasch, 1984). Thus, the question remains to be asked if such an experimental approach has really dissected the natural history (i.e. the history of the process as it takes place really) or if it has dissected a modified history (i.e. the history of an artificial process resulting from unrealistic manipulations) of carcinogenesis.

The mouse skin and the rat liver are the classical targets to study chemical carcinogenesis. Within the frame of such operational concepts, initiation of carcinogenesis has been defined as "a change in a target tissue or organ, induced by exposure to a carcinogen, that can be promoted or selected to develop focal proliferations, one or more of which can act as sites of origin for the ultimate development of malignant neoplasms". Whereas promotion appears as "the process whereby an initiated tissue or organ develop focal proliferations (such as nodules, papillomas, polyps...) one or more of which act as precursors for subsequent steps in the carcinogenic process".
And progression is the "process whereby one or more focal proliferations, such as papillomas, polyps and nodules undergo a slow cellular evolution to malignant neoplasms" (Farber,1982)

1. THE MOUSE SKIN CARCINOGENESIS PROCESS

The multistep nature of a carcinogenic protocol has been first demonstrated on skin . Papillomas are the benign neoplastic lesions which appear before malignant tumors (most often squaneous cell carcinomas). Rous and Kidd (1941) were the first to demonstrate that wounding of the skin of the rabbit's ear previously treated with a carcinogenic polycyclic aromatic hydrocarbon (PAH) resulted in the rapid appearance of neoplastic growth compared with the ears of animals treated only with the hydrocarbon. These experiments suggested to the authors that the application of a PAH to mouse skin had begun a process in skin cells that they termed initiation whereas the wounding had begun a second process which they termed promotion (in other words an action or a proceeding contributing to or helping the progress, development or growth of "initiated cells or tissues").
A few years later Mottram (1944), using mice, demonstrated similarly that the application of a PAH on the shaved skin resulted in the rapid appearance of neoplasms only in those animals subsequently treated with another agent, the vesicant croton oil.
In 1947, Berenblum and Shubik extended the Mottram's study and demonstrated that two distinct stages analogous if

not identical with those of initiation and promotion could be shown in mouse skin carcinogenesis. Furthermore they reported that the administration of the promoting treatment must follow the application of the initiating agent. Moreover the application of croton oil could be delayed for many months after the application of the PAH without significantly affecting the yield of neoplasms at the end of the experiment.

For the next four decades following these pioneering experiments, numerous studies based on the mouse skin system confirmed but also extended these observation demonstrating the reversibility of promotion (Boutwell, 1964) as opposed to the irreversibility of initiation, the non additivity of the effect of a promoting agent (Boutwell, 1964) and the subdivision of tumor promotion into stage I and stage II (Boutwell, 1964; Slaga et al., 1980; Fürstenberger et al., 1981).

All these data are used to support the two stage theory of (skin) carcinogenesis "that over the years has taken on all the qualities of what is traditionally called a paradigm" (Iversen and Astrup 1984).

CARCINOGENIC PROTOCOLS FOR MOUSE SKIN

MOUSE LIFESPAN   Weeks

0   20   40   60

1. I   Single initiating treatment (high dose)

2. IIIIIII   Repeated "initiating" treatments

3. I PPPPPPPPPPP   Two-step protocol

4. PPPPPPPPPPPPPPPPPPPP   Repeated "promoting" treatments

5. I   PPPPP I' I' I' I'   Single initiating treatment
                              Short term repeated "promoting" treatment
                              Repeated "initiating" treatments
                                              (low doses)

6. PPPPPPP I   Reverse two-step protocol

7. I   Single initiating treatment + "abrasion"

Major historical findings in support of the multistage theory
of mouse skin carcinogenesis
(PAH = Polycyclic Aromatic Hydrocarbon.)

But what these data do in fact demonstrate is that :
- some two-or even three-step protocols are carcinogenic for the skin;
- during the carcinogenic process induced by such two-or three-step protocols , two or three operational stages can be identified which coincide with the different steps;
- these two-or three-step protocols are good (but not the only) methods for the rapid experimental production of skin tumors and cancers;
- compounds or treatments do exist which induce (preferentially) one step or the other.

By no means do they allow to conclude that carcinogenesis is a two-or three-step process. Indeed many experimental evidences that have been repeatedly reported are not at all integrated by the two stage theory.

Among these experimental evidences are the following facts: a single application of a skin carcinogen generally at high dose can induce the appearance both of benign and malignant tumors (Shubik, 1977; Terracini et al., 1960);
- treatment with a "promoter" before initiation can, in some experimental conditions, increase the tumor yield the way it does when given after (Iversen and Iversen, 1982);
- feld wheel abrasion alone works as a good tumor promotion treatment. It even produces malignant tumors in mice pretreated with a small dose of 7,12 dimethylbenz (a)anthracene (Rous and Kidd, 1941);
- all chemicals with skin cancer promoting activity that have been tested, induce papillomas and/or carcinomas when applied chronically to mouse skin not previously "initiated" (Iversen and Astrup, 1984);
- a pure "initiating treatment" given repeatedly after initiation and short term promotion is a excellent promoting treatment (Hennings et al., 1983).

Eventhough a two step protocol for skin carcinogenesis may be useful for the rapid experimental production of skin tumors and skin cancers mostly in mouse, the two stage/two phase /multistage/multiphase theory of skin carcinogenesis to which that protocol gives support, has not all the qualities of a paradigm.

2. THE RODENT LIVER CARCINOGENIC PROCESS

The second most frequently used model for experimental cancer research is the rodent liver (mainly the rat, sometimes the mouse) (Farber and Sarma, 1987).

That hepatocarcinogenesis may occur in distinct stages equivalent to those seen in skin was first suspected by the demonstration of Farber (1973) that the hyperplastic nodule may, in some instances, be a potential precursor to hepatocellular carcinoma. The study of Teebor and Becker (1971) lessened the impact of this concept by demonstrating that such nodules induced by the intermittent feeding of 2-acetylaminofluorene (2-AAF) were reversible and disappeared after stopping the treatment. That is true for many of the protocols used for hepatocarcinogenesis (P.Bannasch,1984).

The first two step protocol for hepatocarcinogenesis has been described by Peraino et al., (1973), who demonstrated that chronic phenobarbital (PB) feeding "markedly enhanced" the hepatocarcinogenic action of 2-AAF. During the last fifteen years, other protocols for the production of hepatic cancer have been reported by Scherer and Emmelot (1975) Solt and Farber (1976), Pitot (1978), Lans et al. (1983), Préat et al. (1984,1986) and Shivapurkar et al. (1986). The protocol proposed by Scherer and Emmelot is not a two-step protocol but it has been modified by Pitot to become such. Except that proposed by Peraino, all these protocols use the same chemical as the initiating treatment i.e.(diethylnitrosamine) (DEN). When comparing the hepatocarcinogenesis processes induced by these various protocols it appears that the major, difference is in the kinetic of the appearance of malignant tumors (de Gerlache et al. 1984).

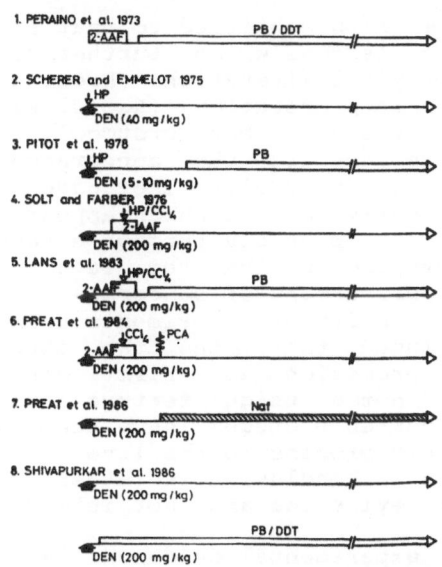

1. PERAINO et al. 1973

2. SCHERER and EMMELOT 1975

3. PITOT et al. 1978

4. SOLT and FARBER 1976

5. LANS et al. 1983

6. PREAT et al. 1984

7. PREAT et al. 1986

8. SHIVAPURKAR et al. 1986

Schematic representation of the experimental protocols used to induce tumors and cancers on mouse skin.

Given as a single dose treatment either alone (high dose) (Shivapurkar et al.,1986, Préat, personal communication) or in combination with partial hepatectomy (low dose) (Scherer and Emmelot,1975), DEN by is itself fully carcinogenic if the rats are allowed to survive for up to 2 years.

Feeding rats chronically with PB after such a single dose treatment with either DEN (high dose) alone (Shivapurkar et al.,1986) or DEN (low dose) + partial hepatectomy or feeding them chronically with a peroxisome proliferator (Nafenopin) after a single dose of DEN (Préat et al., 1986) increases tumor yield and shortens the latency period between the initiating treatment and the appearance of first tumors.

A two week treatment with 2-AAF combined with a stimulus of proliferation in the middle of that treatment results in essentially the same effects (Solt and Farber,1976).According to these authors, that treatment is a "short term promoting treatment". Feeding rats chronically with PB after they had been submitted to a Solt and Farber recipe further increases tumor yield and further reduces the latency period for the appearance of the first cancer (Lans et al., 1983; de Gerlache et al., 1984). In such a three step protocol, the chronic administration of PB can be replaced by a porto-caval shunt (Préat et al.,1984) or high fat diet feeding (de Gerlache et al., 1987) to give essentially the same results.

The chronic administration of 2-AAF, DEN (as well as other nitrosamines), PB or Nafenopin is tumorigenic for rats.

In the liver of the rats treated according to either one of these protocols, whenever it has been analyzed, enzyme altered foci, preneoplastic lesions and/or hyperplastic nodules have been identified and characterized histologically, histochemically or even biochemically. One major exception has however been reported by Préat et al.(1986) using the "promoting effect" of Nafenopin. Indeed the livers of the rats submitted to that protocol have very rare preneoplastic lesions which furthermore show unusual patterns of phenotypical alterations (Préat et al. and Hacker et al. manuscripts in preparation) (Rao et al.,   )

Using the Solt and Farber protocol, Farber and his colleagues have demonstrated the appearance of nodule in nodule or even cancer in nodules. They have also demonstrated that most of the early lesions which appear soon after 2-AAF release disappear most probably through a remodeling process. They favor the hypothesis that the late persistent nodules could be the true precursors of cancers.

Based on the results of experiments using such protocols it has been concluded that "the two stage mechansim of initiation and promotion as first described for skin carcinogenesis is not a unique feature of this system, and that entirely comparable stages have now been demonstrated for the carcinogenic process in the liver"...(Pitot, 1980).

However, such a conclusion is rather surprising because many experimental evidences are not integrated by the two stage theory.

Among these experimental evidences are the following facts   - a single application of a hepatocarcinogen to young rats or to previously hepatectomized adult rats (high dose) induces both benign and malignant tumors provided the period of observation is long enough (Scherer and Emelot,1975; Shivapurkar et al. 1986).
- portocaval shunt or high fat diet are promoting treatment (Préat et al. 1984; de Gerlache et al., 1987)
- all chemicals with liver cancer promoting activity that have been tested induce preneoplastic lesions and/or carcinomas when given chronically to rats not previously "initiated".
- a pure initiating treatment (dialkylnitrosamine) administered chronically after initiation and short term promotion is a promoting treatment (de Gerlache, personnal communication).
- depending upon either the protocol used (single step, two steps, three steps) or the promoting treatment (PB or Nafenopin or porto caval shunt) the kinetic of "initiated cells" to "cancer" may vary as well as the nature and the diversity of the malignant tumors (de Gerlache et al., 1984; Préat et al., 1986).

Eventhough a two- or a three-step protocol for hepatocarcinognenesis may be useful for the rapid experimental production of tumors and cancers,mostly in rats, the two-stage/two-phase/multistage/multiphase theory of hepatocarcinogenesis to which these protocols give support, has not yet the qualities of a paradigm.

3. CONCLUSION

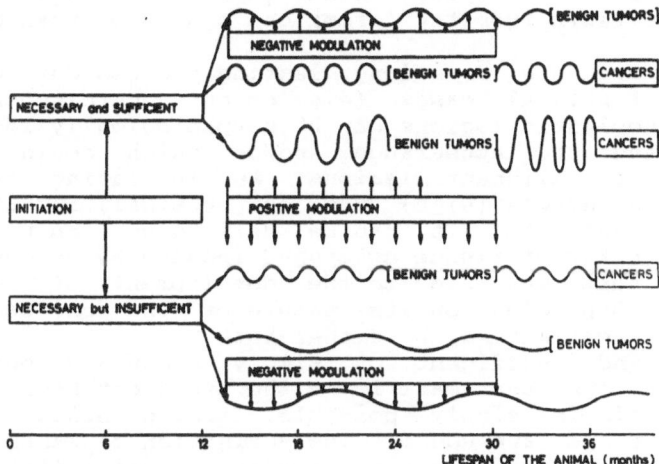

Schematic representation of the process of (chemical)-carcinogenesis introducing the concept of (positive or negative) modulation.

Experimental evidences accumulated over the recent years on mouse skin and rat liver carcinogenesis support the following conclusions which still need to be put together in A THEORY OF CARCINOGENESIS (Fig.3):
1. an initiating treatment is necessary to begin the process;
2. even a single initiating dose of a chemical (high dose), a radiation or a single viral infection may be a fully carcinogenic treatment;
3. sequential administrations of chemicals with initiating or "promoting" activity (whatever the sequence may be), show synergism between the effects of the two (three) classes of chemicals;
4. the consequence of that synergism is either a reductionof the latency period between the initiating treatment and the appearance of cancers or an increased number of cancers;
5. often that consequence is also a modification of the field or incidence of cancers from initiated cells to cancers;
6. even the repeated administration of low doses of an initiating treatment has the effects of a promoting treatment.

Beyond the initiating treatment for which, in some cases, a single (high) dose may be enough, the tissue/the cells slowly become malignant. In most cases the appearance of malignancy is preceded by premalignant lesions from which cancers seem to arise. Additional exogenous treatments can be used to modify or accelerate that history.

A single step protocol begins a "natural" carcinogenic process. We do not know yet how multiphase/multistage that process is.

A multi-step protocol induces a modified carcinogenic process which has the characteristic of a multiphase

35

/multistage process. We do not know for sure if that modified process simply mimics the "natural process". We do not know if what we learn from the former can simply be transposed to the later.

Carcinogenesis is a long lasting process during which, in many but not all cases (e.g. colonic carcinogenesis in rat), preneoplastic lesions can be morphologically identified which preceed the appearance and/or which could be the precursor of malignant lesions. An initiating treatment (sometimes a single (high) dose of chemical) is the only necessary treatment. It can be defined as **"an persistent change in a target tissue or organ, induced by exposure to a carcinogen that may lead to the development of malignant neoplasms"**. Depending on its nature or the dose used, that initiating treatment may be either both
necessary and sufficent or simply necessary but still unsufficient. In that case it is the treatment beyond which carcinogenesis is simply possible, taking place only if additional steps are added. The definition of FARBER (1982) quoted above covers thus a particular type of initation that produces potentially tumorigenic cells that can proliferate if stimulated differentially.

In experimental animals, various means have been discoverd which applied mainly after but also before an **initiating treatment** may:
- shorten the latency period for the appearance of the first tumor;
- accelerate the evolution to malignancy;
- amplify the intensity (increased number of tumors and/or cancers);
- change the phenotypical morphological nature of cancers.

The classical term **promotion** which, as defined above, means "to complete" "to contribute to", "to help" and not "to induce" (Farber, 1982) applies to only part of these effects. It deserves particular meaning when it is used to characterize the mean to potentiate a sub-treatment to make it able to induce a fully carcinogenic process. Besides for such particular situations, promotion may not be the correct word to characterize the effects of the treatments mostly when they are applied to an animal in which a fully carcinogenic process is already ongoing on by itself. Rather than promotion, such treatment should be called.**Modulation**" i.e. the process of varying the frequency, the amplitude, the intensity of ...

With that in mind the carcinogenic process can be viewed as follows (Fig.7): **The "natural history of cancer development** is the one which starts after the initiating treatment. It is a long story which probably goes through various stages/phases. If, initiation is necessary and sufficient the process is going on up to malignancy without any further exogenous treatment. That story can be modified by using **modulating treatments.** If that treatment **shortens the latency period** for the appearance of malignancy, **increases the intensity** and **speeds up** the carcinogenic process it induces a positive modulation part of which being equivalent to what has been called up to now a **promotion.** Such positive modulation (promotion) may be the consequence of the chronic administration of chemical, but also of dietary unbalances, surgeries, or repeated initiation. If that treatment increases the latency period for the appearance of malignancy, decreases the intensity and slows down the carcinogenic process it causes a negative modulation which is the aim of cancer chemoprevention. Such a negative modulation can be realized by administration of free radical scavengers, or antioxidants and by rebalancing dietary habits such as e.g. by increasing fiber and/or reducing fat intakes.(M.Wilpart).

REFERENCES

1.   BANNASCH,P.,(1984) Sequential cellular changes during chemical carcinogenesis.
      J.Cancer Res. Clin.Oncol. 108,11-22.

2.   BOUTWELL, R.K.,(1964) Some biological aspects of skin Carcinogenesis.
      Prog.Exp.Tulmor Res.4,207-250.

3.   de GERLACHE J., LANS M.,PREAT V.,TAPER H. and ROBERFROID M. (1984) Comparison of different models of rat liver carcinogenesis: conclusions from a systemic analysis.
      Toxicol.Pathol.12,374-382.

4.   de GERLACHE J.,TAPER,H.,LANS.M., PREAT.V., and ROBERFROID M.,(1987), Dietary modulation of rat liver carcinogenesis.
      Carcinogenesis, 8,B37 -340.

5.   FARBER E., (1973) Carcinogenesis- cellular evolution as a unifying theory.
      Cancer Res., 33, 2537-2550.

6.   FARBER E., and D.S.R. SARMA,(1987), From the normal cell to cancer: The multistep process: the liver model in: A.MASKENS ed. Concepts and theories in carcinogenesis, Excepta Medica Congress Series, Elsevier Scientific Publ. Amsterdam, in press.

7.   FARBER,E. (1982), Sequential events in chemical carcinogenesis in : F.F.Becker (ed.)Cancer, A Comprehensive Treatise, 2nd edition, Plenum Public.Corp. N.Y., pp 485-506.

8.   FURSTENBERGER G., BERRY D.L. SORG B.,and F.MARKS (1981) Skin tumor promotion by phorbol esters is a two stage process.
      Proc.Natl.Acade.Sci., USA 78, 7722-7726

9.   HENNINNGS,H. SHORES,R., wENCK, M.L.,SPRANGLER,E.F., TARONE R and S.H. YUSPA (1983), Malignant conversion of mouse skin tumours is increased by tumour initiators and unaffected by tumour promoters.
      Nature, 304, 67-69

10. IVERSEN, O.H., and U.IVERSEN (1982) Must initiatiors come first? Tumorigenic and carcinogenic effects on skin of 3 methylcholanthrene and TPA in various sequences. Brit.J.Cancer, 45, 912-920

11. IVERSEN,O.H. and E.G.ASTRUP (1984), The paradigm of two-stage carcinogenesis: a critical attitude. Cancer Investig., 2,51-60

12. LACEY,M., ALPERT,S. and D.HANAHAN (1986) Bovine papilloma virus genome induce skin tumours in transgenic mice Nature 322, 609-612.

13. LANS,M., de GERLACHE,J., TAPER H., PREAT V; AND ROBERFROID   M. (1983),Phenobarbital as a promoter in the initiation/selection process of experimental rat hepatocarcinogenesis. Carcinogenesis, 4,141-144

14. MOTTRAM,J.C.(1944) A developing factor in experimental blastogenesis J.Pathol.Bacteriol., 56,181-187

15. PERRAINO,C., FRY R.J.M.,STAFFELD E. and W.E.KISIELESKI (1973) Effect of varying the exposure to phenobarbital on   its enhancement of 2-acetylaminofluorene induced hepatic tumorigenesis in the rat. Cancer Res., 31, 1506-1512

16. PITOT,H.C., BARSNESS,L. GOLDSWORTHY,T. and K;KITAGAWA (1978). Biochemical characterisation of stages of hepatic carcinogenesis after a single dose of diethylnitrosamine. Nature, 271, 456-458

17. PITOT,H.C.,(1983), Contribution to our understading of the natural history of neoplastic development in lower animals to the cause and control of human cancer. Cancer Surveys, 2, 519-538

18. PREAT V., PECTOR J.C.,TAPER H., LANS M., DE GERLACHE J. and ROBERFROID M. (1984) Promoting effect of portocaval anastomosis in rat hepatocarcinogenesis. Carcinogenesis, 5, 1151-1154

19. PREAT V.,LANS M., DE GERLACHE J., TAPER H., AND ROBERFROID M.(1986) Comparison of the biological effects of phenobarbital and nafenopin in rat hepatocarcinogenesis Japan.J. Cancer Res.,(GANN), 77, 629-638

20. RAO M.S.,LALWANI N.D.,SCARPELLI D.G. AND REDDY J.K.(1986) The absence of g-glutamyl transpeptidase activity in putative preneoplastic lesions and in hepatocellular carcinomas induced in rats by the hipolipidemic peroxisome proliferator Wy-14,643. Carcinogenesis.3,1231-1233.

21. ROBERFROID M.B.(1987), From normal cell to cancer: an
     overview introducing the concept of modulation of
     carcinogenesis, in: A.Maskens (ed.) Concepts and
     Theories
     in Carcinogenesis, Excepta Medica Congress Series,
     Elsevier-Scientific Publishers. 157-167.

22. ROUS,P. and J.G.KIDD (1941) Conditional neoplasms and
     subthreshold neoplastic states. A study of tar tumors in
     rabbits
     J.Exp.Med. 73,365-376.

23. SCHERER,E. and P. EMMELOT (1975), Kinetics of induction
     and growth of precancerous liver cell foci and liver
     tumor formation by dimethylnitrosamine in the rat.
     Europ.J.Cancer, 11, 145-154

24   SHIVAPURKAR,N.HOOVER,K.L. and L.A. POIRIER (1986),
     Effect of methionine and choline on liver tumor
     promotion by phenobarbital and DDT in diethylnitrosamine
     -initiated rats.
     Carcinogenesis, 7, 547-550

25   SHUBIK,P (1977),The implication of multiple tumor
     induction in rodent skin for the biologic nature of
     neoplasia
     Cancer, 40,1821-1824

26. SLAGA J.T.,FISHER,J.M., NELSON,K. and G.L.GLEASON
     (1980),Studies on the mechanism of skin tumor promotion:
     evidence for several stages in promotion
     Proc.Natl.Acad.Sci.USA, 77,3659-3663

27. SOLT,D.B. and E.FARBER (1970) New principle for the
     analysis of chemical carcinogenesis.
     Nature 263, 702-703

28. TEEBOR G.w. AND F.F.BECKER (1972),Regression and
     persistence of hyperplastic nodules induced by N-2
     fluorenylacetamide and their relationship to
     hepatocarcinogenesis.
     Cancver Res., 31,1-3

28. TERRACINI,B., SCHUBIK,P AND G. DELLA PORTA (1960). A
     study of skin carcinogenesis in the mouse with single
     application of 9,10-dimethyl-1,2-benzanthracene at
     different dosages.
     Cancer Res., 20,1538-1542

MODULATING FACTORS OF HEPATOCARCINOGENESIS

Véronique Préat, Nathalie Delzenne

Unité de Biochimie Toxicologique et Cancérologique,UCL 7369

Avenue Mounier 73, 1200   Bruxelles, Belgium

INTRODUCTION

Initiation is a necessary event without which nothing happens and beyond which everything is possible. Indeed, after a sufficient initiating treatment, the carcinogenic process can either evolve naturally or operationally be modulated. The factors that modulate an initiated carcinogenesis can have positive or negative effects. When the incidence and/ or the yield of cancer is increased and/or the latency period is decreased by the modulating treatment, the modulation is considered as positive whereas a treatment which decreases the incidence and/or the yield of cancer and/or increases the latency period is considered as a negative modulator. (Roberfroid, 1987)

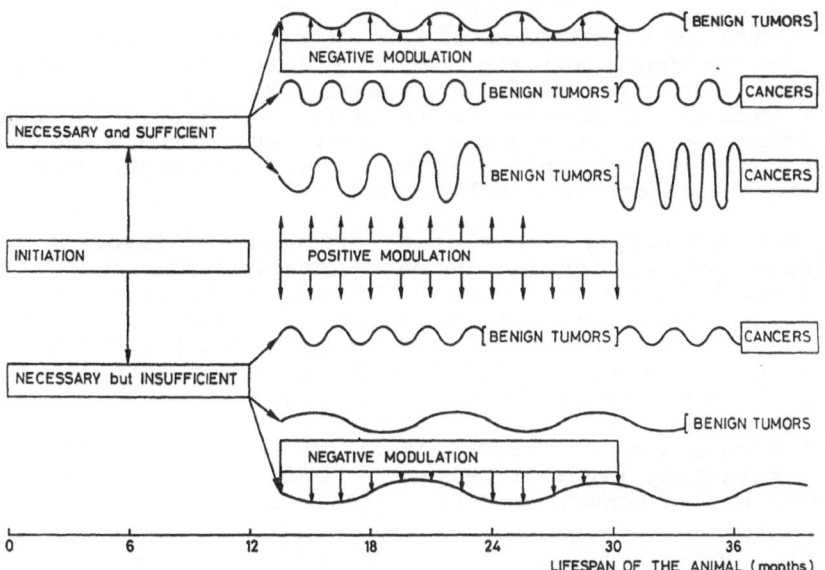

Figure 1 : Schematic representation of the positive and negative modulation of carcinogenesis.

41

The figure 1 schematizes this concept of modulation. If the initiation is not sufficient, no cancer will develop whereas if the initiating treatment is sufficient, cancer will appear without any further treatment. If a positive modulation is applied, more cancers will appear earlier and can develop even after a subcarcinogenic initiating treatment. Inversely, when a negative modulation is applied, less cancers will develop later.

The aim of the present paper is to review positive modulation of rat liver carcinogenesis by focusing on the nature of the modulating factors and their effects on the hepatocarcinogenic process.

I NATURE OF THE MODULATING FACTORS OF RAT HEPATOCARCINO-GENESIS

In liver carcinogenesis, the modulating factors can be:
- chemical or viral carcinogens
- non genotoxic xenobiotics
- endogenous or endogenous like compounds
- dietary factors
- surgery

In the first part of this paper, the modulation of hepatocarcinogenesis will be analyzed with respect to the appearance of the end stage, namely liver cancers rather than with respect to the development of foci and nodules.

I.a Modulation of rat hepatocarcinogenesis by carcinogens

After a single dose or a short treatment with a carcinogen, cancers develop if the dose is sufficiently high and provides a latency period shorter than the life span of the animal.

If the administration of the carcinogen is prolonged, both the incidence and the yield of liver cancer increase whereas the latency period decreases. Therefore, according to the concept of modulation (Roberfroid, 1987), prolonged administration of a carcinogen modulates positively the carcinogenic process initiated by a short treament, even if both treatments are chemically identical.

This modulating effect of a carcinogen on liver carci-nogenesis operates during **chronic administration** or **"stop experiments"** (Bannasch, 1968). Indeed, prolonging the du-ration of the administration of 2-acetylaminofluorene (2-AAF) (Teebor & Becker, 1971), N-nitrosomorpholine (NNM) (Bannasch, 1968) or diethylnitrosamine (DEN) (Barbason et al, 1979) increases the incidence of cancer.

A second dose or **"hit"** with a carcinogen given after a first initiating treament enhances liver cancer development as shown by Van Renselaer Potter (1984) or Scherer (1984).

The **"selection"** procedure of Solt & Farber (1976) consists in a short term 2-AAF administration coupled with a stimulus for cell proliferation. The concept of "selection" is based on the resistance of "initiated" cells to the effects of cytotoxic agents (Farber et al, 1976). Applied after a single dose of an initiating treatment, such a selection procedure increases the incidence and yield of liver cancers and decreases the latency period preceeding their appearance (Solt et al, 1983, Shivapurkar et al, 1986). It is thus a positive modulation of carcinogenesis.

Thus , carcinogens positively modulate the hepatocarcinogenic process initiated by a short term initiating treatment.

I.b Modulation of rat hepatocarcinogenesis by non genotoxic xenobiotics

Among the modulating factors, the **"promoters"** have been the most extensively studied. Indeed, after the initial paper of Peraino et al (1971) which demonstrated the promoting effect of phenobarbital on 2-AAF induced hepatocarcinogenesis, a large number of reports have shown that some non genotoxic xenobiotics promote liver cancer development when administered chronically after a (sub)carcinogenic treatment. These compounds have been initially defined as "promoters". They belong to various chemical classes and exert different biological activities.

Table 1 : Incidence of liver cancer observed after initiation by one dose of 200 mg/kg of DEN, selection with 2 weeks of 0.03% of 2-AAF in the diet and 2 ml/kg of CCl4 in the middle of this treatment followed by chronic feeding with a non genotoxic xenobiotic or basal diet in the reference group.

XENOBIOTIC		INCIDENCE OF LIVER CANCER	REFERENCE Préat et al
----	-Basal diet	10%	1986a,b, 87
DRUG	-Phenobarbital 0.05%	66%	1986a,b, 87
	-Oxazepam 0.1%	62%	1987a
	Diazepam 0.005%	0%	
	-Nafenopin 0.1%	90%	1986a,b, 87
	-Clofibrate 0.5%	20%	1987b
PESTICIDE	-DDT 0.05%	60%	1986a
FOOD ADDITIVE	-Butylated hydro-xy toluene 0.5%	10%	1986a
CONTA-MINANT	-Diethylhexylphtalate 1%	10%	1987b

As an example, Table 1 summarizes the results obtained in our laboratory using a slightly modified Solt & Farber (1976) protocol (Lans et al, 1983). This protocol is carcinogenic by itself since without any further modulating treatment, it induces 75% of cancer incidence after 13 months (Préat et al, 1986b). However, various drugs, pesticides or food additives enhance the incidence and the yield of liver cancer and decrease their latency period when administered chronically for 5 months after such a protocol (Préat et al, 1986a, 1986b, 1987a, 1987b).

I.c Modulation of rat hepatocarcinogenesis by endogenous or endogenous like compounds

As shown in Table 2, several endogenous or endogenous like compounds like sexual hormones, bile acids or intermediate metabolites have been reported to enhance the development of liver cancers when administered chronically after initiation at relatively high doses.

Table 2 : Modification of the incidence of liver cancer observed after chronic administration of endogenous or endogenous like compounds to initiated rats.

TREATMENT	EFFECT ON THE IN- CIDENCE OF CANCER	REFERENCE
DEN/2-AAF+CC14		
cholesterol 0.5%	↗	Delzenne
deoxycholic acid 0.5%	↗	Delzenne
NNM+ovariectomy		
estradiolphenylpropionate	↗	Taper 1978
DEN:		
ethinylestradiol 0.5ppm	↗	Yager 1984
mestranol 0.5ppm	↗	Yager 1984
DEN/2-AAF+PH		
orotic acid 1%	↗	Rao 1983

These results suggest that endogenous compounds like sexual hormones, bile acids and maybe growth factors or peptidic hormones could act as endogenous modulators (positive or negative) of rat liver carcinogenesis. To check this hypothesis, an experimental approach would be to manipulate their physiological levels by surgery, dietary factors or chemicals administration with the aim to analyze the effect of the change in the homeostasis of endogenous factors on cancer development.

I.d Modulation of rat hepatocarcinogenesis by dietary factors

Table 3 : Effect of choline methionine deficient and high fat diets on the incidence of cancer induced by the initiation-selection protocol.

TREATMENT	EFFECT ON THE IN- CIDENCE OF CANCER	REFERENCE
Choline methionine deficient diet	↗	Sells 1979
High fat diet	↗	de Gerlache 87

Epidemiologic studies have concluded of an important role of diet in the development of various cancers. Besides well known carcinogens such as mycotoxins, polycyclic aromatic hydrocarbons or aromatic amines which might be present in the food, dietary factors such as high caloric intake, high fat or high protein, low fiber contents are clearly involved in these epidemiological data.

In rat liver carcinogenesis, a deficiency or an excess in some dietary factors has been reported to modulate the carcinogenic process. As shown in Table 3, a choline methionine deficient diet enhances the development of liver cancer induced by DEN Selles et al, 1979). It can even induce cancer after long term administration without any previous initiation (Goshal Farber, 1984). Recently, we showe th a high fat diet (20%) also exerts a positive modulation on rat hepatocarcinogenesis (de Gerlache et al, 1987).

I.e Modulation of rat hepatocarcinogenesis by surgery

A surgical operation like portocaval shunt positively modulates liver carcinogenesis. When performed after a hibitiond-selection, such a modification of liver blood supply clearly exerts a promoting effect on liver cancer development since it increases cancer incidence as compared to a control group (Préat et al, 1984). However, this effect might be due to a direct hemodynamic effect i.e a decrease in venous blood supply since a portocaval transposition does not have the same effect (Pector, personnal communication).

Besides its effect on initiation through cell proliferation (Cayama et al, 1978), partial hepatectomy may have a slight enhancing effect on liver carcinogenesis induced by DEN (Barbason et al, 1983).

Table 4   Effect of portocaval shunt, portocaval transposition and partial hepatectomy on liver carcinogenesis initiated by DEN.

TREATMENT	EFFECT ON THE IN-CIDENCE OF CANCER	REFERENCE
DEN/2-AAF+CCl4		
portocaval shunt	↗	Préat 84
portocaval transpositio	=	Pector
Chronic DEN		
partial hepatectomy	↗	Barbason 84
Partial hepatectomy		
chronic DEN	↗	Bartsch 87
DEN/2-AAF+CCl4	↗	Bartsch 87

Besides that modulating effect when performed after initiation, partial hepatectom can also modify the carcinogenic process when performed several weeks before initiation. Indeed, we have recently reported that partial hepatectomy performed 8 to 10 weeks before chronic DEN administration or initiation-selection, enhances the incidence of cancers as compared to sham operated animals (Bartsch et al, 1987).

Surgeries which may modify the homeostasis of various
endogenous factors or of the metabolism and/or the cell
proliferation have thus been shown to modulate
hepatocarcinogenesis. Such treatments seem to act not only
if they are applied after but also, at least in some
circumstances, before the initiation of the carcinogenic
process. If confirmed or extended, such observations may
broaden the concept of modulation.

I.f Conclusions on the nature of the modulating factors of rat hepatocarcinogenesis

1.   While studying liver cancer modulation, it should not
be forgotten that initiation with a short term "carcinogen"
treatment is not only necessary but can be sufficient
(Figure 1). In that case, the carcinogenic process evolves
naturally per se without the need of any further "modulating
factors".

2.   The nature of the modulating factors can be very
different since it varies from carcinogens or xenobiotics
administration to dietary factors or surgery.

3.   The mechanisms by which these modulating factors act is
largely unknown. Most likely, they might act through
different mechanisms. Due to the diversity of the modulators as well as to their pleitropic effects, the identification of the relevant factors involved in cancer modulation
and maybe in cancer progression will be very difficult.
Whether nuclear (oncogenes, mutations, ploidy...) or other
cellular alterations (membranes, enzymes activities....),
cell proliferation and/or more systemic perturbations
(metabolism, hormones...) are really involved in the process
and are a cause or only a consequence, remains to be proven.

II.   EFFECT OF THE MODULATING FACTORS ON RAT HEPATO-
CARCINOGENESIS.

It is generally believed that after the administration
of a carcinogen, so called "preneoplastic" and "neoplastic"
lesions which might be precursors of cancer develop in the
liver (Bannasch, 1986). Namely, foci can grow into nodules
which can transform in hepatocellular carcinomas. Even
though never proven, this concept has become generally
accepted as a paradigm.

One of the consequences of this paradigm is that the
effect of the modulating factors are usually analyzed on the
development of foci and nodules rather than on the development of liver cancers (Williams,1982, Bannasch, 1986).
However, this approach can be misleading since the modulating factors can modulate differently the carcinogenic
process (Préat et al, 1986a).

As shown in Table 5, we have compared the effect of
several xenobiotics on the development of foci and nodules
in early stages (1-3 months) and on the development of liver
cancers in later stages (6-7 months) in a carcinogenic
process induced by the Solt & Farber protocol (1976). The
results indicate that various modulating factors can

modulate differently the carcinogenic process. Indeed, compounds like phenobarbital and DDT increase the development of foci, nodules as well as liver cancers. Nafenopin slightly inhibits foci and nodules development but strongly enhances cancer incidence whereas butylated hydroxytoluene increases nodules formation but has no effect on liver cancer incidence (Préat et al, 1986a,b, 1987a).

Table 5   Effect of xenobiotics on the development of foci, nodules and liver cancer induced by the initiation-selection protocol (Préat et al, 1986a,b, 1987a).

TREATMENT	INCIDENCE OF FOCI AND NODULES	INCIDENCE OF CANCER
Phenobarbital		
DDT	↑	↑
Oxazepam		
Nafenopin	↓	↑
Butylatedhydroxytoluene	↑	=

Whether the nature of the modulating factors influences the histological type of liver cancer remain to be analyzed systematically. However, our results tend to indicate that different modulating factors might promote more specifically certain type of cancers. For example, after nafenopin administration, only well differentiated hepatocellular carcinomas are observed whereas with butylated hydroxytoluene, none of the cancers were of the hepatocellular type.

In conclusion, it appears that the modulating factors can modulate differently :
- the evolution of an "initiated" liver to cancer
- the ratio number of foci and nodules per liver
- the ratio number of foci and nodules in early stages per cancer in end stage.

CONCLUSIONS

Cancer development is a complex, long lasting process in which steps have been identified operationnally on the base of specific treaments, biologically on the base of the biological effects of these treatments or pathologically on the base of the formation of "precancerous" stages like focal proliferations or dysplasia preceeding the appearance of cancers (Hicks, 1983).
Experimental liver carcinogenesis is a useful tool for the study of carcinogenesis. Various models have been described. They consist of a single dose or short term treatment with a carcinogen. This "initiating" treatment is necessary and can be sufficient for the induction of liver cancer, the end stage of the carcinogenic process. However, this treatment can be unsufficient and it can be modulated positively by several factors which increase the incidence

and the yield of liver cancer or decrease the latency period preceeding their appearance. Indeed, after the short term carcinogen administration, liver carcinogenesis can be enhanced through a second dose of carcinogen (medium term chronic treatment, selection....) (I.a), chronic administration of non genotoxic xenobiotics (I.b), changes in the homeostasis of endogenous factors (I.c), dietary unbalances (I.d) or surgery (I.e). Importantly, some treatments applied long before initiation can also act as positive modulators. These data fit with earlier reports on skin carcinogenesis (Iversen & Iversen, 1982)

With regard to liver carcinogenesis, the modulating factors can modify not only the development of cancer, the end point, but also the development of foci and nodules (II).

Modulation of carcinogenesis could be an essential factor in the etiology of human cancer. Therefore, their identification and the understanding of its-their mechanism(s) of action(s) would be of importance to prevent that pathology.

Aknowledgement : Véronique Préat is "Chargé de recherches" du Fonds National de la Recherche Scientifique (Belgium). Nathalie Delzenne is a research fellow of I.R.S.I.A (Belgium)

REFERENCES

Bannasch, P. (1968), , The cytoplasm of Hepatocytes during Carcinogenesis, Rec. Results Cancer Res., 19, 1-105.

Bannasch, P., (1986), Preoplastic Lesions as End Points in Carcinogenecity Testing I. Hepatic Neoplasia, Carcinogenesis, 7, 689-695

Barbason,H., Smoliar,V., Fridman-Manduzio,A. and Betz, E. (1979), Effect of Discontinuation of Chronic Feeding of Diethylnitrosamine on the Development of Hepatomas in Adult rats, Br.J. Cancer, 40,260-267

Barbason,H., Rassenfosse,C. and Betz, E., (1983), Promotion Mechanism of Phenobarbital and Partial Hepatectomy in DENA Hepatocarcinogenesis and Cell Kinetics Effect, Br.J.Cancer, 47, 517-525

Bartsch,H., Préat,V.,Aitio,A., Cabral J.and Roberfroid,M., (1987), Partial Hepatectomy of Rats Ten Weeks before Carcinogen Administration Enhances Liver Carcinogenesis Carcinogenesis, in press

Cayama,E., Tsuda,H., Sarma,D.S.R. and Farber, E. (1978), Initiation of Chemical Carcinogenesis Requires Cell Proliferation, Nature, 273, 60-62

Delzenne, N., personnal communication

de Gerlache,J., Taper., H.S., Lans,M., Préat,V. and Rober-
    froid,M., (1987), Dietary Modulation of Rat Liver
    Carcinogenesis, Carcinogenesis, 8, 337-340

Goshal, A. and Farber, E. (1984), The Induction of Liver
    Cancer by Dietary Deficiency of Choline and Methionine
    without Added Carcinogens, Carcinogenesis, 5, 1367-1370

Farber, E., Parker S. and Gruenstein M., (1976), The Resis-
    tance of Putative Premalignant Liver Cell Populations,
    Hyperplastic Nodules to the Acute Cytotoxic Effects of
    Some Hepatocarcinogens, Cancer Res., 3879-3887

Hicks, M., (1983), Pathological and Biochemical Aspects of
    Tumour Promotion, Carcinogenesis, 4, 1209-1214

Iversen,O. and Iversen U. (1982) Must Initiators Come First?
    Tumorigenic and Carcinogenci effects on Skin of 3-Me-
    thylcholanthrene and TPA in Various Sequences., Br.J.
    Cancer, 45, 912-920

Lans,M., de Gerlache,J., Préat,V., Taper,H.S. and Roberfroid
    M., (1983), Phenobarbital as a Promoter in the initi-
    ation/selection Process of Experiemntal Rat Hepatocar-
    cinogenesis, Carcinogenesis, 4, 141-144

Pector,J.Cl, Presonnal communication

Peraino,C., Fry,R. and Staffeld,E. (1971), Reduction and En-
    hancement by Phenobarbital of Hepatocarcinogenesis In-
    duced in Rats by 2-acetylaminofluorene, Cancer Res,31,
    1506-1512

Préat,V., Pector J.CL., Taper,H.S., Lans,M., de Gerlache,J.
    and Roberfroid,M. (1984), Promoting Effect of Portoca-
    val Anastomosis in Hepatocarcinogenesis, Carcinogenesis
    5, 1151-1154

Préat,V., de Gerlache,J., Lans,M., Taper,H.S. and Roberfroid
    M., (1986a), Comparative Analysis of the Promoting Ef-
    fect of Phenobarbital, DDT, Nafenopin and Butylated
    hydroxytoluene in Rat Hepatocarcinogenesis, Carci-
    nogenesis, 7, 1025-1029

Préat,V., Lans,M., de Gerlache,J., Taper,H. and Roberfroid
    M. (1986b), Comparison of the Biological Effect of Phe-
    nobarbital and Nafenopin on Rat Hepatocarcinogenesis,
    Jp..J.Cancer Res., 77, 629-638

Préat,V., de Gerlache,J., Lans,M. and Roberfroid,M., (1987a)
    Promoting Effect of Oxazepam in Rat Hepatocarcinogene-
    sis, Carcinogenesis, 8, 97-100

Préat, V. and Roberfroid M., (1987b) Modulation of rat hepa
    tocarcinogenesis by Peroxisome Proliferators, 2nd In-
    ternational   Conference   on   Anticarcinogenesis   and
    Radiation Protection

Rao,P.M., Wagamine K., Ho,K., Roomi,W., Lairier,C., Rajalak-
    shmi S. and Sarma, D.S.R. (1983), Dietary Orotic Acid
    Enhances the incidence of Gamma-glutamyl-transferase
    Positive Foci in Rat Liver Induced by Chemical Carcino-
    gens, Carcinogenesis, 4, 1541-1545

Roberfroid,M. (1987), From Normal Cell to Cancer : an Over-
    view introducing the Concept of Modulation of Carcino-
    genesis, in A. Maskens (ed), Concepts and Theories in
    Carcinogenesis, Excepta Medica Congress Series, Else-
    vier-Scientific Publishers, 157-167

Shivapurkar,N., Hoover,K.L. and Poirier, L. (1986), Effect
    of Methionine and Choline on Liver Tumor Promotion by
    Phenobarbital and DDT in Diethylnitrosamine-initiated
    Rats, Carcinogenesis, 7, 547-550

Sells, Katyal, S., Sell,S., Shinozuka, H., Lombardi,B.(1979)
    Induction of Foci of Altered Gamma-Glutamyl-Transpepti-
    dase Positive Hepatocytes in Carcinogen Treated Rats
    Fed a Choline Deficient Diet, Br.J.Cancer, 40, 274-283

Solt,D. and Farber,E., (1976), New Principle for the Analy-
    sis of Chemical Carcinogenesis, Nature, 263, 701-703

Solt,D., Cayam,E., Tsuda,H., Enomoto,K, Lee,G. and Farber,E.
    (1983), Promotion of Liver Cancer Development by Brief
    Exposure to Dietary 2-acetylaminofluorene plus Partial
    Hepatectomy or Carbon Tetrachlride, Cancer Res.,43, 188
    -191

Taper,H.S. (1978), The effect of Oestradiol-17-phenyl-
    propionate and Oestradiol benzoate on N-nitrosomorpho-
    line Induced liver Carcinogenesis in Ovariectomised
    female rats, Cancer, 42, 462-467

Teebor,G. and Becker,F., (1971), Regression and Persistance
    of Hyperplastic Nodules Induced by N-2-fluorenylaceta-
    mide and their Relationship to Hepatocarcinogenesis,
    Cancer Res., 31, 1-3

Van Rensselaer Potter (1984), Use of Two Sequetial Applica-
    tions of Initiators in the Production of Hepatomas in
    the Rat, Cancer Res., 44, 2733-2736

Yager,J., Campbell,H., Longnecker,D., Roebuck; B. and M.
    Benoit, Enhancement of Hepatocarcinogenesis in Female
    Rats by Ethinyl Estrodiol and Mestranol but not Estra-
    diol, Cancer Res., 44, 3862-3869

Williams G. (1982), Phenotypic Properties of Preneoplastic
    Rat Liver Lesions and Applications to Detection of Car-
    cinogens and Tumor Promoters, Toxicol. Pathol.,10, 3-10

SEX HORMONES AS MODULATORS OF LIVER TUMOR DEVELOPMENT

Stan D. Vesselinovitch, Nikola Mihailovich and
Silvana Negri

Departments of Radiology and Pathology
University of Chicago
5841 S. Maryland Ave., Chicago, Ill. (60637)

INTRODUCTION

The induction of hepatocellular tumors depends upon the nature of
the chemical agent (1), its requirement for activation to ultimate carcinogenic moiety (2), enzymatic competence of tissue(s) to activate the
procarcinogen (3-5), the interaction of ultimate carcinogenic moiety with
specific macromolecular site(s) (6,7), the rate of removal of the formed
adduct(s) (8), the degree of macromolecular repair (9,10), caloric intake
(11-13), immune competence, and hormonal environment of the host (14-17).
The interplay of all these factors contribute in varying degrees to the
neoplastic expression in the liver. The species, strain (18), age at
treatment (19), and sex (19) of the animals may influence the degree of
the agent's activation. In addition, the age at treatment may affect the
macromolecular damage-repair ratio and consequently the degree of fixation
of the residual macromolecular lesion(s) (20).

However, independent of differences in the metabolic competence between males and females, which may influence the degree of the primary
event of hepatocarcinogenesis or initiation (21), the sex hormonal environment can influence the development or the expression of the originally initiated cells. The latter role of sex hormones in hepatocarcinogenesis was investigated in our laboratory. However, in order to address
this problem it was necessary to establish several experimental conditions
which would allow such a study. Thus, in the course of the preliminary
interpretations, it was necessary to define the experimental model which
would meet the following three experimental requirements: (a) the capa-
bility to respond to a single carcinogenic dose by development of the
early and late hepatocellular lesions culminating in the emergence of the
hepatocellular carcinomas, (b) possesses equal degree of activation of
carcinogen in both sexes, and (c) similar morphologic response pattern in
males and females.

The above requirements were met by $B6C3F_1$ (C57BL/6JxC3HeB/FeJ F_1)
mice which when treated with low dose levels of diethylnitrosamine (DEN)
at 15 days of age developed same morphologic endpoints (tinctorial foci
and hepatocellular nodules, adenomas, and carcinomas)(22). The stereo-
morphometric quantitation of the above lesions was achieved by trans-
lating images from 2-dimensional planes into 3-dimensional space (23-25).

Such quantitation resulted in dose-dependent response and dose-dependent latent periods regarding the development of tinctorial foci, hyperplastic nodules, hepatocellular adenomas, and hepatocellular carcinomas (26).

MATERIALS AND METHODS

In order to clarify the role of sex hormonal environment upon the development of hepatocarcinogenesis, hormonally intact animals (sham-gonadectomized) and sex hormone deficient mice (gonadectomized animals) were used in conjunction with the above-referred experimental conditions. Gonadectomies were performed at various intervals following carcinogenic treatment. The modifying effect of sex hormones was evaluated by comparing kinetics of hepatocarcinogenesis (a) between intact males and females, (b) following progressively delayed orchidectomies (at 20, 30, and 38 weeks of age) and ovariectomies (at 4, 28, and 40 weeks), and (c) after induction by 1.25, 2.5, and 5.0 µg of DEN/g body weight in hormonally intact (4-week sham-orchidectomized) and hormonally deficient (4-week orchidectomized) males. DEN was administered intraperitoneally once at 15 days of age. Details of each experiment are presented, in turn, in Results. Liver tissues were stained with hematoxylin and eosin and the lesions were quantitated as described (26).

RESULTS AND COMMENTS

The original studies utilizing DEN as a hepatocarcinogen and the incidence of tumor-bearing animals as the endpoint showed that B6C3F1 female mice responded similarly to male animals, although after a longer period of time (19). This observation has been substantiated more recently in a study in which the numbers of adenomas per liver were used as the endpoint (Fig. 1).

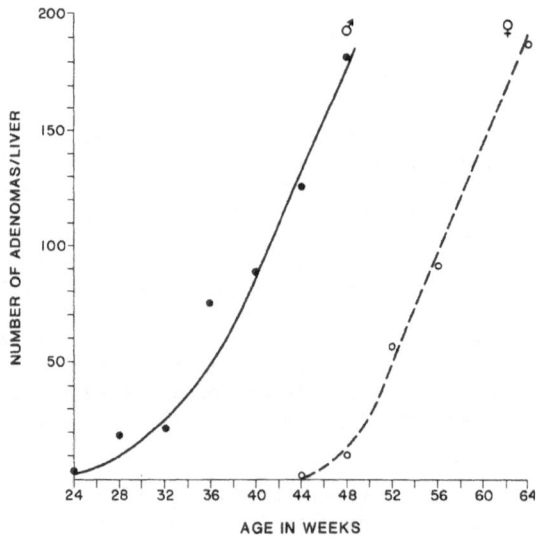

Fig. 1. Development of liver adenomas induced by 10 µg DEN/g body weight.

This figure shows that the expression of hepatocellular adenomas was delayed in females by an average of 16 weeks. This indicated the same degree of initiation of hepatocellular adenomas in both sexes whose rate of expression was modulated by sex hormonal environment.

Early in the investigations we were concerned to find out how much the age at gonadectomy would modify hepatocarcinogenesis. Data in Table 1 are suggestive that orchidectomy performed at 4 weeks might be more effective in delaying hepatocarcinogenesis than when orchidectomy was carried out at 24 weeks (12 vs. 24%). In females, early ovariectomy appeared to be more effective in accelerating hepatocarcinogenesis than if ovariectomy was delayed (44 vs. 32%). The reason for not detecting clearly the role of age at gonadectomy upon hepatocarcinogenesis was that the incidence rather than the multiplicity of lesions was used as the response indicator and the tumor response was measured at a single time point (60 weeks). This explanation is substantiated by more recent studies. In the course of those studies, 15-day-old mice were administered a single dose of DEN (males 2.5 µg/g and females 10.0 µg/g body weights). Groups of males were orchidectomized at 20, 30, and 38 weeks and groups of females were ovariectomized at 4, 28, and 40 weeks of age. Subgroups of each gonadectomized group and the sham-gonadectomized animals were killed at 4-week intervals. Observations made in this study are highlighted in the next three figures (Figs. 2, 3, and 4).

Table 1. Incidence of Hepatocellular Carcinomas 60 Weeks Following DEN Treatment[a]

	Males[b]		Females	
	Ratio	Percent	Ratio	Percent
Sham-gonadectomized	25/25	100	0/23	0
Gonadectomized at age in weeks:				
4	3/25	12	11/25	44
14	5/25	20	11/25	44
24	6/25	24	8/25	32

[a]Diethylnitrosamine: 2.5 µg/g body weight in males and 10.0 µg/g body weight in females at 15 days of age.
[b]C57BLxC3H F_1 mice.

Fig. 2 illustrates that time at orchidectomy (20, 30, or 38 weeks of age) differentially delayed the emergence of hepatocellular adenomas. Thus, the intact males reached their maximal response at 44 weeks and then plateaued. Animals, which were orchidectomized at 20 weeks, showed significantly lower multiplicity of expressed adenomas through the 54th week (18 adenomas per liver in orchidectomized vs. 51 adenomas in hormonally intact males). However, by 58 weeks of age the orchidectomized mice developed all initiated adenomas. Delay in orchidectomy was increasingly less effective in delaying the emergence of hepatocellular adenomas. Thus a similar neoplastic expression of approximately 18 adenomas per liver was observed at 54, 50, and 46 weeks of age in mice orchidectomized at 20, 30, and 38 weeks, respectively. However, similar to the 20-week orchidectomized males, the 30- and 38-week orchidectomized mice expressed all initiated adenomas by 58 weeks of age.

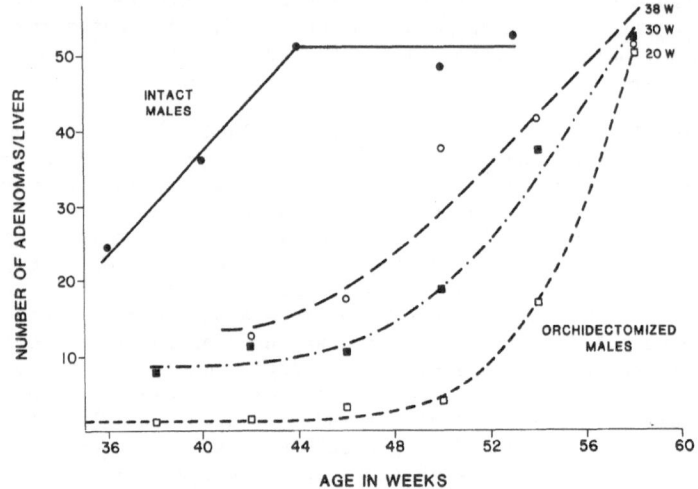

Fig. 2. Effect of orchidectomy on development of hepatocellular adenomas induced by DEN. All males were
treated with 2.5 µg DEN/g body weight at 15 days
of age; orchidectomies were carried out at 20, 30,
or 38 weeks of age. One group of animals was only
sham-orchidectomized at 20 weeks (hormonally intact males).

The temporal distribution of the development of hepatocellular adenomas in hormonally competent and in 20-week orchidectomized males is
illustrated in Fig. 3. The mean difference in the development of adenomas
between those two groups was 19 weeks. The plot of temporal distribution
of 30- and 38-week orchidectomized males would be located between the
above two distributions of which the 38-week orchidectomized plot would
be next to the hormonally intact males.

Fig. 4 demonstrates that time at ovariectomy (4, 28, and 40 weeks of
age) differentially accelerated the emergence of hepatocellular adenomas.
Thus, the adenomas were first observed in the hormonally intact females
at 48 weeks, reaching the multiplicity of 55 adenomas per liver by 56
weeks of age. However, the females which were ovariectomized at 4 weeks
of age showed adenomas first at 32 weeks of age (16 weeks earlier than
intact females) and continued to express neoplasia at a relatively slow
rate, reaching multiplicity of 55 adenomas per liver at 52 weeks (only 4
weeks earlier than hormonally intact females). The acceleration of development of adenomas was somewhat less prominent in females which were
ovariectomized at 28 and 40 weeks, respectively. In the latter two instances, the slope of development of adenomas was greater than in the
4-week ovariectomized animals, occurring within 8 (from 44 to 52 weeks)
and 4 (from 48 to 52 weeks), respectively. However, all three ovariectomized groups reached multiplicity of 55 adenomas per liver by 52 weeks,
4 weeks earlier than the intact females. This figure also illustrates
that the main acceleration of the expression of adenomas in 4-week
ovariectomized females was related to the emergence of the early occurring tumors. The mean number of adenomas per liver (multiplicity of
28 adenomas per liver) has been observed in 4-week ovariectomized females
by 43 weeks and in hormonally intact females by 54 weeks, a median
acceleration of 11 weeks of tumor development triggered by ovariectomy.

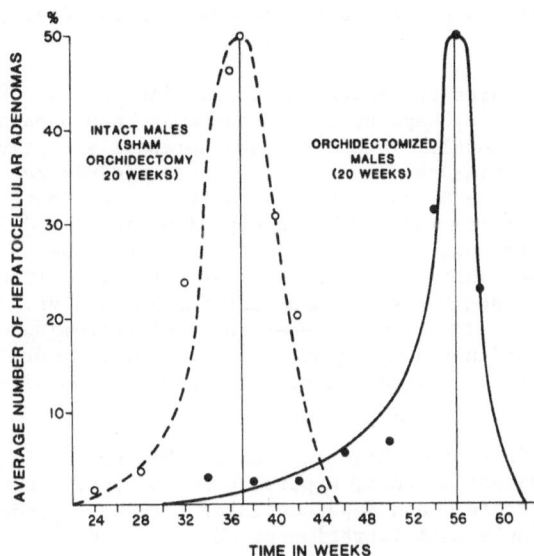

Fig. 3. The effect of orchidectomy on the temporal
distribution of hepatocellular adenomas.
The mice were either sham-orchidectomized
(hormonally intact males) or orchidectomized (hormonally deprived males) at 20
weeks of age.

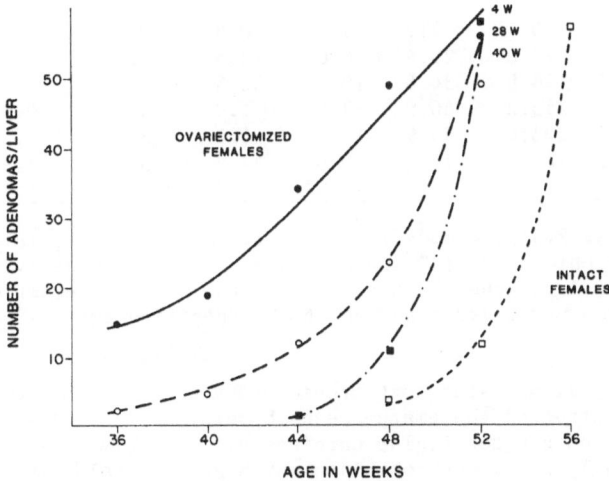

Fig. 4. Effect of ovariectomy on development of hepatocellular adenomas. All females were treated
with 10 µg DEN/g body weight at 15 days of age;
ovariectomies were carried out at 4, 28, and 40
weeks of age (hormonally deprived females). One
group of animals was only sham-ovariectomized at
4 weeks (hormonally intact females).

The estimated median times for 28- and 40-week ovariectomized females were 49 and 51 weeks, respectively. This shows that the acceleration of development of the hepatocellular adenomas was inversely related to the age at ovariectomy.

Table 2 compares the emergence of the intermediate basophilic foci, hyperplastic nodules, hepatocellular adenomas, and hepatocellular carcinomas between hormonally intact (A) and hormonally deprived males (B) Hepatocarcinogenesis was induced by a single administration of DEN (2.5 µg/g body weight) to infant mice. Orchidectomy was performed at 20 weeks. The table illustrates that orchidectomy significantly delayed the emergence of the intermediate basophilic foci up to 40 weeks of age (136.8 vs. 197.5), and hyperplastic nodules (20.6 vs. 36.0), hepatocellular adenomas (16.8 vs. 52.8), and hepatocellular carcinomas (0.4 vs. 7.3) through the 52nd week of age. Thus, by 52 weeks the orchidectomized males developed 17.2 combined benign and malignant hepatocellular tumors per liver in contrast to 60.1 liver tumors expressed in the hormonally intact males.

Table 2. Effect of Orchidectomy on the Emergence of Intermediate Basophilic Foci, Hyperplastic Nodules, Hepatocellular Adenomas, and Hepatocellular Carcinomas Induced by Single Administration of DEN at Infancy[a]

Weeks	Intermediate Basophilic Foci		Hyperplastic Nodules		Hepatocellular Adenomas		Hepatocellular Carcinomas	
	A	B	A	B	A	B	A	B
24	85.2	29.1	217	1.9	0.8	0.0	...	...
32	153.7	75.0	25.4	6.0	12.5	1.6	...	...
40	197.5	136.8	34.6	10.2	36.5	1.4	...	...
44	235.7	255.2	46.9	17.8	51.8	3.1	0.8	...
48	157.4	203.6	38.9	19.1	44.0	3.7	3.5	...
52	85.5	126.9	36.0	20.6	52.8	16.8	7.3	0.4

[a]DEN given at 2.5 µg/g body weight to 15-day-old B6C3F$_1$ male mice. A = sham-orchidectomy (20 weeks of age); B = orchidectomy (20 weeks of age). Body of the table represents the average number of specified lesions per liver observed at the specified age.

This study illustrated that orchidectomy performed at 20 weeks of age significantly affected the emergence of hyperplastic nodules, hepatocellular adenomas, and hepatocellular carcinomas. Recently terminated studies showed that following 4-week orchidectomy a greater delay in hepatocarcinogenesis occurred.

The above series of studies showed that gonadectomy was more effective in modifying hepatocarcinogenesis when performed early in life, and that, in spite of the hormonal modulation, gonadectomized animals developed in time the same number of tumors per liver as the hormonally intact animals. It is obvious that the hormonal environment controlled the rate of the neoplastic expression but had no effect upon the final number of tumors which developed. Therefore, it may be concluded that gonadectomy had no effect upon the final expression of the initiated and neoplastically committed cells.

Fig. 5 presents the dose-response relationship observed at 44 weeks of age in regard to the development of hepatocellular adenomas. Dose-response curves were given for hormonally intact (upper, broken line) and for hormonally deprived male mice (lower, solid line). The sham-orchidectomies and orchidectomies were performed at 4 weeks of age. The lines were fitted to data which were plotted on a double logarithmic scale transforming the exponential into a linear dose-response. The fitted lines were parallel, since in both instances the slopes were the same (tan., 1.2). However, the intercepts differed, being lower in hormonally deprived (0.85) than in the hormonally intact males (20.0). This illustrates clearly a significantly lower expression of hepatocellular adenomas in the hormonally deprived males than in the hormonally competent animals at 44 weeks of age, regardless of the dose.

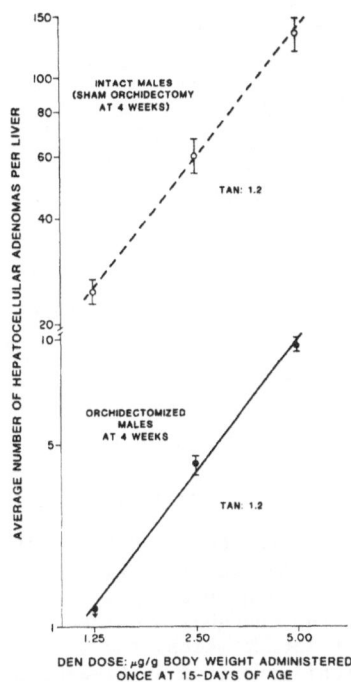

Fig. 5.   Comparative dose response between hor-
          monally intact and hormonally deprived
          males at 44 weeks.   Fifteen-day-old
          B6C3F$_1$ mice received specified dose
          levels of DEN.   Sham-orchidectomies
          and orchidectomies were performed at
          4 weeks of age.

Similar dose response curves (tan., 1) were observed earlier in the case of the intermediate basophilic foci at 20 and 30 weeks of age and hepatocellular carcinomas at 50 and 60 weeks of age. This indicated a common dose-response rate for hepatocellular foci, adenomas, and carcinomas when taken during their development (foci at 20 weeks and carcinomas at 50 weeks) and at the time of their maximal response (foci at 30 weeks, adenomas at 44 weeks, and carcinomas at 60 weeks). The intercepts of these curves were progressively lower for the more advanced lesions (from foci to adenomas to carcinomas). The shift of dose-response curves to later age with the emergence of the more advanced lesions indicated temporal relationship in regard to the development of the above hepatocellular lesions. The latter observation, when considered together with previously reported time-dose relationship studies (26) points out that progressively more events are required for the development of foci, adenomas, and carcinomas, respectively.

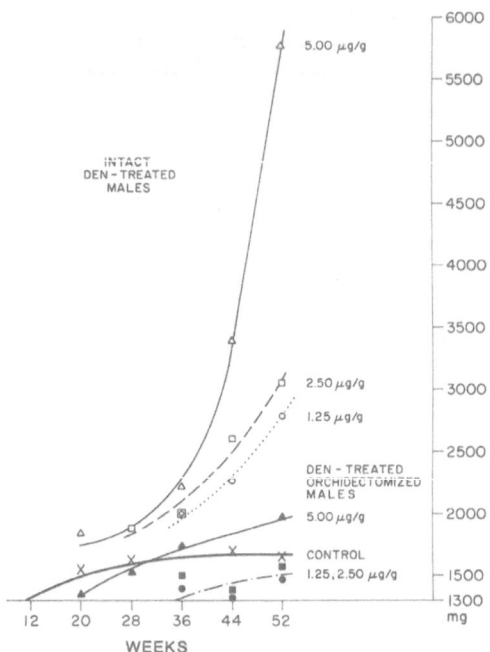

Fig. 6. Liver weights inclusive of neoplastic
lesions. Animals received specified amount
of DEN at 15 days of age. One-half of each
dose group was sham-orchidectomized (hormonally intact males) and the other half
was orchidectomized at 4 weeks of age
(hormonally deprived males). One group was
sham-treated and sham-orchidectomized
(control group).

Fig. 6 and Table 3 show that dose- and time-response was also causally related to liver weights as manifestation of neoplastic growth. The latter endpoint was also significantly affected by orchidectomy carried out at 4 weeks of age. Thus, regardless of age at which the animals were killed, the liver weights containing neoplastic lesions in the hormonally intact males were 2367 mg, 2553 mg, and 3800 mg following treatment with 1.25, 2.5, and 5.0 μg DEN/g body weight, respectively. The corresponding weights in the hormonally deprived mice were 1442 mg, 1390 mg, and 1737 mg, respectively. It may be, therefore, concluded that the level of endogenous androgen controls the growth rate of neoplastic lesions. The growth may represent also the factor underlying the emergence of all nodular lesions. If so, then the endogenous sex hormones may be considered as modifiers of the growth of both the initiated cells early in the process and the neoplastic cells later in the process.

Table 3. Effect of Orchidectomy on the Growth of DEN-induced Liver Neoplasia

Age in Weeks	Non-treated Controls	DEN Dose: µg/g Body Weight		
		1.25	2.5	5.0
		Sham-orchidectomy at 4 Weeks		
36	1492 ± 54	2024 ± 38	1994 ± 67	2221 ± 51
44	1702 ± 31	2287 ± 91	2602 ± 239	3405 ± 225
52	1660 ± 83	2791 ± 217	3063 ± 325	5776 ± 178
		Orchidectomy at 4 Weeks		
36	1492 ± 54	1370 ± 36	1406 ± 43	1744 ± 159
44	1702 ± 31	1380 ± 32	1275 ± 41	1485 ± 113
52	1660 ± 83	1577 ± 66	1491 ± 75	1982 ± 288

The body of the table gives the average weights of the livers, including weights of the preneoplastic and neoplastic nodular lesions; numbers represent mean liver weight ± S.E.

DISCUSSION

Induction and development of tumors in general and in the liver in particular depend upon the sex in both animals and humans (27-29). The sex difference in carcinogenesis may be due to a difference in the initiating and/or the developing phase of the neoplastic process. Thus, the differences in the metabolic activation of the procarcinogens and the fixation-repair ratio of the primary molecular lesion(s) will result in a different degree of initiation. Using an experimental model in which initiation is of equal degree in males and females, the sex of the animal could influence only the development stage of carcinogenesis by modulating either one or several of the following: the degree of the expression of the initiated cells, the time of onset, the rate of neoplastic expression, and the rate of neoplastic progression. Our infant mouse model, utilizing DEN as hepatocarcinogen and gonadectomy, performed at various times following DEN treatment as modifier of hormonal environment of the host, aimed at elucidating the role of sex hormones upon the development phase of carcinogenesis. The obtained data pointed out that sex hormonal environment did not affect the number of initiated cells as measured by the number of focal and nodular lesions per liver. However, the sex hormonal environment influenced the time of onset of the various lesions, the rate of their expression and neoplastic progression. The early and late emerging lesions were associated with cell replication as indicated by an increase in the labeling indices of tinctorial foci (30) and in tumor weights, respectively. Thus, one can assume that sex hormonal environment was a regulator of preneoplastic and neoplastic growth. Predominantly androgenic environment (sham-orchidectomized males) accelerated and the predominantly estrogenic environment (sham-ovariectomized females) delayed neoplastic growth and progression. The shift in the hormonal environment of the host from the hormonally intact state delayed hepatocarcinogenesis following orchidectomy and accelerated carcinogenesis following ovariectomy. Because the process of carcinogenesis occurred regardless of sex hormonal environment and the same number of lesions developed, the sex hormones can not be considered as promoting (androgen) or anti-promoting (estrogen) agents, but rather as modifiers of post-initiation or development stage of hepatocarcinogenesis.

SUMMARY

Following identical induction of hepatocarcinogenesis by single administration of diethylnitrosamine (DEN) to 15-day-old B6C3F$_1$ mice, both sexes developed in time the same multiplicity of various non-neoplastic (intermediate basophilic foci and hyperplastic nodules) and neoplastic (hepatocellular adenomas and carcinomas) lesions. The males, however, developed the same number of lesions within a significantly shorter period of time than females and orchidectomized males. When assessment of the morphologic endpoints was made at the time the response plateaued in the hormonally intact males, the average multiplicities of lesions per liver were significantly lower in the orchidectomized animals. At the time the response reached maximal level in the ovariectomized females, the multiplicity of lesions was significantly lower in the hormonally intact females. Orchidectomy delayed and ovariectomy accelerated the emergence of the hepatocellular foci, hyperplastic nodules, adenomas, and carcinomas without having any effect upon the final multiplicities of these lesions. This indicated that eventually the same numbers of originally initiated cells were expressed as hepatocellular lesions regardless of the sex hormonal environment of the host. Thus, sex steroids should be considered as the modulators of the rate of the genic and morphologic expression and the progression of the neoplastic lesions.

REFERENCES

1. Vesselinovitch, S. D., Liver tumor induction, Toxicol. Path. 10:110-120, 1982.
2. Remmer, H. Metabolism of carcinogens: Its significance for the initiation of liver tumors, in: Primary Liver Tumors, ch. 3, pp. 31-49, H. M. Bolt, P. Bannasch, and H. Popper, eds., M.T.P. Press, Lancaster, UK, 1978.
3. Miller, E. C., and Miller, J. A., Mechanisms of chemical carcinogenesis, Cancer 47:1055-1064, 1981.
4. Miller, E. C., and Miller, J. A., Searches for ultimate chemical carcinogens and their reactions with cellular macromolecules. Cancer 47:2327-2345, 1981.
5. Gelboin, H. V., Wiebel, F. J., and Kinoshita, N., Microsomal aryl hydrocarbon hydroxylases. On their role in polycyclic hydrocarbon carcinogenesis and toxicity and the mechanism of enzyme induction, Biochem. Soc. Symp. 34:103-133, 1972.
6. Becker, R. A., and Shank, R. C. Kinetics of formation and persistence of ethylguanine in DNA of rats and hamsters treated with diethylnitrosamine, Cancer Res. 45:2076-2084, 1985.
7. Brambilla, G., Martelli, A., Pino, A., and Robbiano, L., Sequential analysis of DNA damage and repair during the development of carcinogen-induced rat liver hyperplastic lesions, Cancer Res. 46:3476-3481, 1986.
8. Scherer, E., Steward, A. P., and Emmelot, P. Kinetics of formation of O^6-ethylguanine in, and its removal from liver DNA of rats receiving diethylnitrosamine, Chem.-Biol. Interact. 19:1-11, 1977.
9. Stich, H. F., Laishes, B. A., DNA repair and chemical carcinogens, in: Pathobiology Annual, vol. 3, pp. 341-376, H. L. Ioachim, ed. Appleton-Century-Crofts, New York, 1973.

10. Kleihues, P., Cooper, H. K., and Buecheler, J., Involvement of DNA repair in the organ-specific carcinogenicity of alkylating agents, in: Primary Liver Tumors, ch. 26, pp. 319-326, H. Remmer, H. M. Bolt, P. Bannasch, and H. Popper, eds., M.T.P. Press, Lancaster, UK, 1978.

11. Tucker, M. J. The effect of long-term food restriction on tumors in rodents, Int. J. Cancer 23:803-807, 1979.

12. Conybeare, G., Effect of quality and quantity of diet on survival and tumor incidence in outbred Swiss mice, Food Cosmet. Toxicol., 18:65-75, 1980.

13. Rogers, A. E., and Newberne, P. M., Dietary effects on chemical carcinogenesis in animal models for colon and liver tumors, Cancer Res. 35:3427-3431, 1975.

14. Vesselinovitch, S. D., and Mihailovich, N., The effect of gonadectomy on the development of hepatomas induced by urethan, Cancer Res. 27:1788-1791, 1967.

15. Vesselinovitch, S. D., Itze, L., Mihailovich, N., and Rao, K.V.N., Modifying role of partial hepatectomy and gonadectomy in ethylnitrosourea-induced hepatocarcinogenesis, Cancer Res. 40:1538-1542, 1980.

16. Vesselinovitch, S. D., and Mihailovich, N., Modifying effect of the sex hormonal environment on the growth of basophilic foci and hepatocellular carcinoma, in: The Control of Tumour Growth and Its Biological Bases, pp. 282-286, W. Davis, C. Maltoni, and St. Tanneberger, eds., Akademie-Verlag, Berlin, 1983.

17. Vesselinovitch, S. D., Mihailovich, N., Rao, K.V.N., and Goldfarb, S., Relevance of basophilic foci to promoting effect of sex hormones on hepatocarcinogenesis, in: Carcinogenesis, vol. 7, pp. 127-131, E. Hecker, N. Fusenig, F. Marks, and W. Kunz, eds., Raven Press, New York, 1982.

18. Vesselinovitch, S. D., Koka, M., Mihailovich, N., and Rao, K.V.N., Carcinogenicity of diethylnitrosamine in newborn, infant and adult mice, J. Cancer Res. Clin. Oncol. 108:60-65, 1984.

19. Rao, K.V.N., and Vesselinovitch, S. D., Age and sex-associated diethylnitrosamine dealkylation activity of the mouse liver and hepatocarcinogenesis, Cancer Res. 33:1625-1627, 1973.

20. Vesselinovitch, S. D., Factors modulating response to carcinogenic mutagens, in: Progress in Environmental Mutagenesis, M. Alacevic, ed., Biomedical Press, Elsevier/North Holland, 1980.

21. Yee Chu Toh, Effect of neonatal castration on liver tumor induction by N-2-fluorenylacetamide in suckling BALB/c mice carcinogenesis, Carcinogenesis 2:1219-1221, 1981.

22. Vesselinovitch, S. D., Mihailovich, N., and Rao, K.V.N., Morphology and metastatic nature of induced hepatic nodular lesions in C57BLxC3H F_1 mice, Cancer Res. 38:2003-2010, 1978.

23. Fulmann, R. L., Measurement of particle sizes on opaque bodies. Trans. AIME 197:447-452, 1953.

24. Campbell, H. A., Pitot, H. C., Potter, V. R., and Laishes, B. A., Application of quantitative stereology to the evaluation of enzyme-altered foci in rat liver, Cancer Res. 42:465-472, 1982.

25. Moore, M. R., Drinkwater, N. R., Miller, E. C., Miller, J. A., and Pitot, H. C., Quantitative analysis of the time-dependent development of glucose-6-phosphatase-deficient foci in the livers of mice treated neonatally with diethylnitrosamine, Cancer Res. 41:1585-1593, 1981.

26. Vesselinovitch, S. D., and Mihailovich, N., Kinetics of diethylnitrosamine hepatocarcinogenesis in the infant mouse, Cancer Res. 43:4253-4259, 1983.

27. Higginson, J., The epidemiology of primary carcinoma of the liver, in: Tumors of the Liver, pp. 38-52, G. T. Pock and A. H. Islami, eds., Springer-Verlag, Berlin, 1970.

28. Higginson, J., Geographical pathology of primary liver cancer, Cancer Res. 23:1624-1633, 1963.

29. Toh, Y. C., Physiological and biochemical review of sex differences and carcinogenesis with particular references to the liver, Adv. Cancer Res. 18:155-209, 1973.
30. Vesselinovitch, S. D., Hacker, H. J., and Bannasch, P., Histochemical characterization of focal hepatic lesions induced by single diethyl-nitrosamine treatment in infant mice, Cancer Res. 45:2774-2780, 1985.

These investigations have been supported in part by Grant CA-25522 from the National Cancer Institute (U.S.A.).

LIVER CANCER AND VIRUSES

Zsuzsa Schaff and Károly Lapis

I[st] Institute of Pathology and Experimental Cancer Research, Semmelweis Medical University Budapest VIII. Üllői str. 26. H-1o85, Hungary

INTRODUCTION

Primary hepatocellular carcinoma /PHC/ is one of the ten most common malignant tumors in the world /Lancet editorial, 1983/. Mortality rates associated with PHC are different in low incidence areas of the world such as Europe and U.S.A. /Friedman, 1983; Lapis and Johannessen, 1979; Sandler et al., 1983; Schaff et al., 1971/ and in high incidence areas, such as sub-Saharan Africa /Anthony et al., 1973; Kew, 1978; Szmuness, 1978/, Southeast Asia /China, Korea, Thailand, Japan/ /Beasley et al., 1981; Gibson et al., 1980; Lai et al., 1981; Nakashima et al., 1983; Okuda, 1980/.

Etiologic factors associated with human PHC are hepatitis B virus /HBV/ infection, chronic alcohol abuse, mycotoxins /Blumberg and London, 1981; Friedman, 1983; Popper, 1979; Sherlock et al., 1970/, sex hormons /Williams, 1982/, occupational risk factors, medication /Stemhagen et al., 1983/ and metabolic alterations /Bannasch et al., 1980/.

Liver cancer can be induced in animals by chemicals /Bannasch et al., 1980; Farber, 1982; Farber and Cameron, 1980; Peraino et al., 1973; Pitot and Sirica, 1980; Scherer and Emmelot, 1976/ and by viruses /Beard et al., 1975; Lapis et al., 1975; Summers and Mason, 1982/ as well. In the followings the relationship between certain viruses and PHC is discussed.

HEPADNA /HEPATITIS B-LIKE/ VIRUSES AND PRIMARY HEPATOCELLULAR CARCINOMA

Epidemiology

Evidence suggesting a causual relationship /Sherlock et al., 1970/ between HBV infection and PHC was initially based on epidemiologic observations /Gerin, 1983; Lancet editorial, 1983; Vogel et al., 1970/.

PHC was noted most commonly in regions where chronic carriers of HBV occur, such as sub-Saharan Africa, Southeast Asia, China, Japan /Beasley et al., 1981; Kew, 1978; London, 1981; Okuda, 1980; Okuda et al., 1982; Popper et al., 1982/.

Patients with PHC show significantly higher frequencies of serologic markers /HBsAg, anti-HBc, HBeAg/ of persistent HBV infection than controls /Blumberg and London, 1981; Szmuness, 1978; Tabor et al., 1977/.

In high risk areas of the world, perinatal infection transmitted from chronic carrier mothers to their children are important in the development of carrier state and PHC /Blumberg and London, 1981; Tabor et al., 1983/.

Prospective studies have predicted the risk of PHC in chronic HBsAg carriers /Beasley et al., 1981/.

Localization of HBV antigens in PHC

The virion of hepatitis B virus /known as the Dane particle/ consists of a spherical particle 42nm in diameter /Dane et al., 1970/ with an inner DNA core of 27nm in diameter and a lipid containing hepatitis B surface antigen /HBsAg/. Besides isolation from the sera of HBsAg positive patients, hepatitis B surface antigen /HBsAg/ and core antigen /HBcAg/ have been localized in tumor cells and in the surrounding liver tissue by immunohistochemical methods /Gudat et al., 1975;

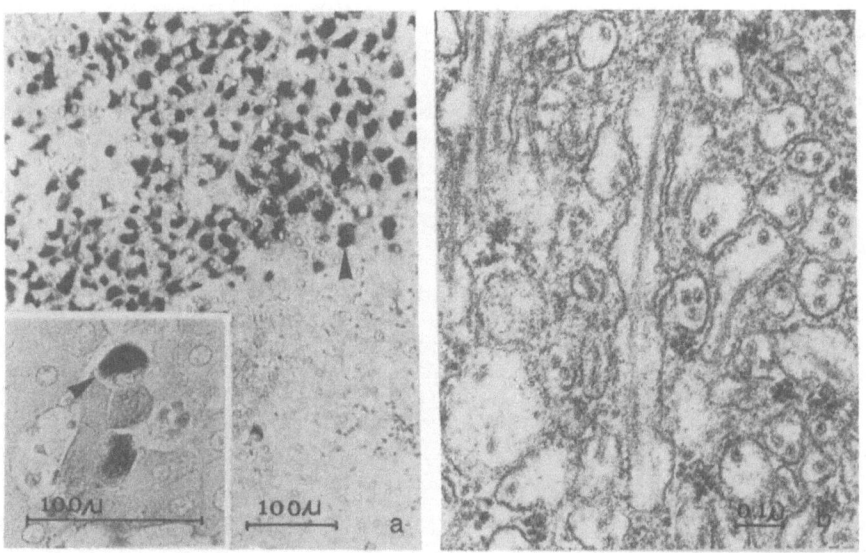

Fig. 1. Localization of HBsAg in hepatocytes. /a/ Immunohistochemical reaction using anti-HBs as primary antibody /avidin-biotin-peroxidase complex method/ for detection of the antigen /arrow/; /b/ Tubules and spherical particles of HBsAg visualized by electron microscopy.

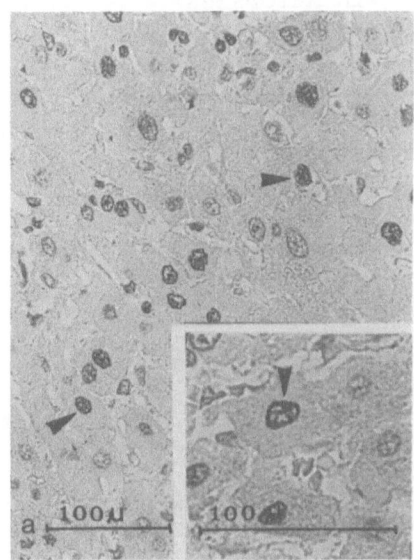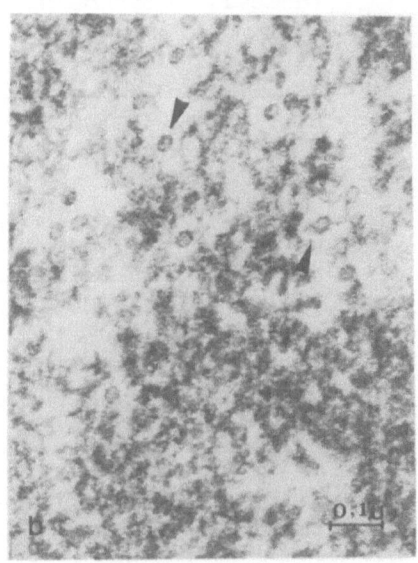

Fig. 2. Localization of HBcAg in the nuclei of hepatocytes.
/a/ Nuclei with dark staining /arrow/ contain the
antigen according to the indirect /peroxidase-
antiperoxidase/ immunohistochemical reaction.
/b/ Core particles 27 nm in diameter /arrow/ can
be seen in the nucleus by electron microscopy.

Hirohashi et al., 1982; Omata et al., 1982/ /Fig. 1., 2./, and
orcein staining /Shikata et al., 1974/. Core particles can be
localized in the nuclei /Fig. 2b./, the tubules of HBsAg in
the endoplasmic reticulum cisternae /Fig. 1b./ of the infected
cells by electron microscopy /Gerber et al., 1974; Schaff et
al., 1986/. Distribution of HBsAg in the nontumorous liver in
in PHC is very irregular, and the amount of antigen varies
from case to case /Shikata, 1976/.

The proportion of liver tumors that express both HBsAg
and HBcAg is relatively small /less than 5%/ /Hirohashi et al.,
1982/. HBsAg was detected in seven of nine serologically HBsAg
-positive PHC /Thung et al., 1979/. A greater number of HBV
antigen-positive hepatocytes were found in the non-tumorous
areas of the liver than in the tumor cells itself /Gudat et
al., 1975; Hirohashi et al., 1982; Nayak and Sachdeva, 1975/.
In 181 autopsies with liver cirrhosis PHC was significantly
more frequent in HBsAg-positive cases than in alcoholic cirrhosis /Bartók et al., 1981/.

Out of 5979 autopsies in the I[st] Institute of Pathology
and Experimental Cancer Research /Budapest, Hungary/ PHC occurred in 87 cases /1,45%/, 65 of them /1,08%/ were associated
with cirrhosis /Table 1./. 5o autopsy cases of cirrhosis and
5o of PHC were studied by immunohistochemical methods /peroxi-
dase-antiperoxidase, avidin-biotin-peroxidase complex/ for localization of five antigens /HBsAg, HBcAg, alpha-fetoprotein

Table 1. Cirrhosis and PHC[a] in Autopsies /1975-1984, over 15 years, I[st] Inst. Path.Exp.Cancer Res., Budapest/

Diagnosis	Number of cases		%	
Cirrhosis	396		6,62	
Cirrhosis and PHC	65	87	1,08	1,45
PHC	22		0,37	
Total number of autopsies	5975		100	

[a]PHC = primary hepatocellular carcinoma

/AFP/, carcinoembryonic antigen /CEA/, alpha-1-antitrypsin /AAT// /Table 2./. HBsAg was located in 10% of cirrhotic and 8% of PHC cases. HBcAg was present in 4% of cirrhosis and 2% of PHC samples studied. Tumor cells of PHC contained AFP in 40% and CEA in 50% of the cases and no AAT was located in the tumor cells.

30 cases of surgically removed benign /adenoma, focal nodular hyperplasia, hemangioma/ and malignant /PHC/ human liver tumors were studied for the same viral /HBV/ and oncofetal /AFP, CEA, AAT/ markers /Table 3./. None of the benign or malignant tumors were positive for HBV markers. AFP and CEA were observed only in malignant tumors, the benign tumors were negative. Activities of enzymes, such as glucose-6-phosphatase /G6Pase/, canalicular adenosine-5'-triphosphatase /ATPase/ and gamma-glutamyl transpeptidase /GGTase/ were studied in the surgically removed human tumors by histochemical methods /Table 3./. Changes in activities of the enzymes were similar in adenomas and focal nodular hyperplasias to those observed during the multistep process of hepatocarcinogenesis in chemically induced neoplasias in experimental animals /Bannasch et al., 1980; Farber, 1980; Lapis et al., in press/. Heterogene-

Table 2. HBV and Oncofetal Antigens[a] in Cirrhosis and PHC

	HBsAg	HBcAg	AFP	CEA	AAT	Total number of cases
Cirrhosis	5/10%/	2/4%/	0	0	0	50
PHC	4/8%/	1/2%/	20/40%/	25/50%/	0	50[b]

[a]Immunohistochemical methods
HBV=Hepatitis B virus, PHC=Primary hepatocellular carcinoma, HBsAg=Hepatitis B surface antigen, HBcAg=Hepatitis B core antigen, AFP=Alpha-fetoprotein, CEA=Carcinoembryonic antigen, AAT=Alpha-1-antitrypsin
[b]Associated with cirrhosis in 44 cases.

Table 3. Immunohistochemical and Histochemical Reaction of Surgically Removed Human Liver Tumors[a]

Diagnosis[b]	HBsAg	HBcAg	AFP	CEA	AAT	G6P	ATP	GGT
FNH /6/	o/6	o/6	o/6	o/6	o/6	4/6	1/6	5/6
Adenoma /4/	o/4	o/4	o/4	o/4	o/4	4/4	o/4	1/4
PHC /15/	o/15	o/15	1o/15	7/15	2/15	6/15	o/15	8/15
Hepato-blastoma /1/	o/1	o/1	1/1	1/1	o/1	o/1	o/1	o/1
Hemangi-oma /4/	o/4	o/4	4/4	o/4	o/4	o/4	o/4	o/4

[a]Positive reaction/total.

[b]Total number of cases is in parenthesis.
FNH=Focal nodular hyperplasia, PHC=Primary hepatocellular carcinoma, HBsAg=Hepatitis B surface antigen, HBcAg=Hepatitis B core antigen, AFP=Alpha fetoprotein, CEA=Carcinoembryonic antigen, AAT=alpha-1-antitrypsin, G6P=Glucose-6-phosphatase, ATP=Adenosine-5'-triphosphatase, GGT=Gamma-glutamyl transpeptidase.

ity in the activity of the enzymes were noted in PHC cases.

In vivo animal studies

Inoculation of different animals with infectious HBV resulted successful transmission of the virus only in chimpanzees and marmosets /Barker et al., 1973; Popper et al., 198o/. No infection was observed in immunosuppressed /Schaff et al., 1982/ or new-born mice /Tabor, 1983/.

Persistent infection with other members of hepadna viruses /Summers, 1981/, such as woodchuck hepatitis virus /WHV/ /Summers et al., 1978/, ground squirrel hepatitis virus /GSHV/ /Marion et al., 198o/, domestic Pekin duck hepatitis B virus /DHBV/ /Mason et al., 198o/ resulted chronic active hepatitis and primary hepatocellular carcinoma in woodchucks only /Table 4./. No PHC was observed in captive ground squirrels infected with DSHV or in Pekin ducks infected with DHBV /Marion and Robinson, 1983/. PHCs in Pekin ducks in China were noted in infected and in uninfected ducks so the relationship of PHC and DHBV is not so evident /Marion et al., 1984/.

Monoclonal antibodies against HBsAg has prevented or suppressed tumor formation in PHC-bearing nude mice /Shouval et al., 1982/.

In vitro studies

Investigation of the expression and replication of the HBV genom has been hampered for a long time by the lack of suitable in vitro cell culture system in which HBV is propagated /Crowley et al., 1983; Sells et al., 1987/.

Table 4.   Viruses Associated with Primary Hepato-
          cellular Carcinoma

Virus	Species	References
Hepadna viruses[a]		
Hepatitis B Virus /HBV/	Human	Sherlock et al. /1970/, Blumberg et al. /1975/
Woodchuck Hepatitis Virus /WHV/	Woodchuck	Summers et al. /1978/
Oncoviruses		
MC29 virus	Chicken	Lapis et al. /1975/ Beard et al. /1975/
	Turkey	Schaff et al. /1978/

[a]Association of PHC and duck hepatitis B virus /Mason
et al., 1980/, and ground squirrel hepatitis virus
/Marion et al., 1980/ is not a strong one.

Some cell lines established from PHC produce HBsAg /Mac-
nab et al., 1976; Marion et al., 1980/. Viral antigen production continues even after injection of the tumor into nude mice /Shouval et al., 1982/. Integration of HBV DNA into the
host cell genome in HBsAg-producing cell lines and cells of
PHC has been detected /Brechot et al., 1980; Charkraborty et
al., 1980; Edman et al., 1980/, but not in carrier chimpanzees
without carcinoma /Shouval et al., 1980/.

HBV sequences were shown to be integrated in at least
eight cellular DNA sites in HBsAg-producing PHC cell line
/Miller et al., 1983/. More extensive methylation of the viral
DNA was detected in tumor cells than in nontumorous liver,
which suggest that methylation of HBV DNA might be involved in
regulation of viral gene expression in PHC /Robinson et al.,
1984/. Up to now there is no evidence that transcription of
known oncogene sequences is altered in PHC cells and HBV or
WHV contain a viral oncogene.

Transfection of several cell lines with cloned HBV DNA
/Dubois et al., 1980; Gough and Murray, 1982; Christman et al.,
1982; Hirschman and Garfinkel, 1982/ did not result the replicative DNA intermediates similar to those identified in the livers of animals infected with hepadna viruses /Buscher et al.,
1985; Summers and Mason, 1982/ or Dane-like viral particles.
More recently Tuttleman et al. /1986/ showed that Pekin duck
liver cells in culture support duck hepatitis virus replication. Sells et al. /1987/ reported production of hepatitis B virus particles in a hepatoblastoma cell line /Hep G2/ transfected with cloned HBV DNA. Components morphologically identical to the 22nm spherical and filamentous HBsAg particles as
well as 42nm Dane particles were visualized /Sells et al.,
1987/. This in vitro system might now be used to study the oncogenic potential of HBV.

ONCOVIRUSES AND PRIMARY HEPATOCELLULAR CARCINOMA

Several members of oncoviruses of the retrovirus family produce tumors in animals /Lowy, 1986/.

Myelocytomatosis virus /MC29/, a C-type oncovirus has been shown to induce liver tumors in chicken, approximately 4o days after inoculation /Beard et al., 1975; Lapis et al., 1975/ and in turkeys after 14 days following inoculation /Schaff et al., 1978/. MC29 virus belongs to the transformation-competent /v-myc+/, replication-defective retroviruses.

The tumor nodules in turkey livers induced by MC29 virus do not contain glycogen, loss of G6Pase and ATPase enzyme activities is similar to the one of chemically induced tumors in rodents. However, no G6Pase reaction was noted in the tumor foci. No premalignant alterations were noted in the animals before development of the malignant tumors /Fig.3./.

NON-A, NON-B HEPATITIS AND PRIMARY HEPATOCELLULAR CARCINOMA

Non-A, non-B hepatitis has been reported for responsible in over 9o% of posttransfusion hepatitis cases in several countries /Alter et al., 1975; Bradley et al., 1981; Feinstone et al., 1983; Gerety et al., 1984/.

No specific test exsist for detection of non-A, non-B hepatitis and the diagnosis is still based in the exclusion of hepatitis A virus, HBV and other causes of hepatitis /Gerety

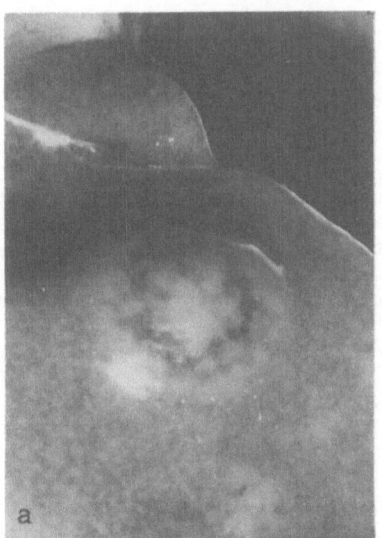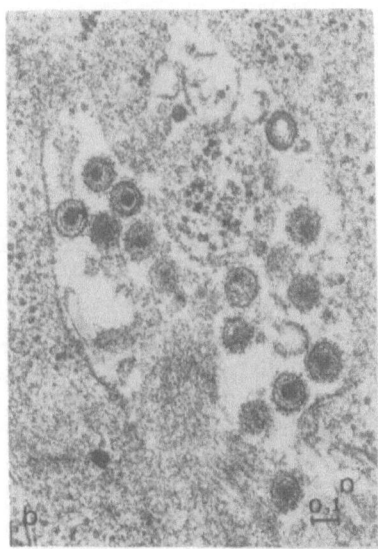

Fig. 3. MC29 virus induced hepatoma in turkey.
/a/ Small tumor in the liver;
/b/ Large number of C-type MC29 virus is found in the bile - canaliculus - like intercellular space formed by the hepatoma cells.

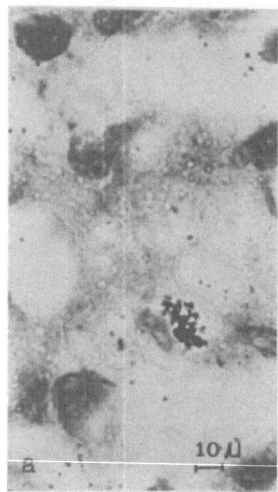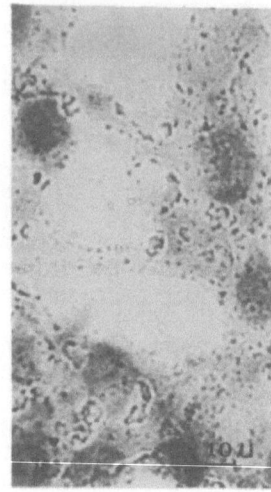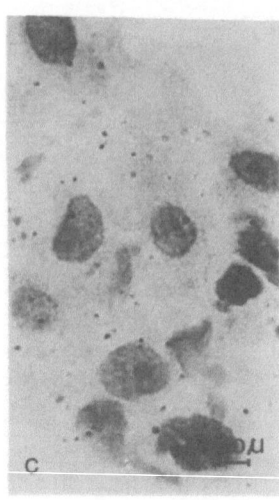

Fig. 4. In situ hybridization using frozen liver biopsy
samples from chimpanzees and radiolabeled /^{35}S/
probes. /a/ ^{35}S-HBV DNA probe hybridazed with
HBV-infected liver cells in spots;
/b/ ^{35}S-NANBH DNA probe hybridized with NANBH-
infected liver diffusely;
/c/ ^{35}S-pBr322 DNA probe did not hybridized with
NANBH-infected liver cells.

et al., 1984/. Chronic hepatitis and cirrhosis develop in high
percentage of non-A, non-B hepatitis cases and recently non-A,
non-B hepatitis has been reported in association with PHC as
well /Gilliam et al., 1984; Kiyosawa et al., 1984; Resnick et
al., 1983/.

A glycoprotein /GP77/ associated with non-A, non-B hepatitis has been isolated from acute phase sera of a patient
with non-A, non-B hepatitis and an antibody was raised against
it /Seto and Gerety, 1985/. The antibody reacted diffusely
with the liver samples of chimpanzees experimentally infected
with non-A, non-B hepatitis and with 11 out of 14 human liver
biopsy materials obtained from patients with non-A, non-B hepatitis /Schaff et al., in press/. Only one liver sample out
of 25 autopsies of PHC reacted with the antibody. This data do
not support the relationship between PHC and non-A, non-B hepatitis, however the possibility can not be ruled out completely.

More recently a 78o pair non-A, non-B hepatitis associated DNA was isolated and cloned in pBr322 plasmic vector /Seto
et al., 1984/. The ^{35}S-NANBH DNA probe in situ hybridized with
the frozen section obtained from non-A, non-B hepatitis infected chimpanzees /Schaff et al., in press/. ^{35}S-pBr322 DNA and
^{35}S-HBV DNA were used as controls /Fig. 4a, b, c/. The use of
the 78o base pair NANBH DNA as a probe might be an other approach for searching non-A, non-B hepatitis viral sequences in human liver tumors.

CONCLUSIONS

Up to now members of hepadna viruses such as human hepatitis B virus /HBV/, woodchuck hepatitis virus /WHV/, and MC29 virus, a member of oncovirus subfamily were found associated with human and animal liver cancers. Initial evidence for a causual relationship between HBV infection and primary hepatocellular carcinoma /PHC/ was based on epidemiological studies. Serological, immunomorphological, cell biological in vivo and in vitro studies support this association. Viral DNA is found integrated in the host DNA of hepatoma cells, exactly how these viruses involved in liver tumor formation and the mechanism of hepatocarcinogenesis by these viruses is still not resolved. In case of MC29 virus the myc-oncogen is probable responsible for the tumor development. The hepadna viruses and retroviruses - at least superficially - seem to share some characteristics. Despite the difference in the nucleic acid of the genom - DNA in hepadna viruses and RNA in retroviruses - the viral messenger RNAs are transcribed from the same DNA strand and in the same direction for viruses of both groups /Robinson, 1986/, and replicate through an RNA intermediate applying the enzyme reverse transcriptase /Summers and Mason, 1982/. No viral oncogen has been detected at this time in hepadna viruses. The clarification of the relationship of non-A, non-B hepatitis and hepatic tumors needs further studies.

REFERENCES

Alter, H.J., Purcell, R.H., Holland, P.V., Feinstone, S.M., Morrow, A.G., Moritsugu, Y., 1975, Clinical and serological analysis of transfusion-associated hepatitis, Lancet, 2:838.

Anthony, P.P., Vogel, C.L., Barker, L.F., 1973, Liver cell dysplasia: a premalignant condition, Am.J.Clin.Pathol., 26:217.

Bannasch, P., Mayer, D., Hacker, H.J., 198o, Hepatocellular glycogenosis and hepatocarcinogenesis, Biochem.Biophys. Acta, 6o5:217.

Barker, L.F., Chisari, F.V., McGrath, P.P., Dulgard, D.W., Kirschstein, R.L., Almeida, J.D., Edgington, T.S., Sharp, D.G., Peterson, M.R., 1973, Transmission of type B viral hepatitis to chimpanzees, J.Infect Dis., 127:648.

Bartók, I., Remenár, É., Tóth, J., Duschanek, P., Kanyár, B., 1981, Clinicopathological studies of liver cirrhosis and hepatocellular carcinoma in a general hospital, Human Path., 12:794.

Beard, J.W., Hillman, E.A., Beard, D., Lapis, K., Heine, U., 1975, Neoplastic response of the avian liver to host infection with strain MC29 leukosis virus, Cancer Res., 35:16o3.

Beasley, R.P., Hwang, L.Y., Lin, C.C., Chien, C.S., 1981, Hepatocellular carcinoma and hepatitis B virus. A prospective study of 22,7o7 men in Taiwan, Lancet, 2:1129.

Blumberg, B.S., Larouzé, B., Thomas, W., Werner, B., Hesser, J.E., Millman, I., Saimot, G., Payet, M., 1975, The relation of infection with hepatitis B agent to primary hepatic carcinoma, Am.J.Pathol., 81: 669.

Blumberg, B.S., London, W.T., 1981, Hepatitis B virus and the prevention of primary hepatocellular carcinoma, N.Engl. J.Med., 3o4:782.

Bradley, D.W., Maynard, J.E., Popper, H., Ebert, J.W., Cook, E.H., Fields, H.A., Kemler, B.J., 1981, Persistent non-A, non-B hepatitis in experimentally infected chimpanzees, J.Infect.Dis., 143:21o.

Brechot, Ch., Pourcel, Ch., Louise, A., Rain, B., Tiollais, P., 198o, Presence of integrated hepatitis B virus DNA sequences in cellular DNA of human hepatocellular carcinoma, Nature, 286:533.

Büscher, M., Reiser, W., Will, H., Schaller, H., 1985, Transcripts and the Putative RNA Pregenome of Duck Hepatitis B Virus: Implications for Reverse Transcription, Cell, 4o:717.

Chakraborty, P.R., Ruiz-Opazo, N., Shouval, D., Shafritz, D. A., 198o, Identification of integrated hepatitis B virus DNA and expression of viral RNA in an HBsAg-producing human hepatocellular carcinoma cell line, Nature, 286:531.

Christman, J.K., Gerber, M., Price, P.M., Flordellis, C., Edelman, J., Acs, G., 1982, Amplification of expression of hepatitis B surface antigen in 3T3 cells co-transfected with a dominant-acting gene and cloned viral DNA, Proc.Natl.Acad.Sci.U.S.A., 79:1815.

Crowley, C.W., Liu, Ch-Ch., Levinson, A.D., 1983, Plasmid-directed synthesis of hepatitis B surface antigen in monkey cells, Mol.Cell.Biol., 3:44.

Dane, D.S., Cameron, C.H., Briggs, M., 197o, Virus-like particles in serum of patients with Australia antigen--associated hepatitis, Lancet, 1:695.

Dubois, M.-F., Pourcel, C., Rousset, S., Chany, C., Tiollais, P., 198o, Excretion of hepatitis B surface antigen particles from mouse cells transformed with cloned viral DNA, Proc.Natl.Acad.Sci.U.S.A., 77:4549.

Edman, J.C., Gray, P., Valenzuela, P., Rall, L.B., Rutter, W. J., 198o, Integration of hepatitis B virus sequences and their expression in a human hepatoma cell line, Nature, 286:536.

Farber, E., 1982, Review article: chemical carcinogenesis. A biologic perspective, Am.J.Pathol., 1o6:271.

Farber, E., Cameron, R., 198o, The sequential analysis of cancer development, Adv.Cancer Res., 32:125.

Feinstone, S.M., Mihalik, K.B., Kamimura, T., 1983, Inactivation of hepatitis B virus and non-A, non-B hepatitis by chloroform, Infect.Immun., 41:816.

Friedman, M.A., 1983, Primary hepatocellular cancer-present results and future prospects, Int.J.Rad:Oncol.Biol. Phys., 9:1841.

Gerber, M.A., Hadziyannis, S., Vissoulis, C., Schaffner, F., Paronetto, F., Popper, H., 1974, Electron microscopy and immunoelectron microscopy of cytoplasmic hepatitis B antigen in hepatocytes, Am.J.Pathol., 75:489.

Gerety, R.J., Tabor, E., Schaff, Zs., Seto, B., Coleman, W. G.Jr., 1984, In: Viral hepatitis and Liver disease, G.N. Vyas, J.L. Dienstag, J.H. Hoofnagle, eds., Grune Stratton Inc. Orlando-San Diego-New York, ch. 3, pp. 23-47.

Gerin, J.L., 1983, Hepatitis B virus and primary hepatocellular carcinoma, Gastroenterology, 84:869.

Gibson, J.B., Wu, P.-C., Ho, J.C.I., Lauder, I.J., 198o, Hepatitis B surface antigen, hepatocellular carcinoma and cirrhosis in Hong Kong, Br.J.Cancer, 42:37o.

Gilliam, J.H., Geisinger, K.R., Richter, J.E., 1984, Primary hepatocellular carcinoma after chronic non-A, non-B post-transfusion hepatitis, Ann.Int.Med., 1o1:794.

Gough, N.M., Murray, K., 1982, Expression of the hepatitis B virus surface, core and E antigen genes by stable rat and mouse cell lines, J.Mol.Biol., 162:43.

Gudat, F., Bianchi, L., Sonnabend, W., Thiel, G., Aenishaenslin, W., Stalder, A., 1975, Pattern of core and surface expression in liver tissue reflects state of specific immune response in hepatitis B, Lab.Invest.,32:1.

Hirohashi, S., Shimosato, Y., Ino, Y., Kishi, K., 1982, Distribution of hepatitis B surface and core antigens in human liver cell carcinoma and surrounding nontumorous liver, J.Natl.Cancer Inst., 69:565.

Hirschman, S.Z., Garfinkel, E., 1982, Replication of hepatitis B virus DNA in transfected animal cell cultures: Synthesis of hepatitis B surface and e antigens, Hepatology, 2:79S.

Kew, M.C., 1978, Hepatocellular cancer in Southern Africa, In: Primary Liver Tumors, H. Remmer, H.M. Bolt, P. Bannasch, H. Popper, eds., University Park Press, Baltimore, pp. 179-183.

Kiyosawa, K., Akahane, Y., Nagata, A., Furuta, S., 1984, Hepatocellular carcinoma after non-A, non-B posttransfusion hepatitis, Am.J.Gastroent., 79:777.

Lai, C.L., Lam, K.C., Wong, K.P., Wu, P.C., Todd, D., 1981, Clinical features of hepatocellular carcinoma: review of 211 patients in Hong Kong, Cancer, 47:2746.

Lancet editorial: 1983, Prevention of primary liver cancer. Report of a meeting of a W.H.O. Scientific Group, Lancet, 1:463.

Lapis, K., Beard, D., Beard, J.W., 1975, Transplantation of hepatomas induced in the avian liver by MC29 leukosis virus, Cancer Res., 35:132.

Lapis, K., Jeney, A., Schaff, Zs., Zalatnay, A., Kovalszky, I., Szécsény, A., /in press/, Enzyme pattern changes in preneoplastic and neoplastic lesions of the liver, Springer Verlag

Lapis, K., Johannessen, J.V., 1979, Pathology of primary liver cancer, In: Liver Carcinogenesis, K. Lapis, J.V. Johannessen, eds., Hemisphere Publishing Corp., Washington, pp. 145-185.

London, W.T., 1981, Primary hepatocellular carcinoma - etiology, pathogenesis, and prevention, Hum.Pathol.,12:1o85.

Lowy, D.R., 1986, Transformation and Oncogenesis: Retroviruses, In: Virology, B.N. Fields, ed., Raven Press, New York, Ch. 13., pp. 235-264.

Macnab, G.M., Alexander, J.J., Lacatsas, G., Bey, E.M., Urbanowicz, K., 1976, Hepatitis B surface antigen produced by a human hepatoma cell line, Br.J.Cancer, 34:5o9.

Marion, P.L., Knight, S.S., Ho, B.K., Guo, Y.Y., Robinson, W.S., Popper, H., 1984, Liver disease associated with duck hepatitis B virus infection of domestic ducks, Proc. Natl.Acad.Sci., 81:898.

Marion, P., Oshiro, L.S., Regnery, D.C., Scullard, G.H., Robinson, W.S., 198o, A virus of Beechey ground squirrels that is related to hepatitis B virus of humans, Proc. Natl.Acad.Sci.U.S.A., 77:2941.

Marion, P.L., Robinson, W.S., 1983, Hepadna viruses: hepatitis B and related viruses, In: Current Topics in Microbiology and Immunology, M. Cooper, P.H. Hofschneider,

H. Koprowski, eds., Springer-Verlag, New York, pp.
  loo-121.
Mason, W.S., Seal, G., Summers, J., 198o, Virus of Pekin ducks
  with structural and biological relatedness to human
  hepatitis B virus, J.Virol., 36:829.
Miller, R.H., Robinson, W.S., 1983, Integrated hepatitis B vi-
  rus DNA sequences specifying the major viral core polypeptide are methylated in PLC/PRF/5 cells, Proc.
  Natl.Acad.Sci.U.S.A., 8o:2534.
Nakashima, T., Kijiro, M., Kawano, Y., Shirai, F., Takemoto,
  N., Tomimatsu, H., Kawasaki, H., Okuda, K., 1982, Histologic growth pattern of hepatocellular carcinoma:
  Relationship to orcein /hepatitis B surface antigen/-
  -positive cells in cancer tissue, Hum.Pathol., 13:563.
Nakashima, T., Okuda, K., Kojiro, M., Jimi, A., Yamaguchi, R.,
  Sakamoto, K., Ikari, T., 1983, Pathology of hepatocel-
  lular carcinoma in Japan, Cancer, 51:863.
Nayak, N.C., Sachdeva, R., 1975, Localization of hepatitis B
  surface antigen in conventional paraffin sections of
  the liver, Am.J.Pathol., 81:479.
Okuda, K., and the Liver Cancer Study Group of Japan, 198o,
  Primary liver cancers in Japan, Cancer, 45:2663.
Okuda, K., Nakashima, T., Sakamoto, K., Ikai, T., Hidaka, H.,
  Kibo, Y., Sakuma, K., Motoike, Y., Okuda, H., Obata,
  H., 1982, Hepatocellular carcinoma arising in non-
  cirrhotic and highly cirrhotic livers: a comparative
  study of histopathology and frequency of hepatitis B
  markers, Cancer, 49:45o.
Omata, M., Mori, J., Yokosuka, O., Iwama, S., Ito, Y., Okuda,
  K., 1982, Hepatitis B virus antigens in liver tissue
  in hepatocellular carcinoma and advanced chronic liver
  disease - relationship, Liver, 2:125.
Peraino, C., Fry, R.J.M., Staffeldt, E., Kisielski, W.E., 1973,
  Effects of varying the exposure to phenobarbital on its
  enhancement of 2-acetylaminofluorene-induced hepatic
  tumorigenesis in the rat, Cancer Res., 33:27o1.
Pitot, H.C., Sirica, A.E.: 198o, The stages of initiation and
  promotion in hepatocarcinogenesis, Biochim.Biophys.
  Acta, 6o5:191.
Popper, H., 1979, Hepatic cancers in man: quantitative perspectives, Environ.Res., 19:482.
Popper, H., Dienstag, J.L., Feinstone, S.M., Alter, H.J., Purcell, R.H., 198o, The pathology of viral hepatitis in
  chimpanzees, Virchows Arch.A., 387:91.
Popper, H., Gerber, M.A., Thung, S.N., 1982, The relation of
  hepatocellular carcinoma to infection with hepatitis
  B and related viruses in man and animals, Hepatology,
  2:1S.
Resnick, R.H., Stone, K., Antonioli, D., 1983, Primary hepatocellular carcinoma following non-A, non-B posttransfusion hepatitis, Dig.Dis.Sci., 28:9o8.
Robinson, W.S., Miller, R.H., Klote, L., Marion, P.L., Lee, S.-
  -C., 1984, Hepatitis B virus and hepatocellular carci-
  noma, In: Viral Hepatitis and Liver Disease, G.N. Vyas,
  J.L. Dienstag, J.H. Hoofnagle, eds., Grune and Strat-
  ton Inc., Orlando - New York, ch. 18. pp. 245-263.
Sandler, D.P., Sandler, R.S., Horney, L.F., 1983, Primary liver cancer mortality in the United States, J.Chronic
  Dis., 36:227.
Schaff, Zs., Lapis, K., Henson, D.E., 1986, Liver, In: The
  pathology of incipient neoplasia, D.E. Henson, J. Al-

bores-Saavedra, eds., W.B. Saunders Co., Philadelphia, Ch. 9. pp. 167-2o2.

Schaff, Zs., Lapis, K., Safrany, L., 1971, The ultrastructure of primary hepato-cellular cancer in man, Virch.Arch. /A/, 352:34o.

Schaff, Zs., Pohl, Ö., Bencsáth, M., Brojnás, J., Lapis, K., Kopper, L., Hollós, I., 1982, HBsAg-like structures in immunosuppressed mice inoculated with human hepatitis virus, Virchows Arch. /Cell Pathol./, 4o:249.

Schaff, Zs., Seto, B., Coleman, W.G.Jr., Lapis, K., in press, Morphology, immunohistochemistry, and in situ hybridization of experimental and human non-A, non-B hepatitis, J.Med.Virol.

Schaff, Zs., Tabor, E., Jackson, D.R., Gerety, R.J., 1984, Ultrastructural alterations in serial liver biopsy specimens from chimpanzees experimentally infected with a human non-A, non-B hepatitis agent, Virchows Arch.B Cell Path., 45:3o1.

Schaff, Zs., Tálas, M., Stóger, I., Lapis, K., Földes, I., 1978, Neoplastic response of turkey liver to MC29 leukosis virus, Acta Morph.Acad.Sci.Hung., 26:325.

Scherer, E., Emmelot, H.P., 1976, Kinetics of induction and growth of enzyme-deficient islands involved in hepatocarcinogenesis, Cancer Res., 36:2544.

Sells, M.A., Chen, M-L., Acs, G., 1987, Production of hepatitis B virus particles in Hep G2 cells transfected with cloned hepatitis B virus DNA, Proc.Natl.Acad. Sci.U.S.A., 84:1oo5.

Seto, B., Gerety, R.J., 1985, A glycoprotein associated with the non-A, non-B hepatitis agent/s/: isolation and immunoreactivity, Proc.Natl.Acad.Sci.U.S.A., 82:4934.

Seto, B., Gerety, R.J., Coleman, W.G.Jr., 1984, Molecular cloning of DNA found in non-A, non-B hepatitis serum, In: Viral Hepatitis and Liver Diseases, G.N. Vyas, J.L. Dienstag, J.H. Hoofnagle, eds., Grune and Stratton Inc., New York, p. 62o.

Sherlock, S., Niazi, S.P., Fox, R.A., Sheuer, P.J., 197o, Chronic liver disease and primary liver cell cancer with hepatitis - associated /Australia/ antigen in serum, Lancet, i:1243.

Shikata, T., 1976, Primary liver carcinoma and liver cirrhosis, In: Hepatocellular Carcinoma, K. Okuda, R.L. Peters, eds., John Wiley and Sons, New York, pp.53-73.

Shikata, T., Uzawa, T., Yoshiwara, N., Akatsuka, T., Yamazaki, S., 1974, Staining methods of Australia antigen in paraffin sections, Jpn.J.Exp.Med., 44:25.

Shouval, D., Chakraborty, P.R., Ruiz-Opazo, N., Baum, S., Spigland, I., Muchmore, R., Gerber, M.A., Thung, S.N., Popper, H., Shafritz, D.A., 198o, Chronic hepatitis in chimpanzee carriers of hepatitis B virus: morphologic, immunologic and viral DNA studies, Proc.Natl. Acad.Sci.U.S.A., 77:6147.

Shouval, D., Shafritz, D.A., Zurawski, V.R., Isselbacher, K.J., Wands, J.R., 1982, Immunotherapy in nude mice of human hepatoma using monoclonal antibodies against hepatitis B virus, Nature, 298:567.

Stemhagen, A., Slade, J., Altman, R., Bill, J., 1983, Occupational risk factors and liver cancer. A retrospective case-control study of primary liver cancer in New Jersey, Am.J.Epidemiol., 117:443.

Summers, J., 1981, Three recently described animal virus models for human hepatitis B virus, Hepatology, 1:179.

Summers, J., Mason, W.S., 1982, Properties of the hepatitis B- -like viruses related to their taxonomic classification, Hepatology, 2:61S.

Summers, J., Smolec, J.M., Snyder, R., 1978, A virus similar to human hepatitis B virus associated with hepatitis and hepatoma in woodchucks, Proc.Natl.Acad.Sci.U.S.A., 75:4533.

Szmuness, W., 1978, Hepatocellular carcinoma and the hepatitis B virus: Evidence for a causal association, Progr.Med. Virol., 24:4o.

Tabor, E., 1983, Animal models, titered inocula, and cell culture systems for hepatitis A, hepatitis B, and non-A, non-B hepatitis. In: Viral Hepatitis. Second Intern. Max von Pettenkofer Symposium, L.R. Oberby, F. Deinhardt, J. Deinhardt, eds., Marcel Dekker, New York, pp. 57-59.

Tabor, E., Bayley, A.C., Cairns, J., Pelleu, L., Gerety, R.J., 1983, Horizontal transmission of hepatitis B virus in children and adults in five rural villages in Zambia, Gastroenterology, 84 /abstr./ 1399.

Tabor, E., Gerety, R.J., Drucker, T.A., Seeff, L.B., Hoonagle, J.H., Jackson, D.R., 1978, Transmission of non-A, non- -B hepatitis from man to chimpanzee, Lancet, 1:463.

Tabor, E., Gerety, R.J., Vogel, C.L., Bayley, A.C., Anthony, P.P., Chan, C.H., Barker, L.F., 1977, Hepatitis B virus infection and primary hepatocellular carcinoma, J.Natl.Cancer Inst., 58:1197.

Thung, S.N., Gerber, M.A., Sarno, E., Popper, H., 1979, Distribution of five antigens in hepatocellular carcinoma, Lab.Invest., 41:1ol.

Tuttleman, J.S., Pugh, J.C., Summers, J.W., 1986, In Vitro Experimental Infection of Primary Duck Hepatocyte Cultures with Duck Hepatitis B Virus, J.Virol., 58:17.

Vogel, C.L., Anthony, P.P., Mody, N., Barker, L.F., 197o, Hepatitis-associated antigen in Ugandan patients with hepatocellular carcinoma, Lancet, ii:621.

Williams, G.M., 1982, Sex hormones and liver cancer, Lab.Invest., 46:352.

MORPHOLOGICAL ALTERATIONS DURING LIVER CARCINOGENESIS

METABOLIC ZONATION OF THE LIVER

Kurt Jungermann

Institut für Biochemie, Georg-August-
Universität, Humboldtallee 23,
D-3400 Göttingen, Germany

INTRODUCTION

The liver is the central service organ of the
organism. First, the liver is the centre of metabolism: it
is responsible, on the one hand, for the maintenance of the
energy supply: 1. it functions as a glucostat supplying
glucose when required and removing it when in excess, 2. it
produces ketone bodies to feed a.o. the central nervous
system, 3. it is the main site of amino acid catabolism, 4.
it removes ammonia operating as a pH-stat, and 5. it
processes nutrient triglycerides and fatty acids. On the
other hand, the organ catalyses important biosynthetic and
biodegradative processes: 1. it has a key position in the
metabolism of phospholipids and cholesterol, i.e. of
lipoproteins, 2. it synthesizes and probably degrades most
plasma proteins, 3. it forms bile for the digestive process,
and 4. it is the main organ of biochemical defense removing
xenobiotics. Second, the liver is a control station of the
hormonal system producing signal substances and degrading
hormones during liver passage thus contributing to the
maintenance of peripheral hormone levels. Third, the liver
is a passive and active blood reservoir.

The manyfold service functions of the liver are provided by
the parenchymal and/or the non-parenchymal (endothelial,
Kupffer, Ito and pit) cells of the organ. The parenchymal
cells can be regulated by six factors: the substrate
concentrations in blood, the circulating hormone levels, the
autonomic innervation of the organ, the zonal hepatocyte
heterogeneity, the non-parenchymal cells and the biomatrix.
The non-parenchymal cells can be controlled similarly by six
factors: the substrate and the hormone concentrations, the
liver nerves, the parenchymal cells, the heterologous non-
parenchymal cells and again the biomatrix. The present short
over-view attempts to summarize the present knowledge of
parenchymal heterogeneity and, thereby, to improve the
understanding of liver functions in normal and pathological
states. The subject has been reviewed previously in more
detail (1-3).

Enzyme histochemical studies had revealed many
years ago that the liver parenchyma showed a zonal
heterogeneity (4,5) (Fig.1). Morevover, the zonal toxicity of xenobiotics had been a well-known phenomenon for
a long time (6). Immuno-histochemical and microbio-
chemical studies of microdissected liver tissue greatly
improved the knowledge of zonal heterogeneity (1-3). It
became possible to develop the understanding of the phenomenon from a more descriptive (4,5) to an increasingly
functional level (1-3).

Zonal heterogeneity of enzyme content and subcellular structures

The periportal hepatocyte has the higher capacity
for oxidative energy metabolism, i.e. the greater
mitochondrial volume and cristae are per cell and the
higher activities of succinate dehydrogenase and cytochrome oxidase (2). The periportal cell possesses also
the higher capacities for gluconeogenesis, fatty acid
utilization and amino acid catabolism, since it contains
greater activities of glucose-6-phosphatase, fructose-1,
6-bisphosphatase, phosphoenolpyruvate carboxykinase,
β -hydroxybutyryl-CoA dehydrogenase, alanine aminotransferase, aspartate aminotransferase and tyrosine aminotransferase (2). Moreover, the periportal cell has the
higher capacities for nitrogen detoxification via ureage-
nesis, for oxidation protection and bile formation as
indicated by the higher activities of carbamoylphosphate
synthetase, ornithine carbamoyltransferase, argini-
nosuccinate synthetase, arginase, glutathione peroxidase,
canalicular ATPase and the greater volume of Golgi-rich
areas and of bile canaliculi per cell (2).

The perivenous hepatocyte has the higher capacities
for glycolysis and liponeogenesis ; it contains higher
activities of glucokinase, pyruvate kinase L. ATP-
dependent citrate lyase, acetyl-CoA carboxylase, fatty
acid synthase, glucose-6-phosphate dehydrogenase and
alcohol dehydrogenase. Furthermore, it possesses the higher capacities for nitrogen detoxification via glutamine formation and of biotransformation ; glutamine
synthetase, most cytochrome P-450 isoenzymes, aryl
hydrocarbon hydroxylase, epoxide hydrolase, UDP-glu-
curonosyl transferase and glutathione-S-transferases
are predominant in perivenous cells (2).

Based on the assumption that different metabolic
capacities indicate different functions for the two major
zones of the parenchyma, the model of "metabolic zona-
ion" (Table1) was proposed, first for carbonhydrate metabolism (7) and later also for the other functions (1,2).

Zonal Heterogeneity of Signals and Signal Transmission

Due to the metabolic activity of the organ gradients
of e.g. oxygen, ammonia and carbon substrates/products
are formed during passage of the blood. The oxygen
tension in periportal blood is about twice that in perivenous blood ; the ammonia concentration is about 5 times
higher upstream than downstream (8) (Fig.2). However,
the concentration gradients

Table 1. Model of metabolic zonation of liver parenchyma:
Predominant localization of major functions as indicated by
the zonal distribution of key enzymes.

Periportal zone	Perivenous zone

Oxidative energy metabolism
    Fatty acid oxidation
    Citrate cycle
    Respiratory chain	

Glucose release
    Gluconeogenesis
    Glycogen synthesis from
        pyruvate
    Glycogen degradation to
        glucose
	Glucose uptake
	    Glycolysis
	    Glycogen synthesis from
	        glucose
	    Glycogen degradation to
	        pyruvate

Amino acid utilization
    Amino acid conversion to
        glucose
    Amino acid degradation
    Ureagenesis from amino acid
        nitrogen	

Cholesterol synthesis	Ketogenesis

NH3 detoxification
    Urea formation
	NH3 detoxification
	    Glutamine formation

Oxidation protection
    GSH-peroxidation
	Biotransformation
	    Monooxygenation
	    Mercapturic acid
	        formation
	    Glucuronidation

Bile formation
    Cholic acid excretion
    Bilirubin excretion	

of most carbon substrates are normally not very steep (2,8).
Due to hepatic degradation the level of hormone such as
insulin, glucagon, adrenaline, noradrenaline, corticosteroids
and T4 is lower in the perivenous zone; other signal
substances such as adenosine and T3 are formed by the liver
so that the perivenous zone receives higher concentrations
(2,8; Miethke and Jungermann, unpublished) (Fig. 2). Due to
the different rates of degradation or formation the signal
ratio changes from the periportal to the perivenous zone.
Morevover, the automatic innervation of the two zones may
also be different (2,8). Finally, the zonal distribution of
the ectocellular receptors for insulin, glucagon or
catecholamines as well as that of the intracellular receptors
for glucocorticoids is unknown; it may well be different. The
heterogeneity of signals and signal transmission will be
important not only for short-term regulation of metabolism
but also for long-term control of enzyme content.

Zonal Heterogeneity of Gene Expression

All hepatocytes have, of course, the same genome. Its
heterogeneous expression must be due to the zonal differences
in signals and/or signal transmission (see above). The
influence of physiological oxygen tensions, insulin and

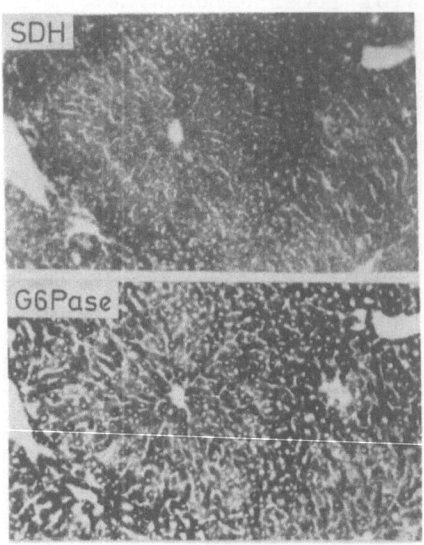

Fig. 1 Distribution of succinate dehydrogenase (SDH) and glucose 6-phosphatase (G6Pase) in liver parenchyma of the rat. SDH and G6Pase were demonstrated histochemically (dark precipitate), both enzymes are predominantly localized in the periportal area.

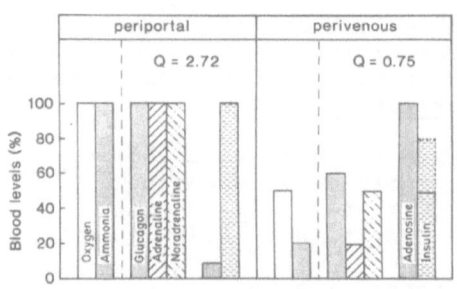

Fig. 2 Zonal heterogeneity of signals. The higher substrate or hormone concentrations either in the portal vein or in the hepatic vein were set equal to 100%. Values are from fed rats (at the shift from the absorptive to the postabsorptive phase), only with insulin the value of eating animals (absorptive phase) is indicated in addition by the dotted line. Since glucagon and the catecholamines can be regarded as antagonists of insulin and adenosine, a normalized ratio Q was defined: Q = (glucagon + adrenaline + noradrenaline)/(insulin + adenosine). (2,8)

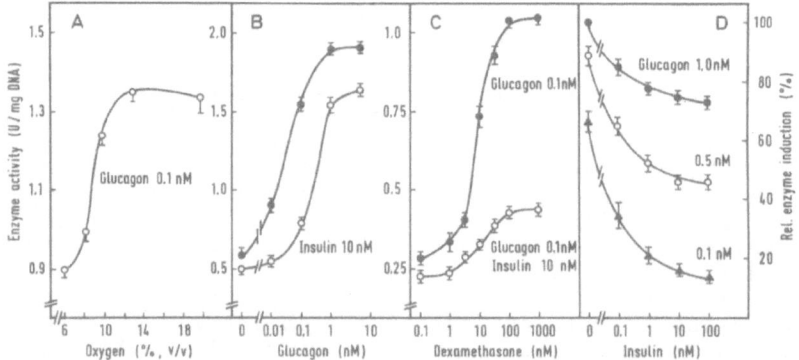

Fig. 3 Induction of phosphoenolpyruvate carboxykinase (PEPCK) by glucagon. Modulation by oxygen, antagonism by insulin and permissive action of glucocorticoids. Rat hepatocytes were cultured for 24 h with 0.5 nM insulin and 0.1 uM or the concentration shown of dexamethasone. Glucagon +/- insulin was added at 24 h under 13% or the percentage shown of Oz: the enzyme activity was measured at 28 h (details in 9,10).

dexamethasone on the glucagon-dependent induction of phosphoenolpyruvate carboxykinase was studied in hepatocyte culture (9,10) (Fig. 3). The results show that under the permissive action of glucocorticoids the decrease of oxygen tension and of the glucagon/insulin ratio during liver passage could be involved in the induction of the enzyme to higher levels in the periportal than in the perivenous zone, and thus in general in the differential zonal gene expression of carbohydrate-metabolizing enzymes. The mechanism of the induction of enzyme zonation is, however, very complex and not really understood.

Zonal Heterogeneity of Functions

The major advantage of the zonal heterogeneity of the parenchymal liver cells consists in the spatial separation of metabolic pathways (Table 1). With respect to carbohydrate metabolism, the model views the _periportal_ (pp) zone as the site of glucose release (via gluconeogenesis and breakdown of glycogen, which is formed from pyruvate rather than from glucose), and the _perivenous_ (pv) zone as the site of glucose uptake (for glycolysis plus liponeogenesis and the synthesis of glycogen) (Fig. 4). with respect to the metabolism of xenobiotics and its adverse side effects the model would predict that the perivenous zone is at higher risk. The model is corrobrated by its dynamic nature, a number of in vivo observations and of in vitro experiments.

Dynamics of zonation. The zonal separation of glucose release and uptake (Fig. 4) appears to be a prerequisite for the effectiveness of the liver as a glucostat; the separation can be quantitated by the capacity index (CI) of the reciprocal distribution of the gluconeogenic phosphoenolpyruvate carboxykinase (PEPCK) and of the glycolytic pyruvate kinase L (PKr) (Fig. 5). A CI around 1 indicates equal capacity for the two antagonistic processes. In the periportal zone gluconeogenesis is predominant: CI_{pp} = 1.7. In the perivenous zone glycolysis is prevalent: CI_{pv} = 0.27. The zonation was found to adapt to longer lasting changes of the metabolic situation, e.g. to the need to "buffer" excess nutritional glucose (8, 11, 12): thus during starvation with no need for glucose buffering the major function of the perivenous zone was changed from glucose uptake to glucose release: CI_{pv} = 2,27. After portocaval anastomosis with a diminished requirement for glucose buffering the perivenous predominance of glucose uptake was reduced: CI_{pv} = 1,04. In the diabetic state with a persisting need for glucose buffering the perivenous function of glucose uptake was not entirely lost as during starvation but severely impaired: CI_{pv} = 1,27 (Fig. 5). Moreover, in the rat the zonal heterogeneity as to carbohydrate metabolism developped only gradually during the second week of life befor weaning, i.e. before the shift from fat-and protein-rich nutrition via maternal milk to carbohydrate-rich nutrition via normal food when the liver takes over the function of a glucostat (8,11).

Flux differences in vivo. The model of metabolic zonation postulates that glycogen in the periportal hepatocytes should be formed from 3-carbon substrates rather than from glucose. This proposal is at variance with the

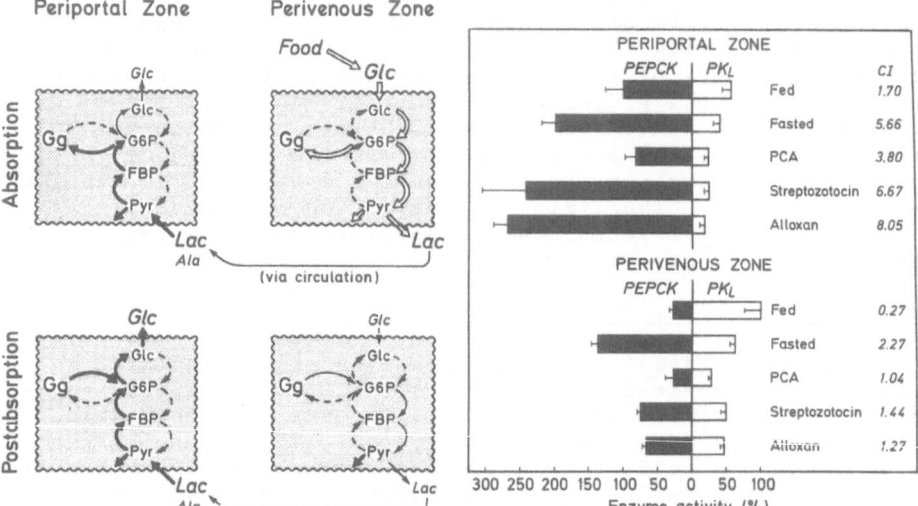

Fig. 4 Hepatic carbohydrate metabolism acc. to the model of metabolic zonation. Absorption: Nutritional glucose is converted in the perivenous zone to lactate, which is transported via the general circulation to the periportal zone, where it is used for the synthesis of glycogen (Gg). Postabsorption: Glycogen, lactate and alanine are converted to glucose in the periportal zone; glycogen is degraded to pyruvate in the perivenous zone.

Fig. 5 Zonal distribution of PEPCK and PK L-type in liver of fed, 48 h fasted, shunted (portocaval anastomosis PCA) and diabetic rats. The higher, either periportal or perivenous value of control fed rats is set equal to 100%. CI = capacity index = zonal ratio of percentage activity of PEPCK (fed periportal = 100% to PK (fed perivenous = 100%): A value 1 indicates a predominance of the gluconeogenic, a value 1 a prevalence of the glycolytic capacity

generally accepted view that intact glucose is the major substrate for glycogen synthesis. However, it has been realized recently that a major portion of hepatic glycogen is formed from pyruvate via gluconeogenesis rather than from glucose. These findings became known under the term "glucose paradox" (13-15); they can be regarded as in vivo evidence for the zonation model.

Lesions in the perivenous zone caused by a number of xenobiotics were difficult to understand for a long time. They may at least in part be explained by hepatocyte heterogeneity. Perivenous necrosis after bromobenzene may be caused by an increased rate of formation of toxic, electrophilic metabolites of the compound due to the higher P-450 content and by the lower level of protective glutathione in perivenous cells (16). Fatty infiltration in the perivenous zone after carbon tetrachloride may be linked to the diminished protection of this zone against hydroperoxides due to the lower content of glutathione peroxidase and glutathione (17). This molecular explanation for zonal toxicity in liver can be regarded as further corroboration of the model of "metabolic zonation".

Table 2. Metabolic rates in cultured hepatocytes resembling periportal and perivenous cells

Enzyme outfit	"Periportal" Cells		"Perivenous" Cells	
	PEPCK	GK	PEPCK	GK
	μmol x min^{-1} x mg DNA^{-1}			
	0.95	0.28	0.19	0.92

Metabolic rates	Gluconeo-genesis	Glyco-lysis	Net glucose balance*	Gluconeo-genesis	Glyco-lysis	Net glucose balance*
	μmol C_6 x min^{-1} x mg DNA^{-1}					
No hormones 5 mM glucose	3.4	0.8		2.2	1.6	
Glucagon 0.3 nM 5 mM glucose	4.2	0.6	+3.6	2.2	0.8	
Insulin 1 nM 5 mM glucose	3.4	1.8		2.2	3.6	−1.4
Glucagon 0.3 nM 10 mM glucose	4.2	1.6	+2.6	2.2	1.2	
Insulin 1 nM 10 mM glucose	3.4	4.2		2.2	8.4	−6.2

Cells were cultured for 48 h under standard conditions. Periportal-like cells were obtained with glucagon, perivenous-like cells with insulin as the major hormone. After a medium change metabolic rates were determined radiochemically under postabsorptive (5mM glucose, 2 mM lactate) and absorptive (10 mM glucose, 2 mM lactate) substrate conditions with varying hormone levels from 1 pM to 100 nM. Half-maximal effects were seen with glucagon at 0.3 nM and with insulin at 1 nM. Enzyme activities were determined both before and after the incubation for the study of metabolic rates. Net rates are given only for conditions that could best be regarded as an extrapolation to the in vivo situation: Since periportal-like or perivenous-like cells, respectively, were obtained by long-term induction with glucagon or insulin, respectively, it can be assumed that their short-term regulation also should be governed predominantly by glucagon or insulin, respectively. Thus in the postabsorptive situation net glucose release in the "periportal" cells would be counterbalanced in part by a net glucose uptake in the "perivenous" cells, resulting in an overall net glucose release. In the absorptive situation net glucose uptake in the "perivenous" cells would be counter-balanced in part by net glucose output in the "periportal" cells leading to an overall glucose uptake.
PEPCK, phosphoenolpyruvate carboxykinase; GK, glucokinase. For details see (20).

Flux Differences in vitro. Since a satisfactory separation of periportal and perivenous cells from isolated hepatocyte suspensions has not been achieved so far (cf.

however 18, 19), the attempt was made to induce periportal-like and perivenous-like hepatocytes in cell culture. With glucagon or insulin, respectively, as the major hormone, the heterogeneous population of freshly isolated cells could be transformed into an apparently homogeneous population, which in a first approximation contained the key enzymes of carbohydrate metabolism in activities as found in vivo in periportal or perivenous cells, respectively (20). Under conditions mimicking the periportal or the perivenous milieu, respectively, gluconeogenesis was the predominant process in the so obtained periportal-like cells, and conversely, in the perivenous-like cells glycolysis was prevalent (Table 2). These cell culture studies can be regarded as further in vitro evidence for the zonation model.

If livers from fasted rats were perfused with only glucose as substrate, glycogen was formed only in the perivenous zone; if livers were perfused with lactate/pyruvate/glutamine as substrates, glycogen was synthesized only in the periportal zone (21). These observations substantiate the model of metabolic zonation.

SUMMARY AND CONCLUSION

Liver parenchymal cells show a zonal heterogeneity as to enzyme content, subcellular structures and possibly translocators and hormone receptor systems.

Cells in the two zones receive different signals due to substrate-, hormone- and mediator gradients and a possibly unequal innervation.

Zonal enzyme and signal heterogeneity is dynamic and functional rather than static and structural. It adapts to longer lasting changes of the metabolic situation.

The spatial, dynamic separation of functions leads to an enhancement of the catalytic and regulatory potential of the liver; it constitutes the major advantage of the phenomenon "zonation".

The apparent decrease of the self-protective capacity of the perivenous zone may be regarded as a major disadvantage.

ACKNOWLEDGEMENTS

This work was supported by grants from the Deutsche Forschungsgemeinschaft, D-5300 Bonn. I would like to thank Drs. I. Probst, H. Bartels, B. Christ, H. Miethke and B. Wittig for their collaboration during various stages of the studies.

REFERENCES

1. Jungermann, K. and Katz, N. (1982) Hepatology 2, 385-395.
2. Jungermann, K. (1986) Enzyme 35, 161-180.
3. Thurman, R.G., Kauffman, F.C. and Jungermann, K. eds. (1986) Regulation of Hepatic Metabolism, Intra- and Intercellular Compartmentation. Plenum Press, New York and London.

4. Novikoff, A.B. (1959) J. Histochem. Cytochem. 7, 240-244.
5. Rappaport, A.M. (1960) Klin. Wochenschr. 38, 561-577.
6. Zimmerman, H.J. (1978) Hepatotoxicity. Appleton-Century-Crofts, New York.
7. Katz, N. and Jungermann, J. (1976) Hoppe-Seyler's Z. Physiol. Chem. 357, 359-375.
8. Jungermann, K. (1986) in op.cit. 3, 445-469.
9. Nauck, M., Wölfe, D., Katz, N. and Jungermann, K., (1981) Eur. J. Biochem. 119, 657-661.
10. Probst, I. and Jungermann, K. (1983) Hoppe-Seyler's Z. Physiol. Chem. 364, 1639-1646.
11. Jungermann, K., (1986) Acta Histochem. Suppl. 32, 89-98.
12. Miethke, H., Wittig, B., Math, A. and Jungermann, K., (1986) Histochemistry 85, 483-489.
13. Katz, J. and McGarry, J.D., (1984) J. Clin, Invest. 74, 1901-1909.
14. Pilkis, S.J., Regen, D.M., Claus, T.H. and Cherrington, A.D., (1985) Bioessays 2, 273-276.
15. Katz, J., Kuwajima, M., Foster, D.W. and McGarry, J.D., (1986) Trends in Biochem. Sci. 11, 136-140.
16. Smith, M.T., Loveridge, N., Wills, E. and Chayen, J., (1979) Biochem. J. 182, 103-108.
17. Yoshimura, S., Komatsu, N. and Watanabe, K., (1980) Biochim. Biophys. Acta 621, 130-137.
18. Quistorff, B., Grunnet, N. and Cornell, N.W., (1985) Biochem. J. 226, 289-291.
19. Lindros, K.O. and Penttilä, K.E., (1985) Biochem. J. 228, 757-760.
20. Probst, I., Schwartz, P. and Jungermann, K., (1982) Eur. J. Biochem. 126, 271-278.
21. Bartels, H. and Jungermann, K., (1987) Z. Gastroenterol. 25, 52-53.

CELLULAR DIFFERENTIATION DURING NEOPLASTIC DEVELOPMENT IN THE LIVER

Peter Bannasch, Harald Enzmann, Youbing Ruan,
Edgar Weber and Heide Zerban

Institut für Experimentelle Pathologie,
Deutsches Krebsforschungszentrum,
D-6900 Heidelberg, Im Neuenheimer Feld 280

INTRODUCTION

Human and experimental liver tumors are classified
according to the similarity in morphology and histological
arrangement of their cells to specific normal counterparts.
Thus, hepatocellular, cholangiocellular and diverse
mesenchymal tumors are distinguished. This histogenetic
classification was established by light microscopy. It has
been supported by many electron microscopical results and
more recently also by immunohistochemical investigations of
certain cytoskeletal components, especially the so-called
intermediate filaments.

In spite of this generally accepted and reliable
morphological basis of tumor classification many aspects of
the morphogenesis of liver neoplasms are still open to a
controversial discussion. Is neoplastic development in the
liver a unicentric or a multicentric process ? Do the tumors
descend from single or a few initiated cells or do they
rather emerge from larger fields of altered cells ? Are the
altered cells mature normal cells which undergo dedifferen-
tiation during neoplastic transformation or do the tumor
cells originate from undifferentiated stem cells which
might be blocked at different levels of maturation ? What is
the relation of hyperplasia and metaplasia to neoplasia in
the liver ? We are not able to give new answers to all of
these old questions. However, the great progress in our
understanding of tumor development in the liver, which has
been achieved during the past two decades, apparently
provides a sound basis for solutions of many problems in the
near future.

In human pathology, the discussion on the pathogenesis of
primary liver tumors is dominated by two concepts, namely the
relatively new idea that the hepatitis B virus (HBV) is a
major risk factor for liver cancer, and the old dogma that
regenerative hyperplasia in long standing liver cirrhosis may
eventually lead to hepatic neoplasia. A strong statistical
correlation between the incidence rate of hepatocarcinoma and

HBV infection has indeed been observed in many countries
(Beasly et al., 1981; Hann et al., 1982). However, this
strong correlation has by no means been seen universally
(Melbye et al., 1984; Tu et al., 1987). Moreover, the
precise pathogenetic mechanism by which HBV infection might
lead to neoplastic transformation of the hepatocytes is far
from clear (Tiollais et al., 1985). On the other hand, in a
recent multivariate epidemiological analysis involving 10
smaller subregions of Swaziland, aflatoxin exposure emerged
as a more potent determinant of the variation in liver cancer
incidence than the prevalence of hepatitis B infection (Peers
et al., 1987)

The role of liver cirrhosis in hepatocarcinogenesis has
been discussed in considerable detail recently (Bannasch and
Zerban, 1987). We will not repeat this discussion here but
would like to mention that the combination of liver cirrhosis
and carcinoma as induced by chemicals depends on the dose and
duration of treatment. After administration of high doses
which produce pronounced unspecific-toxic lesions including
parenchymal necrosis, the tumors are frequently combined with
cirrhosis. However, after treatment with low doses not
leading to remarkable necrotic changes the tumors develop
without any concomitant cirrhosis. These experimental
results obtained in a number of laboratories using different
chemicals, clearly show that there is no direct causal
relationship between liver cirrhosis and carcinoma. However,
regenerative cell proliferation in a cirrhotic liver might
certainly modify the action of oncogenic agents on the liver
cells and, thus, indirectly influence the process of tumor
development.

In addition to these findings on the relation of
cirrhosis and cancer, investigations of experimental models,
especially the rat liver treated with various carcinogens,
have contributed much to our present knowledge of the
pathogenesis of primary liver tumors. We learned from these
studies that hepatocarcinogens may have at least four
different types of target cells in the liver, namely the
hepatocytes, the bile ductular epithelia, the sinusoidal, and
the perisinusoidal cells (Fig. 1). All of these cell types
may be specifically altered by chemical carcinogens and give
rise to different types of tumors (Bannasch and Zerban,
1986).
During neoplastic transformation some components of the
respective cells are characterized by a remarkable phenotypic
stability, whereas other cellular constituents such as
metabolites, enzymes or organelles show a puzzling phenotypic
instability.

PHENOTYPIC STABILITY OF CYTOSKELETAL COMPONENTS

One of the most stable cellular components during
neoplastic transformation is the cytoskeleton (Bannasch et
al., 1980b; Ramaekers et al., 1982; Osborn and Weber, 1986).
The cytoskeleton consists of three major parts : The
microtubuli (Ø 25 nm),the actin-containing microfilaments(Ø
6 nm) and the intermediate filaments (Ø 10 nm). The
morphology of the intermediate filaments is very similar in
different cell types but immunological and biochemical

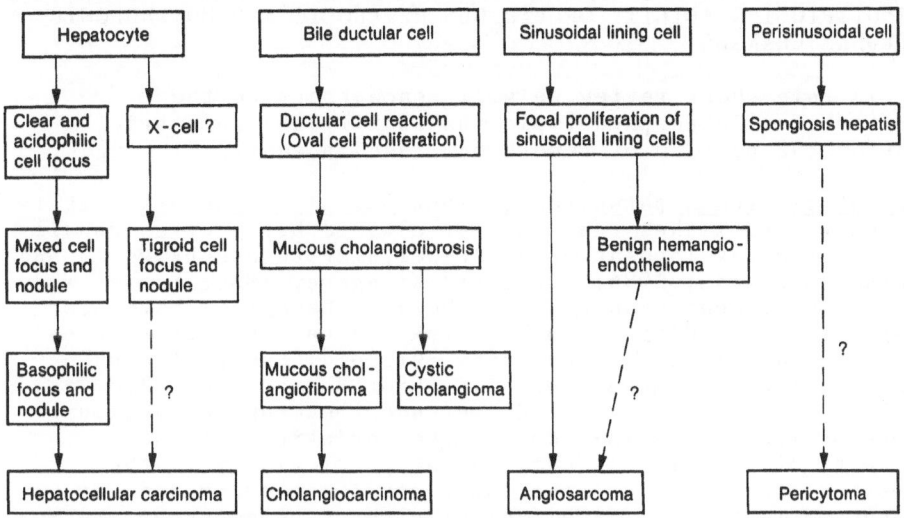

Fig. 1 Schematic presentation of sequential cellular changes in the development of epithelial and mesenchymal liver tumors (from Bannasch and Zerban, 1986).

studies have shown that five classes of intermediate filaments can be distinguished which are characteristic of certain normal tissues, such as epithelia, the mesenchyme of glial cells. In normal liver, antibodies to prekeratin decorate the hepatocytes and the bile duct epithelia but not the mesenchymal cells, while antibodies to vimentin react exclusively with mesenchymal cells, especially the sinusoidal lining cells. In tumors derived from these different cell types the expression of the specific class of intermediate filament is usually maintained. Thus <u>hepatocellular carcinomas</u> show abundant intermediate filaments which react with antibodies to prekeratin but not with antibodies to vimentin. The same holds true for the epithelial component of <u>cholangiocellular tumor</u>. In contrast, <u>angiosarcomas</u> express only vimentin which is characteristic of normal and neoplastic mesenchymal cells. With antibodies to this type of intermediate filament early stages of angiosarcomas can be easily recognized.

There are some rare exceptions to the rules just described (e.g., Ramaekers et al., 1982; Osborn and Weber, 1986) but they do not detract from the fact that certain differentiation markers of the tissue of tumor origin are usually preserved during neoplastic transformation. This finding does not only support the histogenetic tumor classification but it also militates against a biological instability of tumor cells at random. There are indeed many observations which suggest an ordered pattern of phenotypic changes during neoplastic development in the liver. It appeared to be indicated, therefore, to separate the phenotypic instability in unspecific-toxic hepatic lesions from a progression- and a reversion-linked phenotypic instability in specific carcinogen- induced alterations (Bannasch et al., 1985c).

PHENOTYPIC INSTABILITY OF VARIOUS METABOLIC AND MORPHOLOGIC CELLULAR CHANGES

In this short review we will concentrate on the progression-linked phenotypic instability and only briefly mention the problem of reversion-linked phenotypic changes.

Foci of altered hepatocytes and hepatocellular tumors. It is now well established that foci of altered hepatocytes usually precede the development of hepatocellular tumors by weeks and months (Bannasch, 1986; Moore and Kitagawa, 1986; Farber and Sarma, 1987; Montesano et al., 1987). These foci have been classified according to their morphological phenotype into clear, acidophilic, intermediate, tigroid, basophilic and mixed cell foci (Stewart et al., 1980; Bannasch et al., 1985f). The morphological differences between the various types of foci are mainly due to the variations in the quantity of cytoplasmic components, particularly in the amount of the glycogen, the endoplasmic reticulum and the ribosomes (Table 1). The foci of altered hepatocytes are not distributed at random.
They are predominantly localized in the first and second zone of the functional liver acinus as defined by Rappaport. We suppose that the interdependent hemodynamic and metabolic zonation of the liver lobule is responsible for this preferential localization.

Table 1. Morphological phenotype and classification of altered hepatocytes (from Bannasch, 1986).

Type of Focus	GLYCOGEN	SER	RER/RIBOSOMES	MITOSIS
Clear Cell Foci	+ + +	+	+	+
Acidophilic Cell Foci	+ + +	+ +(+)	+	+
Intermediate Cell Foci	+ +	+(+)	+ +	+ +
Tigroid Cell Foci	(+)	+(+)	+ +(+)	+ +(+)
Basophilic Cell Foci	-	-	+ + +	+ + +
Mixed Cell Foci	mixed	mixed	mixed	mixed

From cytomorphological, cytochemical and morphometric studies, we inferred a sequence of cellular changes leading from the clear and acidophilic cell foci storing glycogen in excess through mixed and basophilic cell foci (the latter having little or no glycogen but abundant ribosomes) to neoplastic nodules and hepatocellular carcinomas (Bannasch, 1968; Moore et al., 1982; Enzmann and Bannasch, 1986). A similar developmental sequence has also been described in rat liver after various other hepatocarcinogens and during hepatocarcinogenesis in other species, including primates (Bannasch et al., 1980a; Ward, 1984). The results of dose-response studies in our rat model likewise support the sequence outlined (Moore et al., 1982). It is important, however, to realize that under certain experimental conditions, particularly after repeated administrations of high doses of one or several hepatocarcinogens, reversible foci and nodules may develop that resemble the persistent lesions in their cytology and cytochemical pattern (Farber, 1984; Bannasch, 1986; Goldsworthy et al., 1986; Moore and Kitagawa, 1986). The significance of this reversion-linked phenotypic instability is poorly understood, but this intriguing phenomenon can be largely avoided by appropriate experimental designs, such as the stop experiments mentioned. In this case, the majority of the foci developed after cessation of the carcinogenic treatment in a dose-dependent manner, and acquired phenotypic markers closer to neoplasia without further exposure to the carcinogen (Moore et al., 1982).

Some authors felt that each of the diverse phenotypes might represent the result of a specific set of cellular changes, and that the foci appearing early do not evolve via progressively more deviated forms into tumors. However, the concept of a sequential phenotypic conversion of the altered hepatocytes which we have been pursuing for a number of years, has been further substantiated by studies of the proliferation kinetics, and the behavior of the number and size of the different cell populations emerging during hepatocarcinogenesis. As demonstrated by the incorporation of 3H-thymidine, the early appearing clear or acidophilic glycogen storage foci show a slightly increased proliferation, but they do not differ significantly in their growth from the normal liver parenchyma of untreated controls (Zerban et al., 1985). A pronounced and steadily increasing cell proliferation is only linked with the appearance of mixed and basophilic cell populations in foci, nodules and carcinomas. These findings are consistent with the results, of morphometric studies of the volume of the different types of foci (Enzmann and Bannasch, 1986). When the number of foci was determined from the end of treatment up to 40 weeks after cessation, the total number of all types of foci remained rather constant. However, successive peaks were observed for the glycogen storage, mixed and basophilic cell foci (Fig. 2). The earliest appearing cell population decreased when the subsequently emerging populations increased.

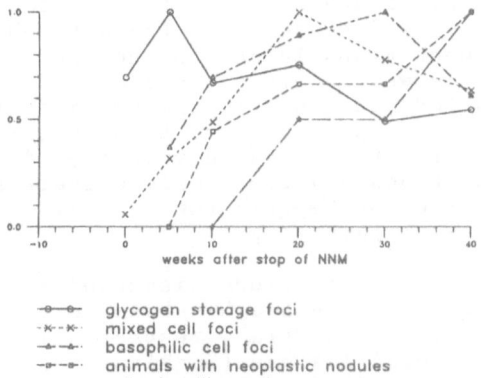

weeks after stop of NNM

- —⊕—⊕— glycogen storage foci
- ·-x--x-· mixed cell foci
- —▲--▲-- basophilic cell foci
- —⊞--⊞— animals with neoplastic nodules
- —+--+— animals with carcinomas

the incidence of the focal lesions is expressed as the fraction
of the highest incidence observed in each type of lesion

Fig. 2 Sequence of preneoplastic and neoplastic lesions induced in rat liver by a 7-week treatment with N-nitrosomorpholine 120 mg/l drinking water) as studied morphometrically from the end of treatment (O) up to 40 weeks after cessation.

93

The increase in number of glycogen storage foci was due to the additional development of small foci of this phenotype, but the increase in total number of mixed and basophilic cell foci was correlated with the appearance of larger lesions of this phenotype. Somewhat later, neoplastic nodules and carcinomas developed in a progressive manner. These results suggest that the phenotypic heterogeneity in preneoplastic foci to a large extent reflects different stages in an ordered sequence of cellular changes during hepatocarcinogenesis (Enzmann and Bannasch, 1986). It is difficult to reconcile our morphometric results with the frequently assumed clonal origin of preneoplastic and early neoplastic foci (Rabes, 1983). The data are more readily compatible with field effects characterized by concurrent alterations in many hepatocytes in larger areas of the liver parenchyma as postulated years ago (Willis, 1953; Bannasch, 1968).

Our schematic presentation of the developmental sequence during hepatocarcinogenesis is certainly too simplistic. We frequently observed morphological transitions between preneoplastic foci and neoplastic lesions which suggested that persistent clear-cell populations might progress to a different type of hepatocellular carcinoma than acidophilic cell foci. A more specific relation of a certain preneo-plastic phenotype to a particular hepatic tumor type has earlier been postulated for the tigroid cell foci which we detected after oral application of a single dose of aflatoxin in rat liver (Bannasch et al., 1985a), and which in the meantime have also been described by Schröter and colleagues (1987). In another experiment in which rats received dihydroepiandrosterone in addition to NNM, we have recently seen highly differentiated carcinomas which contained large numbers of tigroid cells and apparently developed from tigroid cell foci (Heinzelmann, 1986). In the same experiment, we found lesions for which we proposed the descriptive term "amphophilic foci" since they stained with both acidophilic and basophilic dyes (Weber et al., 1986). Preliminary studies have shown, that the amphophilic behavior of these foci is most probably due to the fact that they are rich in ribosomes as well as in peroxisomes and mitochondria. Some observations indicate that the amphophilic foci may progress to nodules and perhaps also to carcinomas. It is intriguing to further study these diversities in preneo-plastic cell populations and to elucidate their relation to the different types of hepatic tumors well known from human and experimental pathology.

In addition to the alterations discussed so far, a large number of other cellular changes has been described as "negative" or "positive" markers", respectively, for the carcinogen-induced focal lesions (Peraino et al., 1983; Farber, 1984; Scherer, 1984; Bannasch, 1986; Goldsworthy et al., 1986; Moore and Kitagawa, 1986). Alterations of enzymes which are involved in the metabolism of drugs and carbohy-drates attracted the greatest attention. From this variety of cytochemical changes, we will only briefly comment on the alterations in the alternative pathway of carbohydrate meta-bolism which will be presented in detail by Hacker et al. (this volume). The primary biochemical lesions leading to the focal hepatic glycogenosis has not been clarified so far,

but it may be speculated that an excess of glucose-6-phosphate plays a key role (Bannasch et al., 1984; see also Mayer, this volume). One of the earliest enzyme histochemical changes observed in the pronounced glycogen storage foci is a loss of activity of adenylate cyclase which is crucial for the regulation of different metabolic pathways, including that of carbohydrate metabolism (Eheman et al., 1986). Adenylate cyclase is the superordinate regulatory enzyme of glycogen degradation since cAMP, which is the product of the adenylate cyclase reaction, activates a cascade of phosphorylation reactions which finally result in the activation of glycogen phosphorylase.
Thus, the decrease in adenylate cyclase activity might explain the reduction in glycogen phosphorylase activity in glycogen storage foci (Hacker et al., 1982; Seelmann-Eggebert et al., 1987). Particularly interesting is the finding that the activity of glucose-6-phosphate dehydrogenase (G6PDH), the key enzyme of the pentose phosphate pathway, is markedly increased in the majority of the glycogen storage foci. More detailed quantitative studies of the glucose-6-phosphate dehydrogenase revealed that there is a gradual increase in enzyme activity from the small glycogenotic foci, which show only a tendency to higher values, over the large glycogenotic to the mixed cell foci (Klimek et al., 1984).

The development of neoplastic nodules and hepatocellular carcinomas from the foci is associated with additional enzyme histochemical changes, such as an increase in the activity of the glycolytic enzyme glyceralde-hyde-3-phosphate dehydrogenase (Hacker et al., 1982). These results are in line with many earlier biochemical findings in transplantable hepatomas (Weber, 1977). They suggest a gradual shift of carbohydrate metabolism from the glycogenotic state to alternative metabolic pathways, such as the pentose phosphate pathway and glycolysis.

Phenotypic alterations of hepatocytes which correspond to those seen in preneoplastic hepatic lesions of laboratory animals have been described in human livers with and without cirrhosis by a number of authors (Altmann, 1978; Cain, 1978; Heine, 1981; Hirota et al., 1982; Mori et al., 1982; Fischer et al., 1986; Karhunen and Penttilä, 1987). Of particular interest are recent observations of Karhunen and Penttilä (1987) who found focal parenchymal lesions composed of clear cells in 11.6% of 95 males studied in a consecutive autopsy series in Helsinki. The possible relevance of the metabolic aberrations discussed for the development of human liver tumors is also underlined by the ever increasing number of reports on patients suffering from inborn hepatic glycogenosis who develop liver cell adenomas and carcinomas when they pass through adolescence (Bannasch et al., 1984; Limmer et al., 1985; Coire et al., 1987).

A few days ago we had the chance of seeing the liver of a transgenic mouse which was sent to us for diagnosis by Dr. Paul from Hannover. The mouse originated from a colony established by Messing and colleagues (1985) who had injected a gene construct composed of the SV40 T antigen gene and the metallothionein-human growth hormone fusion gene into fertilized mouse eggs; the eggs were then transferred to foster mothers for further development. The offspring

carrying the fusion gene developed a high incidence of
hepatocellular carcinomas in addition to pancreatic islet
cell adenomas and peripheral neuropathies. The liver of the
transgenic mouse which we have studied was most remarkable :
multiple and multicentric hepatocellular adenomas and
carcinomas were associated with many prominent clear cell
foci storing glycogen in excess. All transitions between
clear and basophilic cell populations known from chemically
induced hepatocarcinogenesis in animals and from the human
tumor-bearing liver were encountered. If these preliminary
results can be confirmed, the transgenic mice of Messing and
colleagues will become a most interesting tool for further
studies on the mechanism of neoplastic development in the
liver.

In liver tumors of both man and experimental animals,
including the transgenic mice just mentioned, formations
consisting of hepatocyte-like cells are frequently combined
with adenoid structures resembling intra-hepatic bile ducts
(Altmann, 1978; Jones and Butler, 1978). Some observations
in humans favored the concept that tumors or tumor components
exhibiting a cholangiocellular phenotype may not only develop
from cells of the intrahepatic biliary system but also from
hepatocytes which undergo a process of metaplasia or
transdifferentiation during neoplastic development (Altmann,
1984). Recently, this concept has been supported by detailed
electron microscopical and cytochemical studies of adenoid
formations in epithelial liver tumors induced in rats with
NNM (Ruan, 1985). Ruan Youbing from China working as a guest
in our laboratory was able to detect many tumor cells within
adenoid formations which were characterized by fine structural and cytochemical features in between hepatocellular
and cholangiocellular differentiation. Thus, there appears
to be sufficient evidence that tumor components with a cholangiocellular differentiation may develop from hepatocytes
(Altmann, 1984; Ruan, 1985). Such a transdifferentiation
is especially likely when a mixed hepatocholangiocellular
pattern is present.

Ductular (oval) cell proliferation and cholangiocellular
tumors.
In contrast to many adenoid formations in hepatic tumors, the
histogenesis of cholangiocellular tumors usually follows a
different and rather complex sequence (Bannasch et al.,
1985b; Moore et al., 1986; Thamvit et al., 1987). The tumors
develop in particular after application of high doses of
carcinogens, which produce pronounced necrotic alterations of
the liver parenchyma. The changes of the bile duct epithelia
start with a ductular (oval) cell reaction which may progress
to cholangiofibrosis, cystic cholangiomas and eventually also
cholangiocarcinomas. Many ductular cells are converted into
goblet cells storing and secreting abundant mucus substances
which contain PAS-positive neutral glycoproteins and
alcianophilic acid components. This reaction appears to be
specific for carcinogenic liver intoxications. The striking
change in carbohydrate metabolism of the ductular cells,
which might be analogous to the excessive storage of glycogen
in preneoplastic hepatocytes, is associated with changes in
the activity of a number of enzymes, such as an increased
activity of glucose-6-phosphatase or glucose-6-phosphate
dehydrogenase (Bannasch et al., 1985b; Moore et al., 1986),

and with the formation of a prominent brush border. Because
of the obvious similarity of such cells to intestinal
epithelia, the carcinogen-induced changes in ductular
epithelia just described, have been interpreted as intestinal
metaplasia by some authors (Tera and Nakano, 1974; Tatematsu
et al., 1985; Moore et al., 1986; Thamvit et al., 1987).   In
later stages of cholangiocarcinogenesis, the excessive
production of mucus gradually disappears again (Bannasch et
al., 1985b). Surprisingly, the reduction of the mucus
substances may be accompanied by an excessive storage of
glycogen. Apparently transdifferentiations are possible
during neoplastic transformation in various directions.

Peliosis hepatis and hemangioendotheliomas. The pathogenesis
of vascular liver tumors is also linked with characteristic
cellular changes. The sequential histological alterations
that occur during the morphogenesis of angiosarcomas in
rodents and man show many similarities (Popper et al., 1977).

     The sinusoidal lining cells many give rise to three
types of vascular lesions occurring after treatment with
chemical carcinogens, namely peliosis hepatis, benign
angiomas, and angiosarcomas. Peliosis hepatis is
characterized by an irregular focal dilatation of the
sinuses. The classification of this lesion as a neoplastic
disease or a preneoplastic condition is controversial
(Bannasch et al., 1985d). The sinusoidal lining cells may at
best show some minor alterations such as nuclear enlargement.
However, in Mastomys given single or twofold intraperitoneal
injections of 10 or 5 mg/kg body wt. N-nitrosodimethylamine,
Wayss et al. (1979) were able to observe all transitions to
unequivocal angiomas. It is especially interesting that
anabolic androgenic steroids, which have been related to the
liver-cell adenomas frequently developing in association with
peliosis hepatis in man, may induce this lesion in rats, too
(Nadell et al., 1977). In the nitrosamine-treated rodents,
we observed transitions from benign angiomas to angiosarcomas
after very long lag periods, but this seems to be the
exception rather than the rule. Angiosarcomas induced in rat
liver by NNM usually develop without a preceding benign
prestage. Antibodies to vimentin reveal that many cells of
the angiosarcomas accumulate excessive amounts of vimentin
filaments (Bannasch et al., 1981b). These vimentin storage
cells most probably correspond to the polyhedral cells
described in human angiosarcomas by Popper and colleagues
(1978) and are pathognomonic for malignant mesenchymal liver
tumors, especially the angiosarcomas. The cause of
accumulation of the intermediate filaments in sarcoma cells
is not known. However, it may be speculated that metabolic
aberrations similar to those which lead to the storage of
polysaccharides or lipids in epithelial cells hit by chemical
carcinogens might be responsible (Bannasch et al., 1981b).

Spongiosis hepatis and pericytoma. Finally, the
perisinusoidal cells may be the target of chemical
carcinogens. This cell type has only been clearly identified
during the past 20 years and has variously been called Ito
cell, lipocyte, or fat-storing cell (Wake, 1980). The
perisinusoidal cells are located between the sinusoidal

lining cells and the hepatocytes and have been shown to be
involved in the metabolism of vitamin A and most probably
also in the production of collagen. In rat liver treated
with hepatocarcinogens, these cells are considered to be the
site of origin of a cyst-like lesion for which we proposed
the descriptive term "spongiosis hepatis" (Bannasch et al.,
1981a, 1985e). Under the light microscope it is evident
that the holes of the sponge are not lined by epithelial or
endothelial cells. In contrast to peliosis, the multilocular
formations of spongiosis are not filled with blood but with a
finely flocculent material rich in acid mucopolysaccharides.
Electron microscopic analysis of the spongiotic areas reveals
that they are composed of cells which are very similar to
fibroblasts and sometimes even to typical fat-storing cells.
The fibroblast-like cells show extremely elongated
cytoplasmic processes which form the walls of the spongy
lesions and are usually observed in close association with a
thick coat resembling a basement membrane. It is still
unclear whether spongiosis hepatis should be considered as a
preneoplastic or as a neoplastic liver lesion. However,
during the past few years we have observed a considerable
cell proliferation within spongiotic areas in some rats
treated with NNM after long lag periods (Bannasch and
Zerban, 1986). Apparently, there were also transitions into
malignant mesenchymal tumors which we classified as
pericytomas. With respect to the pathogenesis of this tumor
type, it is of particular interest that our experimental
results suggest that the accumulation of acid
mucopolysaccharides within the spongiotic formations seems to
disappear during transformation of spongiosis into
pericytoma. If this surmise can be confirmed, changes in
carbohydrate metabolism of both the intracellular and the
extracellular compartment were closely related to neoplastic
development in the liver.

ACKNOWLEDGEMENTS

This work was supported by the Deutsche Forschungsgemeinschaft. The authors wish to express their appreciation
to B. Pétillon for typing the manuscript. The present
address of Ruan Youbin who worked as a guest research
scientist in our laboratory is Tongji Medical University,
Wuhan, The People's Republic of China.

REFERENCES

Altmann, H.W., 1978, Pathology of human liver tumors, in:
    "Primary Liver Tumors," H. Remmer, H.M. Bolt,
    P. Bannasch, and H. Popper, eds., MTP Press,
    Lancaster.
Altmann, H.W., 1984, Neubildungen der Leber, Verh. Dtsch.
    Krebs.Ges., 5:423.
Bannasch, P., 1968, The cytoplasm of hepatocytes during
    carcinogenesis. Light and electron microscopic
    investigations of the nitrosomorpholine-intoxica-
    ted rat liver, Rec. Res. Cancer Res., 19:1.
Bannasch, P., 1986, Preneoplastic lesions as end points in
    carcinogenicity testing. I. Hepatic preneoplasia,
    Carcinogenesis, 7:689.

Bannasch, P. and Zerban, H., 1986, Pathogenesis of primary
        liver tumors induced by chemicals, Rec. Res.
        Cancer Res., 100:1.
Bannasch, P. and Zerban, H., 1987, Modulation of hepatocellu-
        lar phenotype and proliferation in liver cirrhosis,
        in: "Liver Cirrhosis", MTP Press, Lancaster.
Bannasch, P., Mayer, D., and Hacker, H.J., 1980a, Hepatocel-
        lular glycogenosis and hepatocarcinogenesis,
        Biochim. Biophys. Acta, 605:217.
Bannasch, P., Zerban, H., Schmid, E., and Franke, W.W.,
        1980b, Liver tumors distinguished by immuno-
        fluorescence microscopy with antibodies to
        proteins of intermediate-sized filaments, Proc.
        Natl. Acad. Sci. USA, 77:4948.
Bannasch, P., Bloch, H., and Zerban, H., 1981a, Spongiosis
        hepatis. Specific changes of the perisinusoidal
        liver cells induced in rats by N-nitrosomorpholine,
        Lab. Invest., 44:252.
Bannasch, P., Zerban, H., Schmid, E., and Franke, W.W.,
        1981b, Characterization of cytoskeletal components
        in epithelial and mesenchymal liver tumors by
        electron and immunofluorescence microscopy,
        Virchows Arch. (Cell Pathol.), 36:139.
Bannasch, P., Hacker, H.J., Klimek, F., and Mayer, D.,
        1984, Hepatocellular glycogenosis and related
        pattern of enzymatic changes during hepatocarci-
        nogenesis, Adv. Enzyme Regul., 22:97.
Bannasch, P., Benner, U., Enzmann, H., and Hacker, H.J.,
        1985a, Tigroid cell foci and neoplastic nodules
        in the liver of rats treated with a single dose
        of aflatoxin B1, Carcinogenesis, 6:1641.
Bannasch, P., Benner, U., and Zerban, H., 1985b, Cholan-
        gio fibroma and cholangiocarcinoma, liver, rat,
        in: "Digestive System," T.C. Jones, U. Mohr,
        and R.D. Hunt, eds., Springer Verlag, Berlin-
        Heidelberg-New York-Tokyo.
Bannasch, P., Moore, M.A., Hacker, H.J., Klimek, F.,
        Mayer, D., Enzmann, H., and Zerban, H., 1985c,
        Potential significance of phenotypic instability
        in focal and nodular liver lesions induced by
        hepatocarcinogens, in: "Hepatology: A Fest-
        schrift for Hans Popper, "H. Brunner and H. Thaler,
        eds., Raven Press, New York.
Bannasch, P., Wayss, K., and Zerban, H., 1985d, Peliosis
        hepatis, rodents, in: "Digestive System,"
        T.C. Jones, U. Mohr, and R.D. Hunt, eds.,
        Springer-Verlag, Berlin-Heidelberg-New York-
        Tokyo.
Bannasch, P., Zerban, H., and Fügel, H.J., 1985e, Spongiosis
        hepatis, rat, in: "Digestive System," T.C.
        Jones, U. Mohr, and R.D. Hunt, eds., Springer-
        Verlag, Berlin-Heidelberg-New York-Tokyo.
Bannasch, P., Zerban, H., and Hacker, H.J., 1985f, Foci of
        altered hepatocytes, rat, in: "Digestive
        System," T.C. Jones, U. Mohr, and R.D. Hunt,
        eds., Springer-Verlag Berlin-Heidelberg-New York-
        Tokyo.
Beasly, R.P., Hwang, L.-Y., Lin, C.-C., and Chien C.-S.,
        1981, Hepatocellular carcinoma and hepatitis
        B virus. A prospective study of 22,707 men
        in Taiwan, Lancet, 2:1129.

Cain, H., 1978, Liver cell carcinoma in infancy and child-
    hood, in: "Primary Liver Tumors," H. Remmer,
    H. Bolt, P. Bannasch, and H. Popper, eds., MTP
    Press, Lancaster.
Coire, C.I., Qizilbash, A.H., and Castelli, M.F., 1987,
    Hepatic adenomata in type Ia glycogen storage
    disease, Arch. Pathol. Lab. Med., 111:166.
Ehemann, V., Mayer, D., Hacker, H.J., and Bannasch, P.,
    1986, Loss of adenylate cyclase activity in
    preneoplastic and neoplastic lesions induced
    in rat liver by N-nitrosomorpholine, Carcino-
    genesis, 7:567.
Enzmann, H. and Bannasch, P., 1986, Sequential phenotypic
    conversion of hepatocytes during carcinogenesis,
    Cancer Lett., 30:S67.
Farber, E., 1984, Precancerous steps in carcinogenesis.
    Their physiological adaptive nature, Biochim.
    Biophys. Acta, 738:171.
Farber, E., and Sarma, D.S.R., 1987, Hepatocarcinogenesis:
    A dynamic cellular perspective, Lab. Invest.,
    56:4.
Fischer, G., Hartmann, H., Droese, M., Schauer, A., and Bock,
    K.W., 1986, Histochemical and immunohistochemical
    detection of putative preneoplastic liver foci in
    woman after long-term use of oral contraceptives
    Virchows Arch. (Cell Pathol.), 50:321.
Goldsworthy, T.L., Hanigan, M.H., and Pitot, H.C., 1986,
    Models of hepatocarcinogenesis in the rat -
    contrasts and comparisons, CRC Critical Rev.
    Toxicol., 17:61.
Hacker, H.J., Moore, M.A., Mayer, D., and Bannasch, P., 1982,
    Correlative histochemistry of some enzymes of
    carbohydrate metabolism in preneoplastic and neo-
    plastic lesions in the rat liver, Carcinogenesis,
    3:1265.
Hann, H.L., Kim, C.Y., London, W.T., Whitford, P., and
    Blumberg, B.S., 1982, Hepatitis B virus and prima-
    ry hepatocellular carcinoma: family studies in
    Korea, Int. J. Cancer, 30:47.
Heine, W.D., 1981, Experimentelle und menschliche hepatozel-
    luläre Lebertumoren und ihre Vostufen - histolo-
    gische, histochemische und zellkinetische Charak-
    teristika, in: "Experimentelle und klinische
    Hepatologie," O. Zelder, H.D. Röher, M. Fischer,
    and J. Ch. Bode, eds., F.K. Schattauer Verlag,
    Stuttgart-New York.
Heinzelmann, D., 1986, Modulation der Nitrosamin induzierten
    Hepatocarcinogenese der Ratte durch Dehydroepian-
    drosteron. Inauguraldissertation, Universität
    Heidelberg.
Hirota, N., Hamazaki, M., and Williams, G.M., 1982, Resis-
    tance to iron accumulation and presence of
    hepatitis B surface antigen in preneoplastic
    and neoplastic lesions in human hemochromatotic
    livers, Hepatogastroenterol., 29:49.
Jones, G., and Butler, W.H., 1978, Light microscopy of
    rat hepatic neoplasia, in: "Rat Hepatic
    Neoplasia," P.M. Newberne and W.H. Butler, eds.,
    MIT Press, Cambridge.
Karhunen, P.J., and Penttilä, A., 1987, Preneoplastic
    lesions of human liver, Hepato-gastroenterol.,

      34:10.
Klimek, F., Mayer, D., and Bannasch, P., 1984, Biochemical
      microanalysis of glycogen content and glucose-6-
      phosphate dehydrogenase activity in focal lesions
      or rat liver induced by N-nitrosomorpholine,
      Carcinogenesis, 5:265.
Limmer, J., Mohr, W., Bittner, R., Krautzberger, W., und
      Beger, H.G., 1985, Hepatozelluläres Karzinom auf
      dem Boden einer Glycogenose Typ von Giercke,
      Z. Gastroenterol., 23:303.
Melbye, M., Skinhøj, P., Nielsen, H.H., Vestergaard, B.F.,
      Ebbesen, P., Hansen, J.P.H., and Biggar, R.J.,
      1984, Virus-associated cancers in Greenland:
      Frequent hepatitis B virus infection but low
      primary hepatocellular carcinoma incidence,
      J. Natl. Cancer Inst., 73:1267.
Messing, A., Chen, H.Y., Palmiter, R.D., and Brinster, R.L.,
      1985, Peripheral neuropathies, hepatocellular
      carcinomas and islet cell adenomas in transgenic
      mice, Nature, 316:461.
Montesano, R., Bartsch, H., Vaino, H., Wilbourn, J., and
      Yamasaki, H., eds., 1986, "Long-term and short-
      term assays for carcinogens : A critical apprai-
      sal", IARC Scientifique Publications, N°. 83,
      Lyon.
Moore, M.A., and Kitagawa, T., 1986, Hepatocarcinogenesis in
      the rat; the effect of the promoters and
      carcinogens in vivo and in vitro, Int. Rev. Cytol.,
      101:125.
Moore, M.A., Mayer, D., and Bannasch, P., 1982, The dose-
      dependence and sequential appearance of putati-
      ve preneoplastic populations induced in the
      rat liver by stop experiments with N-nitrosomor-
      pholine, Carcinogenesis, 3:1429.
Moore, M.A., Fukushima, S., Ichihara, A., Sato, K., and Ito,
      N., 1986, Intestinal metaplasia and altered enzyme
      expression in propyl-nitrosamine-induced Syrian
      hamster cholangiocellular and gallbladder lesions,
      Virchows Arch. (Cell Pathol.), 51:29.
Mori, H., Tanaka, T., Sugie, S., Takahashi, M., and Williams,
      G., 1982, DNA content of liver cell nuclei of N-2-
      fluorenylacetamide-induced altered foci and
      neoplasms in rats and human hyperplastic foci,
      J. Natl. Cancer Inst., 69:1277.
Nadell, J., and Kosek, J., 1977, Peliosis hepatis. Twelve
      cases associated with oral androgen therapy,
      Arch. Pathol. Lab. Med., 101:405.
Osborn, M. and Weber, K., 1986, Intermediate filament
      proteins: a multigene family distinguishing
      major cell lineages, trends Biochem. Sci.,
      11:469.
Peers, F., Bosch, X., Kaldor, J., Linselle, A., and Plui-
      jomen, M., 1987, Aflatoxin exposure, hepatitis
      B virus infection and liver cancer in Swaziland,
      Int. J. Cancer, in press.
Peraino, C., Richards, W.L., and Stevens, F.J., 1983,
      Multistage hepatocarcinogenesis, in:
      "Mechanisms of Tumor Promotion," T.J. Slaga,
      ed., CRC Press, Boca Raton.
Popper, H., Maltoni, C., Selikoff, I.J., Squire, R.A., and
      Thomas, L.B., 1977, Comparison of neoplastic

hepatic lesions in man and experimental animals, in: "Origin of Human Cancer," Book C, Human Risk Assessment, H.H. Hiat, J.D. Watson, and J.A. Winsten, eds., Cold Spring Harbor Laboratories, Cold Spring Harbor.

Popper, H., Thomas, L.B., Telles, N.C., Falk, H., and Selikoff, I.J., 1978, Development of hepatic angiosarcoma in man induced by vinyl chloride, thorotrast, and arsenic, Am. J. Pathol., 92:349.

Rabes, H.M., 1983, Development and growth of early preneoplastic lesions induced in the liver by chemical carcinogens, J. Cancer Res. Clin. Oncol., 106:85.

Ramaekers, F.C.S., Puts, J.J.G. Kant, A., Moesker, O., Jap, P.H.K. and Vooijs, G.P., 1982, The use of antibodies directed against intermediate filaments in the characterization of human tumors, Cold Spring Harbor Symposia on Quantitative Biology, 46:331.

Ruan, Y.-B., 1985, Zytochemische und elektronenmikroskopische Charakterisierung des zellulären Phänotyps adenoider Lebertumoren, Inaugural-Dissertation, Universität Heidelberg.

Scherer, E., 1984, Neoplastic progression in experimental hepatocarcinogenesis, Biochim. Biophys. Acta, 738:219.

Schröter, C., Parzefall, W., Schröter, H., and Schulte-Hermann, R., 1987, Dose-response studies on the effects of γ-, β-, and α- hexachlorohexane on putative preneoplastic foci, monooxygenases, and growth in rat liver, Cancer Res., 47:80.

Seelmann-Eggebert, G., Mayer, D., Mecke, D., and Bannasch, P., 1987, Expression and regulation of glycogen phosphorylase in preneoplastic and neoplastic hepatic lesions in rats, Virchows Arch. B (Cell Path.), 53:44.

Stewart, H.L., Williams, G., Keysser, C.H., Lombard, L.S., and Montali, R.J., 1980, Histologic typing of liver tumors of the rat, J. Natl. Cancer Inst., 65:179.

Tatematsu, M., Kaku, T., Medline, A., and Farber, E., 1985, Intestinal metaplasia as a common option of oval cells in relation to cholangiofibrosis in liver of rats exposed to 2-acetylaminofluorene, Lab. Invest., 52:354.

Terao, K., and Nakano, M., 1974, Cholangiofibrosis induced by short-term feeding of 3'-methyl-4-(dimethylamino) azobenzene: an electron microscopic observation, Gann, 65:249.

Thamavit, W., Kongkanuntn, R., Tiwawech, D., and Moore, M.A., 1987, Level of Opisthorchis infestation and carcinogen dose-dependence of cholangiocarcinoma induction in Syrian golden hamsters, Virchows Arch B, submitted.

Tiollais, P., Pourcel, C., and Dejean, A., 1985, The hepatitis B virus, Nature, 317:489.

Tu, J., Gao, R., Zhang, D., Gu, B., Xu, G., Fang, R., Pan, J., Yu, H., Huang, Y., and Zhou, X., 1987, Risk factors of primary liver cancer in the high prevalence area Chongming County - results

from a five years follow up, in: "Cancer of the
Liver, Esophagus, and Nasopharynx," G. Wagner and
You-Hui Zhang, eds., Springer, Berlin-Heidelberg-
New York-Tokyo.

Wake, K., 1980, Perisinusoidal stellate cells (fat-storing
cells, interstitial cells, lipocytes), their related structure in and around the liver sinusoids,
and vitamin A-storing cells in extrahepatic organs,
Int. Rev. Cytol., 66:303.

Ward, J.M., 1984, Morphology of potential preneoplastic
hepatocyte lesions and liver tumors in mice and
a comparison with other species, in: "Mouse
Liver Neoplasia," J.A. Popp, ed., Hemisphere
Publishing Corporation, Washington-New York-London.

Wayss, K., Bannasch, P., Mattern, J., and Volm, M., 1979,
Vascular liver tumors induced in Mastomys (Prao-
mys) natalensis by single dimethylnitrotrosamine,
J. Natl. Cancer Inst., 62:1199.

Weber, E., Heinzelmann, D., and Bannasch, P., 1986, The
The effect of DHEA on peroxisomes in nitrosamine-
treated rat liver, Europ. J. Cell Biol., 41
(Suppl 14):44.

Weber, G., 1977, Enzymology of cancer cells, Parts 1 and
2, New Engl. J. Med., 296:486.

Willis, R.A., 1953, "Pathology of Tumors", 2nd Edition,
Butterworth & Co, London.

Zerban, H., Rabes, H.M., and Bannasch, P., 1985, Kinetics
of cell proliferation during hepatocarcinogenesis,
Europ. J. Cancer Clin. Oncol., 21.:1424.

HISTOCHEMICAL ANALYSIS OF HEPATOCARCINOGENESIS

Hans Jörg Hacker[1], Gabriele Seelmann-Eggebert[1], Fritz Klimek[1],
Peter Peschke[2], and Rolf F. Kletzien[3]

[1]Institut für Experimentelle Pathologie, [2]Inst. f. Nuklear-
medizin, Deutsches Krebsforschungszentrum, D-6900 Heidelberg
[3]Dep. of Biochemistry, West Virginia Univ., Morgantown,
West Virginia 26506-6302

INTRODUCTION

The hybrid discipline of histochemistry, a borderline field between
histology and analytical chemistry or biochemistry is concerned with the
identification, localization and quantification of specific substances,
reactive groups and sites of enzymatic activities in tissues, cells and
cell organelles. Principally metabolic products or enzymes can also be
assessed by biochemical analysis nowadays much more efficiently because of
the development of new sensitive microchemical techniques. However, the
data provided by this approach represent average values and cannot give
any information about the true distribution of certain compounds in individual cells and organells. That individual cells differ markedly in
their metabolic compartimentation is best illustrated by the kidney tu-
bular system[1] and even the liver which looks quite homogeneous uncovers
at closer inspection the well known metabolic zonation[2]. Biochemical
analysis becomes really difficult or cannot be performed at all when
patholologically altered tissue has to be investigated in which cellular
structure as well as metabolic activities may have changed. Because
histochemistry offers a wide spectrum of effective methods to surmount
such serious problems it turned out to be an indispensable tool for scientists in many fields from botany to histopathology which is frequently
applied in toxicology and cancer research. In the following paragraphs
the application of currently most important histochemical techniques is
described in more detail including some pitfalls and difficulties inherent to these methods.

WHOLE-BODY AUTORADIOGRAPHY

When toxic compounds enter the body they undergo different fates
e.g. they are excreted unchanged or they are bioactivated by intestinal
tissue, kidney and predominantly by the liver. This process results in
non-toxic highly water soluble derivatives being easily eliminated from
the body[3]. Unfortunately, liver is also capable of biotransforming many toxic compounds into potent reactants that produce serious lesions in
the hepatic tissue such as necrosis and tumors[4]. N-nitrosomorpholine
(NNM) e.g. is known to be metabolized by the liver[5] subsequently in-

ducing a high incidence of liver[6,7] or kidney[8] tumors in rats and mice. Until recently, organotropy was deduced from biochemical as well as histological investigations on isolated organs. Recently, however, using a modern histochemical technique, namely whole-body autoradiography with [14C-NNM] Löfberg and Tjälve[9] could elegantly demonstrate that apart from the label in the nasal olfactory mucosa and the kidney liver bound most of the radio-labelled NNM (Fig.1). Together with the biochemical data on the high activity of biotransformation in liver these results indicate the liver to be the prevalent site of tumor formation after NNM-treatment. Whole-body autoradiography combined with microautoradiography at the electron microscope level provide also now the possibility to test the tissue distribution of a hepatocarcinogen during chronic dosing in connection with the drug resistance of altered hepatoytes as has been extensively discussed by Farber and Sarma[10].

Oesophageal mucosa   Intestinal contents

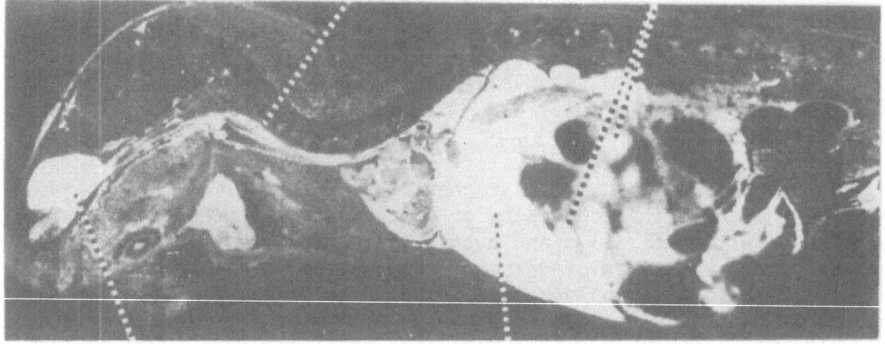

Nasal mucosa   Liver

Fig. 1 Whole-body autoradiogram of Sprague-Dawley rats injected i.v. with N-nitroso[14C]morpholine, with white areas corresponding to radioactivity. Note high level of non volatile metabolites in the liver and the nasal mucosa and considerable labelling of the oesophagal mucosa and intestinal contents. Courtesy of Fd. Chem. Tox.

ANALYTICAL HISTOCHEMISTRY

The first cytopathological phenomenon of hepatocarcinogenesis in rat are foci of altered hepatocytes. In H&E stained paraffin sections these cells depict a clear and/or acidophilic cytoplasm. To answer the question whether the altered liver cells are hydropic or contain some special material a method of analytical histochemistry has to be applied. This discipline identifies chemical compounds in tissues and cells e.g. small molecules such as amino acids, ions like phosphate or iron, but also macromolecules such as proteins, nucleic acids, lipids or polysaccharides[11,12]. The higly water soluble glycogen belongs to the latter class. It can be specifically stained in tissue sections by the PAS-reaction, when the proper control by amylase digestion is performed[13]. Despite optimal retention of glycogen in normal or alterd liver after routine immersion-fixation with Carnoy's fluid two phenomena were encountered that seriously impeded the true intracellular localization of this polysaccharide. First there was an accumulation of glycogen at the cell pole faced to the block center (Fig. 2a). Second after oxydation with aqueous

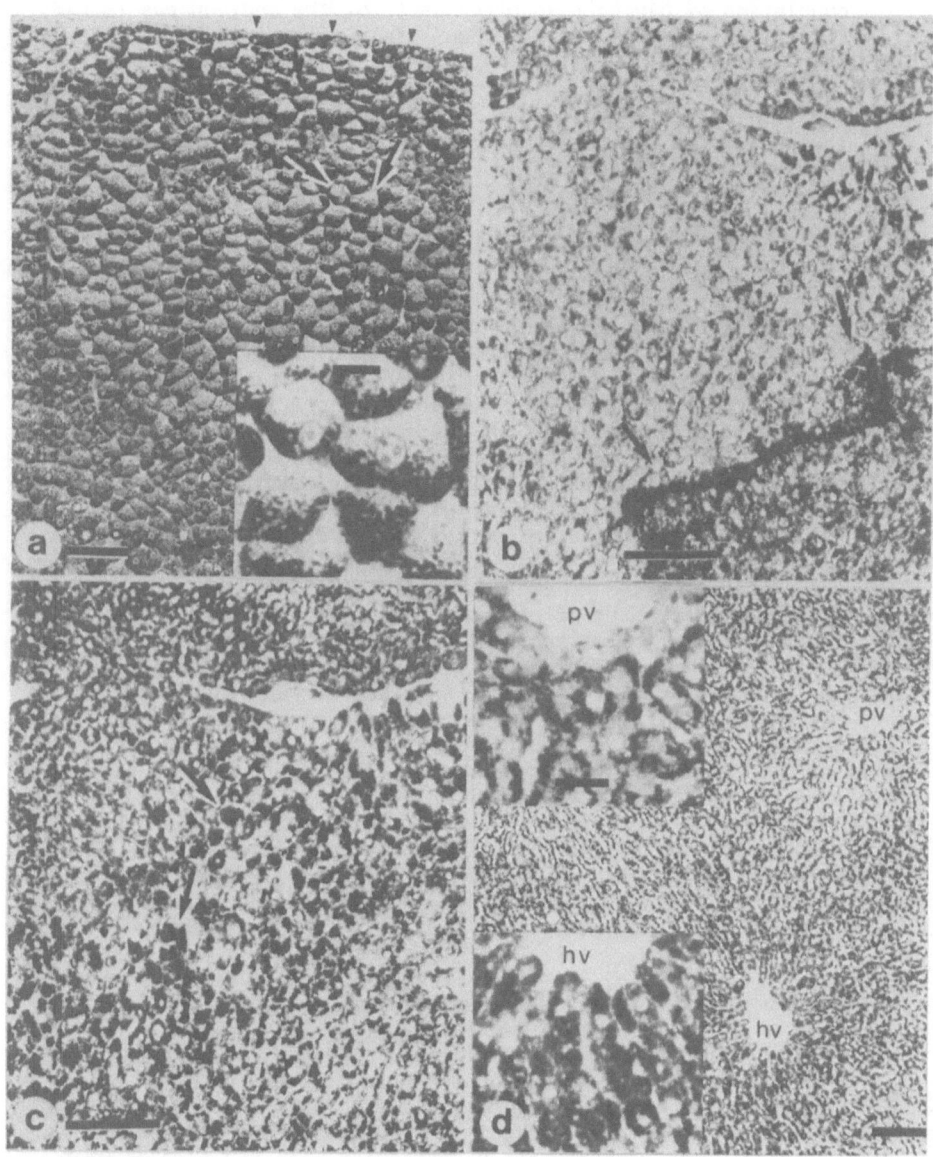

Fig. 2 Demonstration of glycogen under different histochemical conditions.
(a) Polarization of glycogen in hepatocytes of normal rat liver
after block-fixation with Carnoy's fluid at 20° C. Oxydation of
glycogen was performed with alcoholic periodic acid followed by
Schiff's reaction. Arrow heads indicate surface of liver block.
Note glycogen accumulation at the cell pole facing to the centre
of the tissue block (arrows). Bar, 100 µm. Insert shows hepatocytes with pronounced glycogen polarisation. Bar, 20 µm;   (b)
Glycogen distribution in a native cryostat section of a carcinogen-treated rat liver. Oxydation with aqueous periodic acid immediately after mounting. Glycogen polarization is not detectable.

However, tissue structure is blurred because glycogen has partly leaked out of and overlaid the liver cells. Note also massive accumulation of glycogen in other parts of the section due to redistribution (arrows). Bar, 100 µm; (c) Serial section to the section in Fig. 2b. Oxydation with alcoholic periodic acid. Neither polarization nor leaking or redistribution of glycogen is visible Hepatocytes storing glycogen in excess can clearly be identified (arrows). Note remarkable good preservation of tissue structure. Bar, 100 µm; (d) Glycogen distribution in a native cryostat section of normal rat liver. Oxydation with alcoholic periodic acid immediately after mounting. Counterstaining with 0,1% toluidine blue. No intracellular polarization of glycogen is visible. Bar, 100 µm. Inserts show glycogen localization in periportal hepatocytes (upper corner left) and in perivenular hepatocytes (lower corner left). Bar, 25 µm. pv=portal venule; hv=hepatic venule.

periodic acid large quantities of glycogen were lost from the sections. This loss could be prevented when the sections were treated with alcoholic periodic acid[14] (Fig. 2a). However, polarization of glycogen was still visible even after low temperature fixation. This artifact[15] did not occur when liver was fixed either by perfusion[16] or by snap-freezing in isopentane at -150°C[17]. The latter method has several advantages: a lot of material can quickly be processed and most important, all cell components are preserved close to the living state. This holds true especially for the enzymes which often loose their activity during chemical fixation. So, native cryostat sections of snap-frozen liver should render optimal localization of glycogen when aqueous periodic acid (Fig. 2b) is replaced by alcoholic one (Fig. 2c,d). Precise intracellular localization of glycogen is therefore based on two principles: first avoiding of its displacement by cryo-fixation, and second making it insoluble by combination of alcohol and periodic acid. The latter transforms part of the polysaccharide into a polyaldehyde functioning as an intracellular fixative. With an improved PAS-method considering these principles it could be shown in paraffin as well as in native cryostat sections that the clear and/or acidophilic liver cell foci stored glycogen in excess. Because glycogen is very typical for liver cells it can be used as a marker in toxicologic studies testing chemicals for carcinogenicity.

ENZYMEHISTOCHEMISTRY AND IMMUNOHISTOCHEMISTRY

Since the excessive storage of glycogen in the early hepatocellular foci indicates a disturbance in glycogen metabolism the question arises what mechanism at the enzyme level might be the cause. According to the schematic presentation of liver glycogen metabolism (Fig. 3) several possibilities exist which confront the histochemist with the problem what enzyme has to be selected for studying a certain metabolic pathway. As pointed out by Newsholme et al.[18] there are enzymes that catalyse near equilibrium and those which catalyse non equilibrium reactions. Only enzymes of the latter class may provide information of the maximum flux through a given metabolic pathway. For example, glycogen phosphorylase (PHO) controls the maximum flux through the phosphorolytic pathway of glycogen metabolism[19]. A decreased PHO activity favours glycogen accumulation in hepatocytes. Excessive glycogen storage must be expected when in addition another rate limiting enzyme namely glucose-6-phosphatase (G6PASE)[20] shows a reduction in or a lack of activity. On the other hand

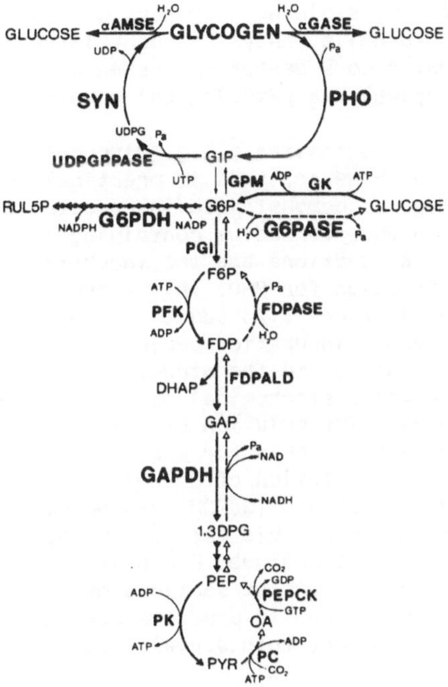

Fig. 3. Simplified schematic presentation of liver carbohydrate metabolism. Glycogen and enzymes investigated histochemically (SYN, PHO,G6PASE, G6PDH and GAPDH) are displayed in particularly large bold letters. = glycogen metabolism, = oxidative pentose phosphate pathway, = glycolysis, = gluconeogenesis; αAMSE = α-amylase; DHAP = dihydroxyacetone phosphate; 1,3DPG = 1,3-diphosphoglycerate; FDP = fructose-1,6-diphosphatase; F6P = fructose-6-phosphate; GAP = glyceraldehyde-3-phosphate; GAPDH = glycer-aldehyde-3-phosphate dehydrogenase; α-GASE = α-glucosidase; GK = glucokinase; GPM = phosphoglucomutase; G1P = glucose-1-phosphate; G6P = glucose-6-phosphate; G6PASE = glucose-6-phosphatase; G6PDH = glucose-6-phosphate dehydrogenase; OA = oxalacetate; Pa = inorganic phosphate; PC = pyruvate carboxylase; PEP = phosphoenolpyruvate carboxykinase; PFK = phosphofructokinase; PGI = phosphoglucoisomerase; PHO = glycogen phosphorylase; PK = pyruvate kinase; PYR = pyruvate; RUL5P = ribulose-5-phosphate; SYN = glycogen synthetase; UDPG = uridine diphosphate glucose; UDPGPPASE = uridinediphosphate glucose pyrophosphorylase; UTP = uridine triphosphate. Courtesy of Adv. Enzyme Reg.

glycogen storage may be caused by an elevated activity of glycogen synthetase (SYN). Thus, when one studies changes in liver glycogen metabolism
SYN, PHO, G6PASE including glycogen should be tested. This strategy
might be called correlative biochemistry (see also [21]) which can also be
applied to histochemsitry now denoted as correlative histochemistry[22].
As already mentioned, conventional biochemical enzyme assays on homogenates cannot detect a possible heterogenous distribution of enzymes in
individual cells and organells. Enzymehistochemistry bridges this gap
and therefore contributes to a deeper understanding of metabolic events
under various physiological and pathological conditions.

It would be ideal to demonstrate e.g. glycogen, SYN, PHO and G6PASE in
the same tissue section. However, this is practical impossible for several reasons. G6PASE e.g. is demonstrated in cryostat sections fixed in
glutaraldehyde using an aqueous medium containing lead ions[23]. It is the
pretreatment of the liver sections and the incubation conditions that
block a simultaneous reaction for PHO. This enzyme is known to be very
sensitive to lead and fixation[24]. In addition there is complete loss of
the enzyme into the aqueous incubation medium for it is highly water soluble like glycogen in contrast to the structurally bound G6PASE. Thus,
conditions optimal for the histochemical detection of one enzyme may be
detrimental for the other. The solution of this problem is to cut serial
sections and to stain each one only for a single enzyme under optimal
histochemical conditions. Diffusion of soluble enzymes like PHO, SYN or
glucose-6-phosphate dehydrogenase (G6PDH) can be considered and effectively prevented using the semipermeable membrane method [25,26]. Figure 4
shows the principle of this technique. Recently, a very promising alternative to the use of serial cryostat sections has been published by
which several enzymes and metabolic products such as glycogen can be histochemically visualized in very thin serial sections of methacrylate
embedded material[27].

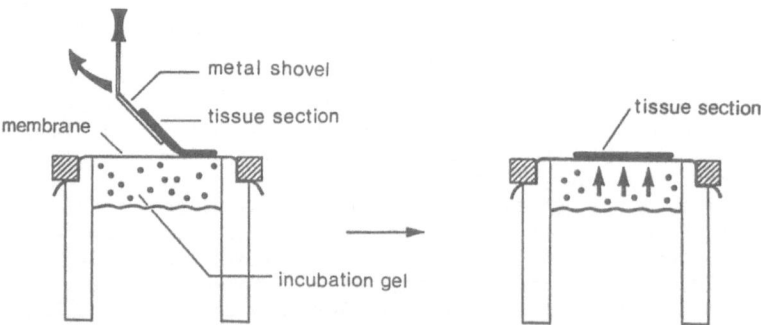

Fig. 4. Principle of the semipermeable membrane technique. All ingre-
dients necessary for the enzyme histochemical reaction are mixed
with gelifying substances such as agar or gelatine. The mixture is
poured into the vessel with dialysis membrane down being stretches
with a ring. After solidifying of the gelmedium cryostat sections
are mounted with the help of a precooled metal shovel in the
cryostat cabinet. The reaction starts as soon as the sections are
thawed up. After removal of the gel and restretching of the membrane they can be fixed very gently by formaldehyde through the
membrane.

Evaluation of individually stained tissue sections is greatly facilitated by the use of a comparison microscope (Fig. 5) which helps to detect histochemical patterns in liver lesions e.g. in glycogen storage foci (Fig. 6a).

Among other enzymehistochemical changes[22] these focal lesions showed a marked decrease in PHO activity (Fig. 6b). Since the histochemical assay detects only the a-form of PHO decrease in enzyme activity may be due to a defect in the activation mechanism or to a loss of the enzyme protein[28]. With the help of immunohistochemistry[29] one or the other alternative could be ruled out. Serial cryostat sections through glycogen

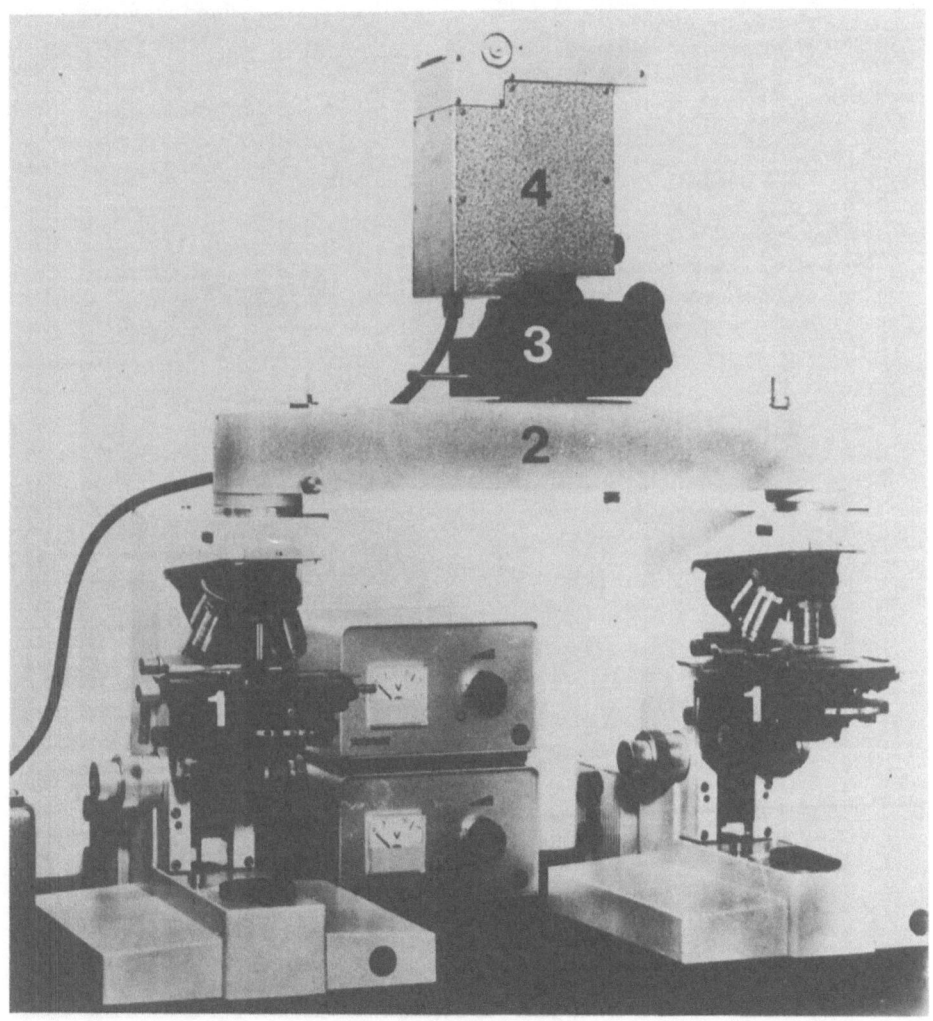

Fig. 5. Comparison microscope.

It consists of two normal microscopes (1) linked by a comparison bridge (2). Pictures of the slides can be looked at (3)/photographed (4) either serially or simultaneously as half frames in the same viewing field.

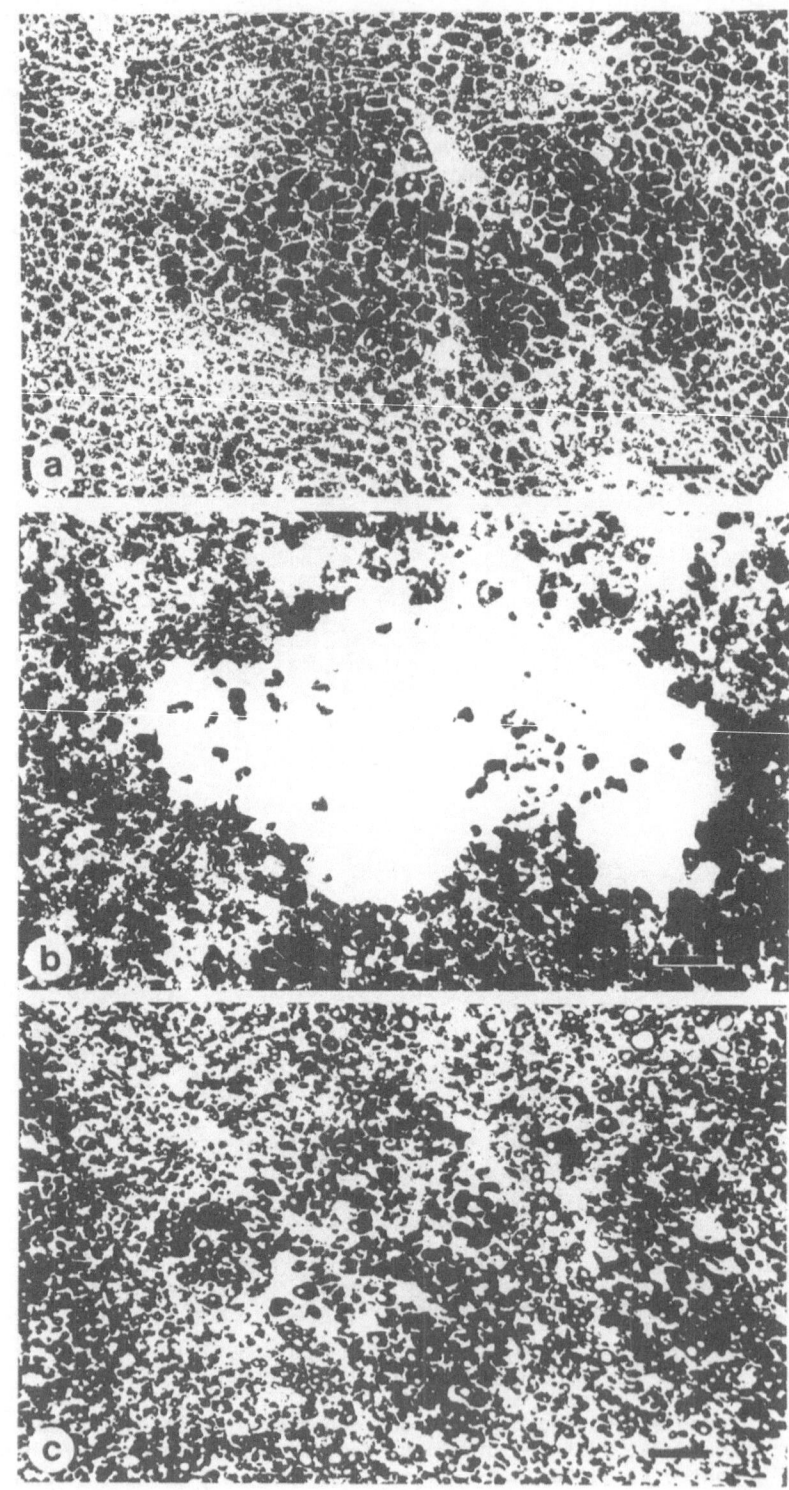

Fig. 6. Serial sections through glycogen storage focus induced in rat liver by NNM. (a) PAS staining for glycogen. BAR, 100 μm; (b) PHO activity (enzyme histochemistry). Bar, 100 μm; (c) PHO protein (immunoperoxydase). Bar, 100 μm.

storage foci were reacted with an antibody directed against the liver type of PHO (L-PHO) i.e. it detects both a- and b-form of PHO. A high content of the PHO-protein could be demonstrated in the glycogen storing hepatocellular foci (Fig. 6c, see also reference [28]). These findings suggest that in glycogen storage foci L-PHO is still expressed but the whole enzyme appears to be converted to the inactive b-form by a yet unknown mechanism possibly involving a sugar phosphate like glucose-6-phosphate[30]. Using more advanced immunochemical methods[31,32] it should be possible to raise antibodies being able to distinguish between a- and b-form of PHO in order to clarify which enzyme species is actually present in the foci.

That glucose-6-phosphate (G6P) most likely plays a role in the imbalance of sugar metabolism of glycogen storage foci is indicated by the high G6PDH activity gained by enzymehistochemical tests (Fig. 7a) (see e.g. reference [33]. In complementary immunocytochemical studies on serial cryostat sections Hacker, Kletzien and Peschke (unpublished) could demonstrate also a high protein content of this key enzyme of pentose phosphate pathway in the foci (Fig. 7b).

If we continue to follow up our strategy of correlative histochemistry we may ask the question whether there are also changes of key enzymes of glycolysis in glycogen storage foci. One of the rate limiting enzymes is pyruvate kinase (PK)[34]. Enzymehistochemical as well as biochemical

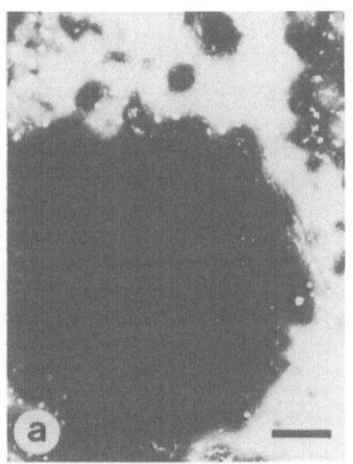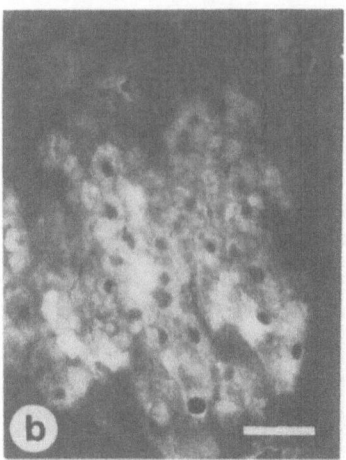

Fig. 7. Demonstration of G6PDH in cryostat sections through a glycogen storage focus. (a) G6PDH activity (enzyme histochemistry). Bar 100 μm; (b) G6PDH protein (immunofluorescence). Bar, 250 μm.

determinations revealed a high PK activity in microdissected material[35]. When the liver type of PK (L-PK) was checked immunohistochemically in the glycogen storage foci no reduction of the enzyme protein content could be observed (Fig. 8a,b,c). This is at variance with the findings of Reinacher et al.[36] who consistently found low L-PK content in focal rat liver lessions.

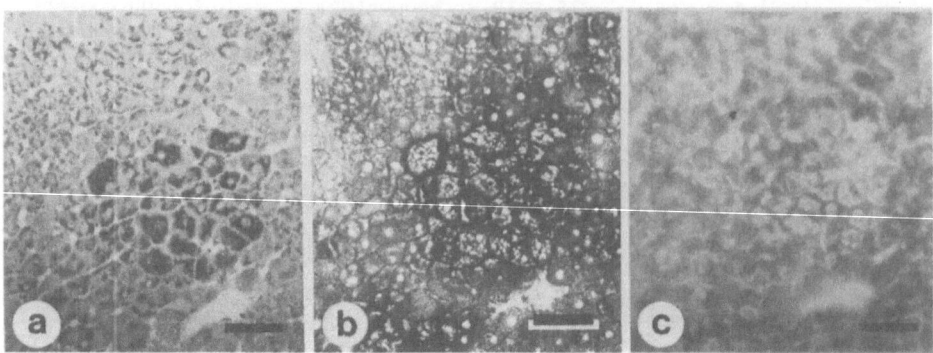

Fig. 8. Serial sections through small glycogen storage focus induced in rat liver by NNM. (a) PAS staining for glycogen. Bar, 100 μm; (b) PK activity (enzyme histochemistry). Bar, 100 μm; (c) L-PK protein (immunoperoxydase). Bar, 100 μm.

We suppose that lesions with low L-PK are corresponding at least partly to the more advanced mixed cell foci showing a clear L-PK reduction also in our material (Fig. 9a,b,c). Further studies are necessary to find the cause for these discrepances.

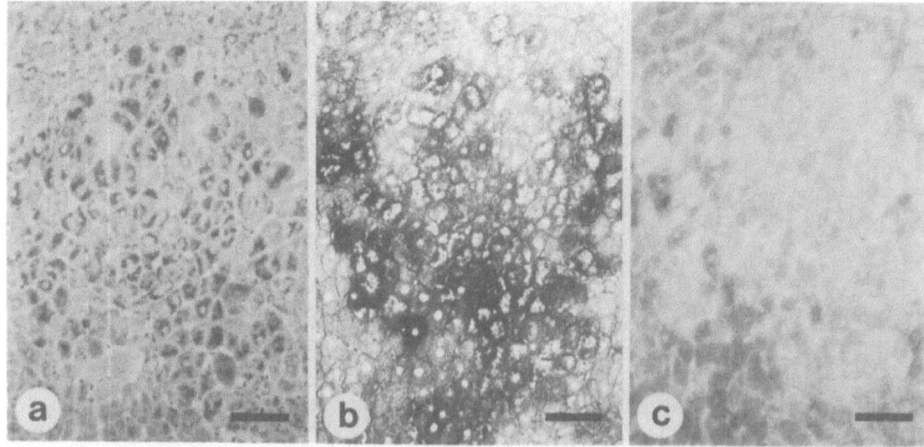

Fig. 9. Serial sections through a mixed cell focus induced in rat liver by NNM. (a) PAS staining for glycogen. Bar, 100 μm; (b) PK activity (enzyme histochemistry). Bar, 100 μm; (c) L-PK protein (immunoperoxidase). Bar, 100 μm.

HEPATOCELLULAR TUMORS

Of course correlative histochemistry can also be used for characterization of the endstages of hepatocarcinogenesis, the hepatocellular tumors and their metastases. However, as Rath[37] emphasized, histochemical patterns of liver tumors may be rather heterogeneous compared to the marked uniformity of their prestages. "Marker enzymes" for hepatocarcinogenesis such as γ-glutamyl transferase should be considered with some reservations for it can be demonstrated in NNM-induced rat liver lesions and tumors[30] whilst lacking in those of Nafenopin treated rats[38] and of DEN-treated mice[39]. In addition, only a minority of human hepatocellular neoplasms showed γGT-activity according to the findings of Cohen[40]. In contrast G6PDH is usually elevated in hepatocellular tumors[30].

QUANTITATIVE HISTOCHEMISTRY

Once the qualitative histochemical pattern of the different stages of hepatocarcinogenesis are established it is necessary to put these findings on a more quantitative basis. Relative quantitative data may be obtained by densitometric measurement of histochemical colorations e.g. PAS staining of glycogen, Feulgen reaction for DNA or evaluation of formazan produced during tetrazolium salt reduction catalyzed by enzymes such as dehydrogenases[41]. However, certain criteria must be satisfied such as preciseness, reproducibility and validity the latter being extensively discussed by Stoward[42]. In comparison to microanalysis these criteria are matched only partly and by a few reactions. This is because - among other reasons - of the difficulties to cut sections of reproducible thickness and to gain a valid relation between final reaction product (FRP) and absorption[42].

Microdissection and biochemical microanalysis on the other hand[43,44] do not only provide absolute quantitative data on activities and content of enzymes even in very small tissue samples such as focal liver lesions[35] but principally any other compound like DNA or RNA. Therefore, detection of possible interrelations between changes in metabolism with those of genetic material is greatly facilitated.

MOLECULAR BIOLOGY AND HISTOCHEMISTRY

Although the molecular mechanism underlying liver tumor development and associated metabolic changes is still unknown histochemistry can make important contribution to the answer of this basic question. With the help of the in situ hybridization technique genomic DNAs and/or mRNAs of important regulatory proteins such as key enzymes of metabolism can be identified[45,46] in early and late stages of hepatocarcinogenesis. By combining this method with immunocytochemistry (protein content) an enzyme histochemistry (enzyme activity) it is possible to show which cells of a hepatic lesion depict a change in activity of a special enzyme and how this is related to its content and the concentration of specific mRNA encoding for this protein.

In summary histochemical methods such as autoradiography, analytical histochemistry, enzymehistochemistry, immuncytochemistry, microdissection followed by by biochemical microanalysis may successfully be applied for studies on the course and mechanism of hepatocarcinogenesis. In contrast to conventional biochemistry the use of histochemistry led to a precise characterization of liver tumors and their precursors that have many features in common e.g. imbalance in carbohydrate metabolism. Transfer of the strategy of correlative histochemistry to other parts of cellular metabolism (proteins, nucleic acids) and use of hybrid thechniques between molecular biology and histochemistry such as in situ hybridisation will help to gain a deeper understanding of how normal liver undergoes neoplastic transformation.

References

1. B.D. Ross and W.G. Guder, Heterogeneity and compartmentation in the kidney, in: "Metabolic Compartmentation", H. Sies, ed., Academic Press, London, New York (1982)
2. K. Jungermann, Dynamics of zonal hepatocyte heterogeneity. Perinatal development and adaptive alterations during regeneration after partial hepatectomy, starvation and diabetes, Acta histochem. Suppl.-Band XXXII, S. 89-98 (1986)
3. R.T. Williams, Chemistry of detoxication, in: "Drugs and the Liver", W. Gerok and K. Sickinger, ed., F.K. Schattauer Verlag, Stuttgart, New York (1975)
4. J.R. Mitchell, D.J. Jollow, Role of metabolic activation in chemical carcinogensis and in drug-induced hepatic injury, in: "Drugs and the Liver", W. Gerok and K. Sickinger, eds., F.K. Schattauer Verlag, Stuttgart, New York (1975)
5. S.S. Hecht and R. Young, Metabolic hydroxylation of N-Nitrosomorpholine and 3,3,5,5-Tetradeutero-N-Nitrosomorpholine in the F344 rat, Cancer Res. 41: 5039-5043 (1981)
6. P. Bannasch and H.A. Müller, Lichtmikroskopische Untersuchungen über die Wirkung von N-Nitrosomorpholin auf die Leber von Ratte und Maus, Arzneimittel Forsch. 14: 805-814 (1964)
7. H. Druckrey, R. Preussmann, S. Ivankovic, D. Schmähl, Organotrope carcinogene Wirkungen bei 65 verschiedenen N-Nitrosoverbindungen an BD-Ratten, Z. Krebsforsch. 69: 103-201 (1967)
8. P. Bannasch, H.J. Hacker, H. Tsuda and H. Zerban, Aberrant regulation of carbohydrate metabolism and metamorphosis during renal carcinogenesis, Adv. Enzyme Reg. 25: 279-296 (1986)
9. B. Löfberg and H. Tjälve, Tissue specificity of N-Nitrosomorpholine metabolism in Sprague-Dawley rats, Fd. Chem. Toxic. 23: 647-654 (1985)
10. E.D. Farber and D.S.R. Sarma, Biology of Disease, Hepatocarcinogenesis. A dynamic cellular perspective, Lab. Invest. 56: 4-22 (1987)
11. J. Chayen, L. Bitensky, R.G. Butcher, "Practical Histochemistry", John Wiley & Sons, London, New York (1973)
12. R.W. Mowry, Contributions of practical carbohydrate histochemistry to the histopathological diagnosis of renal diseases, fungal infections, and some types of cancer, in: "Histochemistry", P.J. Stoward and J.M. Polak, ed., John Wiley & Sons, London, New York (1981)
13. A.G.E. Pearse, "Histochemistry", Vol. 2, Churchill Livingstone, Edinburgh, London, New York (1985)
14. R. Hotchkiss, A microchemical reaction resulting in the staining of polysaccharide structures in fixed tissue preparations, Arch. Biochem. 16: 131-141 (1948)
15. R. Roos, The "chessboard" distribution of glycogen in liver. Artifact of fixation or the effect of an enzyme, Histochem. J. 6: 511-521 (1974)
16. H.D. Fahimi, Perfusion and immersion fixation of rat liver with glutaraldehyde, Lab. Invest. 5: 736-750 (1967)
17. W. Umrath, Rapid freezing in open cooling baths, Arzneim. Forsch. 25: 450-451 (1975)

18. E.A. Newsholme, B. Crabtree, V.A. Zammit, Use of enzyme activities as indices of maximum rates of fuel utilization, in: "Trends in Enzyme Histochemistry and Cytochemistry", Ciba Foundation Symposium 73, Excerpta Medica, Amsterdam (1980)

19. H.G. Hers, the control of glycogen metabolism in the liver, Annu. Rev. Biochem. 45: 167-189 (1976)

20. R.C. Nordlie and K.A. Sukalski, Multiple forms of type I glycogen storage disease: underlying mechanisms, TIBS 11: 85-88 (1986)

21. G. Weber, Carbohydrate metabolism in cancer cells and the molecular correlation concept, Naturwiss. 55: 418-429 (1968)

22. H.J. Hacker, M.A. Moore, D. Mayer and P. Bannasch, Correlative histochemistry of some enzymes of carbohydrate metabolism in preneoplastic and neoplastic lesions in the rat liver, Carcinogenesis 3: 1265-1272 (1982)

23. U. Benner, H.J. Hacker and P. Bannasch, Electron microscopical demonstration of glucose-6-phosphatase in native cryostat sections fixed with glutaraldehyde through semipermeable membranes, Histochemistry 65: 41-47 (1979)

24. L.A. Lindberg, Lead and some other metals in the histochemical demonstration of liver glycogen phosphorylase activity, J. Histochem. Cytochem. 20: 331-335 (1972)

25. H.J. Hacker, Histochemical demonstration of glycogen phosphorylase (EC 2.4.1.1) through the use of semipermeable membranes, Histochemistry 58: 289-296 (1978)

26. A.E.F.H. Meijer and G.P. de Vries, Semipermeable membranes for improving the histochemical demonstration of enzyme activities in tissue sections. IV. Glucose-6-phosphate dehydrogenase and 6-phosphogluconate dehydrogenase (decarboxylating), Histochemistry 40: 349-359 (1974)

27. T.P. Pretlow, R.W. Grane, P.D. Goehring, A.S. Lapinsky and T.G. Pretlow, Examination of enzyme-altered foci with γ-glutamyl transpeptidase, aldehyde dehydrogenase, glucose-6-phosphate dehydrogenase, and other markers in metacrylate-embedded liver, Lab. Invest. 56: 96-100 (1987)

28. G. Seelmann-Eggebert, D. Mayer, D. Mecke and P. Bannasch, Expression and regulation of glycogen phosphorylase in preneoplastic and neoplastic hepatic lesions in rats, Virch. Arch. B 53: 44-51 (1987)

29. W.D. Kuhlmann, "Immuno Enzyme Techniques in Cytochemistry", Verlag Chemie, Weinheim (1984)

30. P. Bannasch, H.J. Hacker, F. Klimek and D. Mayer, Hepatocellular glycogenosis and related pattern of enzymatic changes during hepatocarcinogenesis, Adv. Enzyme Reg. 22: 97-121 (1984)

31. A.C. Nairn, J.A. Detre, J.E. Casnellie and P. Greengard, Serum antibodies that distinguish between the phospho- and dephospho-forms of a phosphoprotein, Nature 299: 734-736 (1982)

32. A.B. Frey, D.J. Waxman and G. Kreibich, The structure of Phenobarbital-inducible rat liver cytochrome P-450 isoenzyme PB-4, J. Biol. Chem. 260:15253-15265 (1985)

33. P. Bannasch, H.J. Hacker, F. Klimek and D. Mayer, Hepatocellular glycogenosis and related pattern of enzymatic changes during hepatocarcinogenesis, Adv. Enzyme Reg. 22: 97-121 (1984)

34. C.G. Hoar. G.W. Nicoll, E. Schiltz, W. Schmitt, D.P. Bloxham, M.F. Byford, B. Dunbar and L.A. Fothergill, Muscle and Liver pyruvate Kinases are closely related; amino acid sequence comparisons, Febs. Lett. 171:

35. P. Bannasch, U. Benner, H.J. Hacker. F. Klimek, D. Mayer, M. Moore and H. Zerban, Cytochemical and biochemical microanalysis of carcinogenesis, Histochem. J. 13: 799-820 (1981)

36. M. Reinacher. E. Eigenbrodt, U. Gerbracht, G. Zenk, I. Timmermann-Trosiener, P. Bentley, F. Waechter and R. Schulte-Hermann, Pyruvate kinase isoenzymes in altered foci and carcinoma of rat liver, Carcinogenesis 7: 227-240 (1981)
37. F.W. Rath, Enzymhistochemie maligner Tumoren - Bedeutung für Forschung und diagnostische Praxis, Z. Klin. Med. 41:1045-1048 (1986)
38. M.S. Rao and J.K. Reddy, Peroxysome proliferation and hepatocarcinogenesis, Carcinogenesis 8: 631 (1987)
39. S.D. Vesselinovitch, H.J. Hacker and P. Bannasch, Histochemical characterization of focal hepatic lesions induced by single diethylnitrosamine treatment in infant mice, Cancer Res. 45: 2774-2780 (1985)
40. M.B. Cohen, J.H. Beckstead, L.D. Ferrell and T.S.B. Yen, Enzyme histochemistry of hepatocellular neoplasms, Amer. J. Surg. Pathol. 10: 789-794 (1986)
41. R.G. Butcher and C.J.F. Van Noorden, Reaction rate studies glucose-6-phosphate dehydrogenase activity in sections of rat liver using 4 tetrazolium salts, Histochem. J. 17: 993 (1985)
42. P.J. Stoward, Criteria for validation of quantitative histochemical enzyme techniques, in: "Trends in enzyme histochemistry and cytochemistry", Excerpta medica, Amsterdam, Oxford, New York (1980)
43. D. Glick, Trends in quantification in histochemistry and cytochemistry, Histochem. J. 13: 227-240 (1981)
44. D. Glick, Fifty years with histochemistry and cytochemistry, J. Histochem. Cytochem. 33: 720-728 (1985)
45. J.I. Morrell, Symposium on in situ hybridization with nucleotide probes: a histochemical tool, J. Histochem. Cytochem. 34: 25-26 (1986)
46. J.P. Coghlan, P. Aldred, J. Haralambidis, H.D. Niall. J.D. Penschow and G.W. Tregear, Hybridization Histochemistry, Anal. Biochem. 149: 1-28 (1985)

CELL PROLIFERATION, CELL DEATH AND LIVER CARCINOGENESIS

CELL PROLIFERATION AND HEPATOCARCINOGENESIS

Hartmut M. Rabes

Institute of Pathology
University of Munich
Munich, F.R.Germany

Carcinogenesis is intrinsically coupled with cell proliferation. Proliferation in excess characterizes a manifest malignant tumor, proliferation plays an important role during the latency period until the neoplastic phenotype emerges, and proliferation is essential during the initiation of transformation. This is apparently true for the development of all kinds of malignant tumors, induced by physical, chemical or viral factors, and applies also to hepatocarcinogenesis. This contribution is aimed at dissecting some critical phases of the carcinogenic process in the liver with respect to cell proliferation.

The adult liver is a stable organ. Under normal conditions it contains only about 1 ^{o}/oo hepatocytes in the cell cycle. The others remain in the G_o phase, are functionally active, but do not proliferate. It is only after cell loss induced by hepatotoxins, infections, wounding or resection of part of the organ that the liver cells are triggered from G_o into the cell cycle (Rabes 1978).

A single small dose of a potential hepatocarcinogenic chemical fails, in normal adult rat liver, to induce a liver tumor. However, if the dose is increased up to an acute toxic level, induction of a hepatoma may occur. The explanation would either be that the genotoxic effect of this dose of a carcinogen is large enough to initiate transformation, or that the carcinogen acts not only specifically as a transforming agent, but also as an indirect stimulus for proliferation because of the high cell loss in the liver after such exposure (Rabes 1979; Ying et al. 1981). An analysis of the role of proliferation during initiation becomes possible using regenerating liver as a model. The first attempts to correlate initiation probability with the proliferative response after partial hepatectomy date back to the early fifties when Glinos et al. (1951) described that a single dose of 4-dimethylaminoazobenzene induced liver tumors in rats when given in combination with partial hepatectomy. In the mean-time many reports were published confirming the increased transformation sensitivity of proliferating adult hepatocytes in rats and mice for a variety of carcinogens (Laws 1959; Hollander and Bentvelzen 1968; Marquardt et al. 1970; Chernozemski and Warwick 1970; Craddock 1971, 1973; Craddock and Frei 1974; Fridman-Manduzio et al. 1977; Pound and McGuire 1978, Cayama et al. 1978).

On the basis of these findings models of rat liver carcinogenesis
were developed which combined the application of a single dose of a
carcinogen with partial hepatectomy, for example diethylnitrosamine and
partial hepatectomy as proposed by Scherer et al. (1972), followed by
phenobarbital as a promotor as shown by Pitot et al. (1978), or, widely
used, the Solt-Farber model (1976) which combines a high dose of diethylnitrosamine, 2-acetylaminofluorene and partial hepatectomy.

All these attempts follow the same principle. It is acknowledged that
a combination of partial hepatectomy or intoxication, for instance with
carbon tetrachloride (Tsuda and Farber 1980; de Gerlache et al. 1982),
with a hepatocarcinogen effectively induces liver tumors and the sequence
of events during the preneoplastic latency period could be analyzed
further in these models with a defined starting point of the process.

If cell proliferation proves to be essential for the initiation of
liver carcinogenesis (Cayama et al. 1978, Rabes 1979, Columbano et al.
1981) the question arises how the increased transformation sensitivity is
brought about. There are a few kinetic studies on the time-relation
between carcinogen exposure, partial hepatectomy and tumorigenic effect.
Craddock and Frei (1974) injected a single dose of N-methyl-N-nitrosourea
(MNU) at 6, 24 or 31 hr after partial hepatectomy and observed the highest
frequency of liver cell adenomas at 24 hr. With 1,2 dimethylhydrazine
injection and partial hepatectomy 12, 24, 48 or 168 hr later the highest
incidence of preneoplastic lesions was observed after partial hepatectomy
at 12 hr. (Ying et al. 1982), while diethylnitrosamine induced most foci
when followed by partial hepatectomy 4 hr later (Ishikawa et al. 1980).

When trying to interprete these results, one has to bear in mind that
the cell kinetics of hepatocytes after partial hepatectomy follow a
peculiar time course. The post-operative G_1 period of the cell cycle
differs in length between 15 and 40 hr depending on the intralobular
localization of hepatocytes (Rabes and Tuczek 1970, Rabes et al. 1976).
It is not easily possible in such system to relate the increased transformation sensitivity to a specific cell cycle period. Kaufmann et al. (1981)
and our group tried therefore to synchronize the liver cell cycle in vivo
in order to be able to pinpoint down the cell cycle periods with the
highest transformation sensitivity. Kaufmann used injections of hydrocortisone to obtain a better synchronization of the S phase of hepatocytes
in regenerating rat liver and found that injection of MNU in S phase
yielded the highest number of hepatic tumors. He repeated these experiments recently with methyl(acetoxymethyl)nitrosamine and came to the same
conclusion (Kaufmann et al. 1987).

We were able to synchronize the start of DNA synthesis by a temporary
inhibition of the G_1-S traverse by means of a continuous infusion of
hydroxyurea (Rabes et al. 1977, 1986). In this system, a single dose of
MNU injected in early or late G_1, at different parts of the S phase or at
G_2M produced the highest number of ATPase-deficient putative preneoplastic
foci after exposure in early S phase, with a rapid decline of transformation sensitivity in the middle or late S phase (Rabes et al. 1986).

Maximum transformation sensitivity in early S phase can further be
substantiated in a non-synchronized regenerating liver system without the
use of hydrocortisone or hydroxyurea where the G_1- S transit rate is
exactly determined at 2 hr intervals after partial hepatectomy. Injection
of MNU at a single dose of 25 mg/kg at these time intervals with a
defined G_1-S transit rate reveals that the transformation probability
runs parallel with the influx rate of hepatocytes into the early S phase
(Maguire and Rabes 1987).

Preferential target cell for liver carcinogenesis is according to these findings a proliferating hepatocyte in early S phase. What is peculiar about this cell cycle phase? Determination of the DNA adduct formation during different phases of the liver cell cycle in hydroxyurea-synchronized regenerating rat liver did not disclose a higher binding of alkylating N-nitroso-compounds during the critical early S phase which could explain the increased transformation (Rabes et al. 1979). However, when the promutagenic DNA lesion O^6-methylguanine (Loveless 1969) was quantified in S phase of regenerating rat liver, a surprizing result was obtained. 2 hr after ^{14}C-dimethyl-nitrosamine injection the radiochromatograms showed substantially less O^6-methylguanine in replicating DNA than during G_1. The ratio O^6-methylguanine/7-methylguanine which corrects for dilution of adducts during DNA replication, was significantly lower in S phase cells than in G_1 cells (Rabes et al. 1984). Further experiments revealed that the promutagenic O^6-methylguanine is repaired more readily during the S phase as compared with G_1.

The enzyme responsible for this reaction, the O^6-methylguanine DNA transferase (Lindahl 1982; Pegg et al. 1983) shows a peak in early S phase after hydroxyurea-synchronization (Schuster et al. 1985). It might be concluded that rat liver potentiates this kind of DNA repair during the critical transformation sensitive phase of the cell cycle, thus providing a means to eliminate small amounts of O^6-methylguanine. However, this repair enzyme is rapidly exhausted during the reaction and does not protect the liver cell after exposure with higher doses of alkylating carcinogens.

It has to be noted that a similar cell cycle related increase of the O^6-methylguanine DNA transferase has not been observed in mouse, gerbil and hamster liver where this enzyme is constitutively expressed at a low level (Saffhill et al. 1985). Human liver shows a high constitutive O^6-methyltransferase activity (Pegg et al. 1982); cell cycle fluctuations have not been reported for human liver.

It is conceivable that unrepaired promutagenic DNA lesions after carcinogen exposure might permanently be fixed in the genome when DNA replication occurs. Miscoding of O^6-methylguanine has been demonstrated by Abbott and Saffhill (1979) using synthetic methylated poly(dC-dG) templates. DNA base mispairing is likely to occur also in vivo during DNA replication. It is known that a preferential site of mutagenesis is the replication point of DNA (Cerda-Olmedo et al. 1968). It is tempting to speculate about the possibility that transformation sensitivity of early S phase might be based on replication and preferred mutation of transformation-related genes during this part of DNA synthesis. In fact, recently it was shown that several proto-oncogenes are indeed early S phase replicating genes (Iqbal et al. 1987). Since these genes are intimately involved in regulation of cell proliferation and differentiation, a point mutation in these genes or in their regulatory sequences might represent the first permanent initiation event of carcinogenesis (Tabin et al. 1982; Reddy et al. 1982). Malignant activation of the Ha-ras proto-oncogene in experimental mammary carcinomas by a specific G-A transition mutation after MNU exposure has been described (Zarbl et al. 1985). This could exactely be the final result of an O^6-alkylguanine-induced G-A base mispairing. Similar mutations of proto-oncogenes are also discussed for hepatocarcinogenesis, but not yet proven.

Other possibilities of genetic cellular changes during early S phase exposure to a carcinogen might be related to the fact that carcinogen exposure may lead to a temporary stop of DNA replication and thus could induce amplification of DNA segments as shown for 2-acetylaminofluorene (Tlsty et al. 1984) by a process similar to the amplification of the dihydrofolate reductase gene by methotrexate treatment (Schimke 1984). The consequences of an amplification of an oncogene in liver carcinogenesis will be discussed later.

Another permanent change of a hepatocyte exposed in early S phase to a carcinogen could be based on a disturbance of the physiological methylation pattern (Riggs and Jones 1983) which could lead to hereditary alterations of the transcriptive activity in the progeny.

The second part of this review shall focus on proliferation of enzyme-aberrant hepatocellular foci which are induced in the liver by carcinogen treatment in a dose-dependent pattern (Bannasch and Müller 1964, Gössner and Friedrich-Freksa 1964, Kunz et al. 1978). A fraction of these subpopulations appears to progress into hepatomas (Kaufmann et al. 1985) depending on the mode of treatment of the animals during the preneoplastic latency period. It is assumed that these cells represent the progeny of cells which have been initiated by the carcinogen treatment. This would imply that these cells are endowed, in contrast to the normal resting adult hepatocyte, during initiation with a potential for proliferation. If this proliferative advantage over normal hepatocytes is an essential consequence of initiation, one would suggest that these putative preneoplastic foci at least in some cases are the progeny of a single initiated cell, that is, that they represent clonal growths. We feel that the decision whether the foci are clonal or multicellular in origin represents a crucial question in the evaluation of their biological role.

The use of phosphoglycerate kinase mosaic mice helped to solve this question. A mouse strain became available with a mutation of the X-chromosomal gene for phosphoglycerate kinase (Nielsen and Chapman 1977). Mating of a male mouse bearing the mutant PGK-1A with a female of wild-type PGK-1B generated a female offspring of mice the cells of which contain both, the paternal mutant and the maternal wild-type X-chromosome. Because of early embryonic random inactivation of one of the two X-chromosomes (Lyon 1974) the adult female mouse consists of a mosaic of cells expressing either the paternal mutant PGK or the maternal wild-type one. Both enzyme allotypes can be separated in electropherograms. Bücher et al. (1980) developed a microelectrophoretic method of separating the enzyme from very small tissue samples. This method was used for the evaluation of samples from normal tissue and from ATPase-deficient foci in mice treated with 2-acetylaminofluorene (Rabes et al. 1982). Even smallest samples from normal liver tissue contained always both allozymes in the microelectropherograms. However, almost all samples punched out from putative preneoplastic foci contained exclusively either the wild-type PGK-1B or only the mutant PGK-1A. This is a strong argument in favour of the hypothesis, that enzyme-aberrant altered hepatic foci originate by clonal growth of a single initiated cell (Rabes et al. 1982).

In the mean-time this observation has been confirmed with histochemical methods using the X-linked enzyme ornithine carbamoyl transferase as a marker in diethylnitrosamine-treated female mice heterozygous for the sparse-fur strain (Howell et al. 1985).

Taking the single cell origin of preneoplastic foci for granted one has to assume an aberrant proliferative behaviour of these subpopulations of initiated cells and their progeny when comparing them with normal adult hepatocytes. There are striking proliferative differences depending on the treatment of the animals during the preneoplastic latency period.

If the carcinogen, as for instance diethylnitrosamine, is administered continuously in the drinking water, proliferation is high and increases with age and number of cells in the foci. Tritiated thymidine labeling indices increase, the duration of DNA synthesis is shortened and the calculated potential population doubling time decreases at late stages of the preneoplastic foci. Finally occuring hepatomas show a very rapid cell cycle time (Rabes 1969; Rabes and Szymkowiak 1979).

A similar effect on the proliferation in preneoplastic foci is observed when rats are exposed, after initiation with a carcinogen, to a promotor of liver carcinogenesis, as for instance phenobarbital. Under conditions of continuous phenobarbital-feeding the tritiated thymidine labeling index in preneoplastic foci is significantly higher than in the surrounding phenotypically normal liver tissue (Schulte-Hermann et al. 1981, Barbason et al. 1983).

A less active proliferation during the preneoplastic latency period is observed when the carcinogen is administered only for a limited period of time with no further treatment following (Barbason and Betz 1981). However, because of the significant augmentation of the size of preneoplastic foci as a function of time (Barbason and Betz 1981, Scherer 1984) an intrinsic growth advantage of these subpopulations even under non-stimulatory conditions is evident, provided clonal origin is accepted (Scherer and Hoffmann 1971, Rabes et al. 1982).

Do preneoplastic foci respond to normal regulatory factors of liver growth? At early stages they react on a stimulus for growth in a similar pattern as do normal hepatocytes. Continuous infusion of tritiated thymidine after partial hepatectomy results in these foci in approximately the same high growth fraction (Rabes et al. 1970; Rabes and Szymkowiak 1975) and mitotic activity (Barbason et al. 1983) as observed in the phenotypically normal parenchyma. However, with prolonged feeding of a carcinogen, the regenerative response decreases in parallel to the higher intrinsic growth potential (Rabes et al. 1970). It is remarkable that the circadian rhythm of proliferation vanishes at this time period indicating a disturbance of the normal homeostatic control (Barbason et al. 1983).

It has to be pointed out that at early stages preneoplastic foci consist of a homogeneous clonal population of phenotypically altered cells with a limited growth advantage over normal hepatocytes. An argument for early homogeneity comes from DNA measurements in these foci (Sarafoff et al. 1986). Small foci show in DNA cytometry either a selective presence of diploid or a homogeneous population of tetraploid hepatocytes, the diploid foci forming the majority. However, when larger foci were measured, a heterogeneous DNA pattern of hepatocellular nuclei was observed which consisted of a mixture of di- and tetraploid cells and other cells with a DNA content in between, which represent aneuploid and DNA synthetizing cells (Sarafoff et al. 1986). Autoradiographic evaluation at the cytological level confirms these observations. At early stages homogeneous clear glycogen-storing hepatocytes show a rather low tritiated thymidine labeling index. With progression of these foci, a heterogeneous intermediate stage with proliferating acidophilic and basophilic cells occurs followed by the period of more rapidly growing basophilic cells finally ending up in hepatomas with the highest labeling index (Zerban et al. 1985).

Determination of the cell kinetics at early and late stages of the preneoplastic latency period reveals an increasing frequency of cells with a shortened cell cycle. At 20 days of a continuous feeding of diethylnitrosamine the majority of hepatocytes shows a cell cycle time of more than 40 hr, in contrast to cells at the boundary period between preneoplasia and tumor manifestation with a preferential cell cycle time of about 20 hr (Rabes and Szymkowiak 1979).

A special situation is found when the cell cycle kinetic of nodules induced with the Solt-Farber (1976) procedure is determined. Cells of these nodules showed during 2-acetylaminofluorene exposure after partial hepatectomy a somewhat longer cell cycle time than normal hepatocytes after partial hepatectomy (Rotstein et al. 1984). The biological significance of these finding remains open.

Cell proliferation during the preneoplastic latency period is different from normal. Initiated cells appear to be partially released from the strict growth restraints of a normal hepatocyte. They are clonogenic and endowed with an elevated intrinsic growth potential. Nevertheless, preneoplastic cells respond quite readily to superimposed growth regulatory influences. With increasing endogeneous proliferative activity this responsiveness to growth regulation appears to be diminished, the cells seem to escape from the homeostatic circuits of the organ.

Aberrations from normal proliferative behaviour are small at first, but appear to rise in parallel with an increasing heterogeneity of preneoplastic foci. Nowell (1976) coined the term of genetic instability of tumor cells. One would tend to apply this hypothesis also to preneoplastic liver cells. They do not appear to be stable. They may revert into phenotypically normal cells (Tatematsu et al. 1983), but also subpopulations may develop with a higher rate of independence from homeostatic control. A good example comes from preneoplastic liver cells in vitro. After initiation in vivo by means of a continuous exposure to diethylnitrosamine for about 50 days liver cells can be kept in vitro (Rabes et al. 1972). From the initial mixture of normal and enzyme-aberrant putative preneoplastic cells normal adult hepatocytes are lost from the culture after about 3 weeks. The remaining cells form, sometimes after a long latency period, foci each of which can then be selectively harvested and separately subcultured (Kerler and Rabes 1986). The cell lines obtained from these populations differ in chromosome number and growth rate (Kerler and Rabes, manuscript in preparation). A few lines reach the final state of tumorigenicity proven by transplantation into nude mice. A cytogenetic evaluation discloses in one of these lines striking aberrations from the normal karyotype (Holecek et al. 1986) coupled with an extremely high rate of proliferation (Kerler and Rabes, manuscript in preparation).

The availability of such cell lines gives the opportunity to investigate the presence and activity of proto-oncogenes which are assumed to be involved in regulating the proliferative state of cells. Goyette et al. (1984) as well as Makino et al. (1984) showed that induction of cell proliferation in normal liver after partial hepatectomy goes along with a rapid increase of the transcriptive acitivity of the proto-oncogene c-myc with a maximum during the middle of G_1. c-Ha-ras transcription follows and reaches a peak when the majority of hepatocytes is in DNA synthesis. In Northern blots of RNA obtained from regenerating rat liver at different intervals after partial hepatectomy this pattern was confirmed in our laboratory. When RNA blots from liver tumors induced by MNU or from tumorigenic hepatocellular lines propagated in vitro were hybridized with radioactive probes, an elevation of transcriptive activity of c-Ha-ras as well as c-myc was observed which exceeded in some tumors the values determined in regenerating rat liver. This is in agreement with reports published recently (Makino et al. 1984; Cote et al. 1985; Zhang et al. 1987). In contrast to regenerating rat liver this increase of transcriptive activity of c-Ha-ras and of c-myc may be based on or combined with amplification of the number of genomic copies of these genes. In the tumorigenic cell line with the most rapid mode of cell proliferation c-Ha-ras was found to be amplified about 2.5fold and c-myc about 14fold. In addition, the Southern blots of c-myc after DNA treatment with the restriction enzymes Eco RI or Hind III disclose that this gene is not only amplified, but rearranged in the genome (Suchy et al. 1987). Southern blots hybridized with various parts of the three exons of c-myc indicate that c-myc is rearranged as a complete gene in this tumorigenic cell line. This suggests that the product of this rearranged and amplified gene might contain the same information for sustained cell proliferation as its counterpart in normal cells. However, the strict cell cycle dependent expression of c-myc as seen in normal proliferating hepatocytes in regenerating rat liver appears likely to be suspended under these conditions of gene amplification, and this could result in a constitutively increased, cell cycle independent overexpression of c-myc with the consequences of retaining cells permanently in the cycle. It was recently observed that normal cell lines lost their cell cycle-dependent fluctuations in the expression of c-myc and c-Ha-ras when transformed by a chemical carcinogen (Kelly et al. 1983). Similar processes might be operative in liver carcinogenesis.

Liver carcinogenesis appears to be a stepwise process with probably repetitive clonal selections of subpopulations and an increasing tendency for progession into malignancy. The main risk factor for progression may reside in an inherent genetic or epigenetic instability. Each round of replication might then include a new risk for the realization of malignant properties.

ACKNOWLEDGMENTS

The author is grateful to Deutsche Forschungsgemeinschaft and to Dr. Mildred Scheel-Stiftung für Krebsforschung for generous support.

REFERENCES

Abbott, P. J. and Saffhill, R., 1979, DNA synthesis with methylated poly (dC-dG) templates: evidence for a competitive nature to miscoding by 0^6-methylguanine.
Biochim. Biophys. Acta, 562:51-61

Bannasch, P. and Müller, H. A., 1964, Lichtmikroskopische Untersuchungen über die Wirkung von N-Nitrosomorpholin auf die Leber von Ratte und Maus.
Arzneimittelforsch., 14:805-814

Barbason, H. and Betz, E. H., 1981, Proliferation of preneoplastic lesions after discontinuation of chronic DEN feeding in the development of hepatomas in rat.
Br. J. Cancer, 44:561-566

Barbason, H., Rassenfosse, C. and Betz, E. H., 1983, Promotion mechanism of phenobarbital and partial hepatectomy in DENA hepatocarcinogenesis cell kinetics effect.
Br. J. Cancer, 47:517-525

Bücher, Th., Bender, W., Fundele, R., Hofner, H. and Linke, I., 1980, Quantitative evaluations of electrophoretic allo- and isozyme patterns.
FEBS Lett., 115:319-324

Cayama, E., Tsuda, H., Sarma, D. S. R., and Farber, E., 1978, Initiation of chemical carcinogenesis requires cell proliferation.
Nature (Lond.), 275:60-62

Cerda-Olmedo, E., Hanawalt, P. C., and Guerola, N., 1968, Mutagenesis of the replication point by nitrosoguanidine: map and pattern of replication of the Escherichia coli chromosome.
J. Mol. Biol., 33:705-719

Chernozemski, N. and Warwick, G. P., 1970, Liver regeneration and induction of hepatomas in BGAF[1] mice by urethan.
Cancer Res., 30:2685-2690

Columbano, A., Rajalakshmi, S., and Sarma, D. S. R., 1981, Requirement of

cell proliferation for the initiation of liver carcinogenesis as assayed by three different procedures.
Cancer Res., 41:2079-2083

Cote, G. J., Lastra, B. A., Cook, J. R., Huang, D. P. and Chiu, J. F., 1985, Oncogene expression in rat hepatomas and during hepatocarcinogenesis.
Cancer Lett., 26:121-127

Craddock, V. M., 1971, Liver carcinomas induced in rats by single administration of dimethylnitrosamine after partial hepatectomy.
J. Nat. Cancer Inst., 47:899-907

Craddock, V. M., 1973, Induction of liver tumors in rats by a single treatment with nitroso compounds given after partial hepatectomy.
Nature, 245:386-388

Craddock, V. M., and Frei, J. V., 1974, Induction of liver cell adenomata in the rat by a single treatment with N-methyl-N-nitrosourea given at various times after partial hepatectomy.
Br. J. Cancer, 30:503-511

Fridman-Manduzio, A., Gol-Winkler, R., and Goutier, R.,1977, Tumor frequency and characteristics after a single dose of dimethylnitrosamine or diethylnitrosamine in partially hepatectomized rats.
Z. Krebsforsch., 90:13-24

deGerlache, J., Lans, M., Taper, H., Préat, V. and Roberfroid, M., 1982, Promotion of the chemically initiated hepatocarcinogenesis. in: "Mutagens in our environment", p. 35-46
M. Sorsa, H. Vaina (eds), Liss, New York

Glinos, A. D., Bucher, N. L. R., and Aub, J. C., 1951, The effect of liver regeneration on tumor formation in rats fed 4-dimethylaminoazobenzene.
J. Exp. Med., 93:313-324

Gössner, W., Friedrich-Freksa H., 1964, Histochemische Untersuchungen über die Glucose-6-Phosphatase in der Rattenleber während der Cancerisierung durch Nitrosamine.
Z. Naturforsch., 19b:862-864

Goyette, M., Petropoulos, C. J., Shank, P. R., and Fausto, N., 1984, Regulated transcription of c-Ki-ras and c-myc during compensatory growth of rat liver.
Mol. Cell. Biol., 4:1493-1498

Holecek, B., and Rabes, H. M., 1986, Cytogenetic analysis of normal and diethylnitrosamine-initiated preneoplastic hepatocytes.
J. Cancer Res. Clin. Oncol., 111 (Suppl.): S95

Hollander, C. F., and Bentvelzen, P., 1968, Enhancement of urethan induction of hepatomas in mice by prior partial hepatectomy.
J. Nat. Cancer Inst., 41:1303-1306

Howell, S., Wareham, K. A., Williams, E. D., 1985, Clonal origin of mouse liver cell tumors.
Am. J. Pathol., 121:426-432

Iqbal, M. A., Chinsky, J., Didamo, V. and Schildkraut, C. L., 1987, Replication of proto-oncogenes early during the S phase in mammalian cell lines.
Nucl. Acids Res., 15:87-103

Ishikawa, T., Takayama, S., and Kitagawa, T., 1980, Correlation between time of partial hepatectomy after a single treatment with diethylnitrosamine and induction of adenosine triphosphatase-deficient islands in rat liver.
Cancer Res., 40:4261-4264

Kaufmann, W. K., Kaufman, D. G., Rice, J. M., and Wenk, M. L., 1981, Reversible inhibition of rat hepatocyte proliferation by hydrocortisone and its effect on cell cycle-dependent hepatocarcinogenesis by N-methyl-N-nitrosourea.
Cancer Res., 41:4653-4660

Kaufmann, W. K., Mackenzie, S. A., Kaufman, D. G., 1985, Quantitative

    relationship between hepatocytic neoplasms and islands of cellular
    alteration during hepatocarcinogenesis in male F344 rat.
    Am. J. Pathol., 119:171-174

Kaufmann, W. K., Rice, J. M., Wenk, M. L., Devor, D., and Kaufman, D. G.,
    1987, Cell cycle-dependent initiation of hepatocarcinogenesis in
    rats by methyl(acetoxymethyl)nitrosamine.
    Cancer Res., 47:1263-1266

Kelly, K., Chochran, B. H., Stiles, C. D., and Leder, Ph., 1983, Cell-
    specific regulation of the c-myc gene by lymphocyte mitogens and
    platelet-derived growth factor.
    Cell, 35:603-610

Kerler, R., and Rabes, H. M., 1986, In vitro propagation of preneoplastic
    hepatocytes initiated in vivo by diethylnitrosamine.
    J. Cancer Res. Clin. Oncol., 111 (Suppl.): S46

Kunz, W., Appel, K. E., Rickart, R., Schwarz, M., Stöckle, G., 1978,
    Enhancement and inhibition of carcinogenic effectiveness of
    nitrosamines. In: "Primary liver tumors",
    H. Remmer, H.M. Bolt, P. Bannasch and H. Popper, eds., p.261-283
    MTP Press, Lancaster

Laws, J. O., 1959, Tissue regeneration and tumor development.
    Br. J. Cancer, 13:669-674

Lindahl, T., 1982, DNA repair enzymes.
    Annu. Rev. Biochem., 51:61-87

Loveless, A., 1969, Possible relevance of 0^6-alkylation of deoxyguanosine
    to the mutagenicity and carcinogenicity of nitrosamines and
    nitrosamides.
    Nature, 233:206-207

Lyon, M. F., 1974, Mechanisms and evolutionary origins of variable
    X chromosome activity in mammals.
    Proc. R. Soc. Lond. B, 187:243-268

Maguire, S., and Rabes, H. M., 1987, Transformation sensitivity in early
    S phase and clonogenic potential are target cell characteristics
    in liver carcinogenesis by N-methyl-N-nitrosourea.
    Int. J. Cancer, 39:385-389

Makino, R., Hayashi, K., and Sugimura, T., 1984, c-myc transcript is
    induced in rat liver at a very early stage of regeneration or by
    cycloheximide treatment.
    Nature, 310:697-698

Makino, R., Hayashi, K., Sato, S., and Sugimura T., 1984, Expressions of
    the c-Ha-ras and c-myc genes in rat liver tumors.
    Biochem. Biophys. Res. Comm., 119:1096-1102

Marquardt, H., Sternberg, S. S., and Philips, F. S., 1970, 7,12-dimethyl-
    benz(a)anthracene and hepatic neoplasia in regenerating rat liver.
    Chem.-Biol. Interactions, 2:401-043

Nielsen, J. T., and Chapman, V. M., 1977, Electrophoretic variation for
    sex-linked phosphoglycerate kinase (PGK-1) in the mouse.
    Genetics, 87:319-325

Nowell, P. C., 1976, The clonal evolution of tumour cell populations.
    Science, 194:23-28

Pegg, A. E., Roberfroid, M., Bahr, C., Foote, R. S., Mitra, S., Bresil
    H., Likhachev, A., Montesano, R., 1982, Removal of 0^6-methylgua-
    nine from DNA by human liver fractions.
    Proc. Natl. Acad. Sci.(US), 79:5162-5165

Pegg, A. E., Wiest, L, Foote, R. S., Mitra, S., Perry, W., 1983, Purifi-
    cation and properties of 0^6-methylguanine-DNA transmethylase from
    rat liver.
    J. Biol. Chem., 258:2327-2333

Pitot, H. C., Barsness, L., Goldsworthy, F., Kitagawa, T., 1978, Bioche-
    mical characterisation of stages of hepatocarcinogenesis after a
    single dose of diethylnitrosamine.
    Nature, 271:456-458

Pound, A. W., and McGuire, L. J., 1978, Repeated partial hepatectomy as a promoting stimulus for carcinogenic response of liver to nitrosamines in rats.
Br. J. Cancer, 37:585-594

Rabes, H., 1969, Bestimmung der Zellzyklusphasen in heterogenen Tumorzellpopulationen.
Z. Naturforsch., 24b:468

Rabes, H., Hartenstein, R., and Scholze, P., 1970, Specific stages of cellular response to homeostatic control during diethylnitrosamine-induced liver carcinogenesis.
Experientia, 26:1356-1359

Rabes, H., and Tuczek, H.-C., 1970, Quantitative autoradiographische Untersuchung zur Heterogenität der Leberzellproliferation nach partieller Hepatektomie.
Virchows Arch., Abt. B Zellpath., 6:302-312

Rabes, H. M., Scholze, P., and Jantsch, B., 1972, Growth kinetics of diethylnitrosamine-induced, enzyme-deficient "preneoplastic" liver cell populations in vivo and in vitro.
Cancer Res., 32:2577-2586

Rabes, H. M., Wirsching, R., Tuczek, H.-V., and Iseler, G., 1976, Analysis of cell cycle compartments of hepatocytes after partial hepatectomy.
Cell Tissue Kinet., 9:517-532

Rabes, H. M., Iseler, G., Czichos, S., and Tuczek, H.-V., 1977, Synchronization of hepatocellular DNA synthesis in regenerating rat liver by continuous infusion of hydroxyurea.
Cancer Res., 37:1105-1111

Rabes, H. M., 1978, Kinetics of hepatocellular proliferation as a function of the microvascular structure and functional state of the liver. in:"Ciba Foundation Symposium 55 (new series): Hepatotrophic Factors", p.31-59.
Elsevier-Excerpta Medica-North Holland, Amsterdam-Oxford-New York

Rabes, H. M., 1979, Proliferative Vorgänge während der Frühstadien der malignen Transformation.
Verh. Dtsch. Ges. Path., 63:18-39

Rabes, H. M., Kerler, R., Wilhelm, R., Rode, G., and Riess, H., 1979, Alkylation of DNA and RNA by ^{14}C-dimethylnitrosamine in hydroxyurea-synchronized regenerating rat liver.
Cancer Res., 39:4228-4236

Rabes, H. M., and Szymkowiak, R., 1979, Cell kinetics of hepatocytes during the preneoplastic period of diethylnitrosamine-induced liver carcinogenesis.
Cancer Res., 39:1298-1304

Rabes, H. M., Bücher, Th., Hartmann, A., Linke, I., and Dünnwald, H., 1982, Clonal growth of carcinogen-induced enzyme-deficient preneoplastic cell populations in mouse liver.
Cancer Res., 42:3220-3227

Rabes, H. M., Kerler, R., Rode, G., Schuster, Ch., and Wilhelm, R., 1984, O^6-methylguanine repair in liver cells in vivo: Comparison between G_1- and S-phase of the cell cycle.
J. Cancer Res. Clin. Oncol., 108:36-45

Rabes, H. M., Müller, L., Hartmann, A., Kerler, R., and Schuster, Ch., 1986, Cell cycle-dependent initiation of ATPase-deficient populations in adult rat liver by a single dose of N-methyl-N-nitrosourea.
Cancer Res., 46:645-650

Reddy, E. P., Reynolds, R. K., Santos, E., Barbacid, M., 1982, A point mutation is responsible for the acquisition of transforming properties by the T24 human bladder carcinoma oncogene.
Nature, Lond., 300:149-152

Riggs, A. D., Jones, P. A., 1983, 5-Methylcytosine, gene regulation and cancer. Adv. Cancer Res., 40:1-30

Rotstein, J., MacDonald, P. D. M., Rabes, H. M., and Farber, E., 1984, Cell cycle kinetics of hepatocytes in early putative preneoplastic lesions in hepatocarcinogenesis.
Cancer Res., 44:2913-2917

Saffhill, R., Margison, G. P., O'Connor, P. J., 1985, Mechanisms of carcinogenesis by alkylating agents.
Biochim. Biophys. Acta, 823:111-145

Sarafoff, M., Rabes, H. M., and Dörmer, P., 1986, Correlations between ploidy and initiation probability determined by DNA cytophotometry in individual altered hepatic foci.
Carcinogenesis, 7:1191-1196

Scherer, E., Hoffmann, M., 1971, Probable clonal genesis of cellular islands induced in rat liver by diethylnitrosamine.
Eur. J. Cancer, 7:369-371

Scherer, E., Hoffmann, M., Emmelot, P., Friedrich-Freska, H., 1972, Quantitative study on foci of altered liver cells induced in the rat by a single dose of diethylnitrosamine and partial hepatectomy.
J. Natl. Cancer Inst., 49:93-106

Scherer, E., 1984, Neoplastic progression in experimental hepatocarcinogenesis.
Biochim. Biophys. Acta, 738:219-236

Schimke, R. T., 1984, Gene amplification, drug resistance, and cancer.
Cancer Res., 44:1735-1742

Schulte-Hermann, R., Ohde, G., Schuppler, J., Timmermann-Trosiener, J., 1981, Enhanced proliferation of putative preneoplastic cells in rat liver following treatment with the tumor promoters phenobarbital, hexachlorocyclohexane, steroid compounds, and nafenopin.
Cancer Res., 41:2556-2562

Schuster, Ch., Rode, G., and Rabes, H. M., 1985, O^6-methylguanine repair of methylated DNA in vitro: Cell cycle-dependent action of rat liver methyltransferase.
J. Cancer Res. Clin. Oncol., 110:98-102

Solt, D., Farber, E., 1976, New principle for the analysis of chemical carcinogenesis.
Nature, 263:702-703

Suchy, B., Sarafoff, M., Kerler, R., and Rabes, H. M., Amplification and enhanced expression of c-myc in chemically induced liver tumors in vivo and in vitro.
Bioengineering, in press

Tabin, C. J., Bradley, S. M., Bargmann, C. I., Weinberg, R. A., Papageorge, A. G., Scolnik, E. M., Dhar, R., Lowy, D. R., Chang, E. H., 1982, Mechanism of activation of a human oncogene.
Nature, Lond., 300:143-149

Tatematsu, M., Nagamine, Y., and Farber, E., 1983, Redifferentiation as a basis for remodeling of carcinogen-induced hepatocyte nodules to normal-appearing liver.
Cancer Res., 43:5049-5058

Tlsty, T. D., Brown, P. C., Schimke, R. T., 1984, UV radiation facilitates methotrexate resistance and amplification of the dihydrofolate reductase gene in cultured 3T6 mouse cells.
Mol. cell. Biol., 4:1050-1056

Tsuda, H., Lee, G., Farber, E., 1980, Induction of resistant hepatocytes as a new principle for a possible short term in vivo test for carcinogenes.
Cancer Res., 40:1157-1164

Ying, T. S., Sarma, D. S. R., and Farber, E., 1981, Role of acute hepatic necrosis in the induction of early steps in liver carcinogenesis by diethylnitrosamine.
Cancer Res., 41:2096-2102

Ying, T. S., Enomoto, K., Sarma, D. S. R., and Farber, E., 1982, Effects of delays in the cell cycle on the induction of preneoplastic and neoplastic lesions in rat liver by 1,2-dimethylhydrazine. Cancer Res., 42:876-880

Zarbl, H., Sukumar, S, Arthur, A. V., Martin-Zanca, D., and Barbacid, M., 1985, Direct mutagenesis of Ha-ras-1 oncogenes by N-nitroso-N-methylurea during initiation of mammary carcinogenesis in rats. Nature, Lond., 315:382-385

Zerban, H., Rabes, H. M., and Bannasch, P., 1985, Kinetics of cell proliferation during hepatocarcinogenesis. Eur. J. Cancer Clin. Oncol., 21:1424

Zhang, X.-K., Huang, D.-P., Chiu, D.-K., and Chiu, J.-F., 1987, The expression of oncogenes in human developing liver and hepatomas. Biochim. Biophys. Res. Comm., 142:932-938

INITIATION OF CHEMICAL HEPATOCARCINOGENESIS: COMPENSATORY CELL PROLIFERATION VERSUS MITOGEN INDUCED HYPERPLASIA

A.Columbano, G.M.Ledda-Columbano, P.Coni, D.S.R.Sarma, P. Pani

Istituto di Farmacologia e Patologia Biochimica, Università di Cagliari, Cagliari, Italy, and Department of Pathology, University of Toronto, Canada

Cell proliferation has often been implicated in the carcinogenic process and cell transformation induced by chemicals, radiation, and viruses (1-7). Compelling evidence to support the role of cell proliferation in the carcinogenic process has come from the observation that several carcinogens that do not induce liver cancer in adult animals become hepatocarcinogenic when given coupled with liver cell proliferative stimuli such as partial hepatectomy (PH) or a necrogenic dose of carbon tetrachloride (CCl_4) (2,3,5,7,8). Using foci of enzyme altered hepatocytes as the end point and several selection and/or promoting procedures, it was demonstrated that cell proliferation is a necessary prerequisite for the initiation phase of liver carcinogenesis (9-11). Although the mechanism by which cell proliferation plays a crucial role in initiation of the carcinogenic process is not clearly understood, it is believed that replication of DNA with carcinogenic-induced miscoding lesions such as 0^6-alkylguanine (12-14), 0^4-alkylthymine (15-17), or non-coding lesions such as apurinic sites (18,19) or certain types of gap filling mechanisms (20,21), may be the critical events involved in initiation step.

In all these studies, the proliferative stimulus for cell proliferation was of compensatory type following PH or necrosis. On the contrary, although it is known that liver cells may be stimulated to divide also by a variety of agents that do not induce previous cell death (mitogens), the effect of liver hyperplasia induced by mitogens on initiation of liver carcinogenesis has not been studied.

Recently, during a study on liver cell proliferation induced by the mitogen lead nitrate (22), we have found that following the initial hyperplasia there was a rapid regression of the liver mass to its normal size. During the regression phase there was

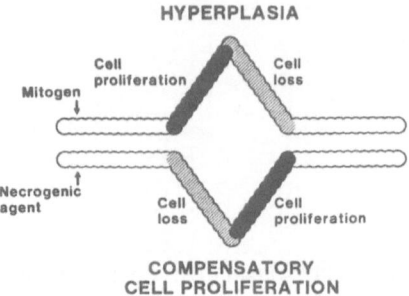

Fig.1.   Schematic representation of induction of liver cell proliferation induced by mitogens and necrogenic agents.

also a rapid disappearance of excess DNA together with the occurrence
of a type of cell death, namely apoptosis (23), which has been
found to occur in a wide variety of normal circumstances (24).
The finding that apoptosis also occurred during the induction of
liver hyperplasia following cessation of treatment with the mitogen
cyproterone acetate (CPA) (25) seems to suggest that apoptosis
may be triggered anytime there is an overgrowth of the liver mass
such as that induced by mitogen treatment. Thus, at least 2 major
differences between the compensatory type of cell proliferation
and that induced by mitogens exist (Figure 1): while in the former
case cell loss is the primary event and cell proliferation is needed
to replace the cells that have been lost, in the latter case, the
mitogenic effect which is the primary event results in an excess
of cells which are removed within days or weeks by apoptosis. In
addition, unlike the compensatory cell proliferative stimulus,
the mitogen-induced direct cell proliferative stimulus has to overcome
the growth control mechanism normally operating in the organ.

Since it is not known whether these differences could mean
anything in terms of the role of cell proliferation in initiation
of liver carcinogenesis, we have performed studies aimed to establish
whether cell proliferation induced by hepatic mitogens could play
the same role of the compensatory cell proliferation in supporting
initiation of liver carcinogenesis (Figure 2).

Initial results have indicated that unlike compensatory cell
proliferation, liver hyperplasia induced by two hepatic mitogens,
lead nitrate (22) and ethylene dibromide (26), could not result
in the formation of γ-glutamyltransferase (GGT) positive foci when

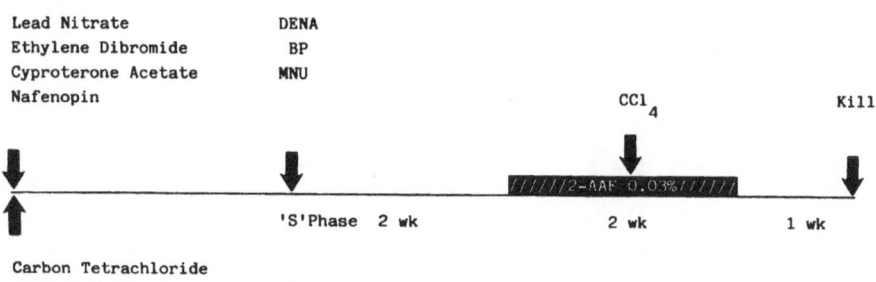

MITOGENS

Lead Nitrate   DENA
Ethylene Dibromide   BP
Cyproterone Acetate   MNU
Nafenopin

                                          CCl$_4$ Kill

                      'S'Phase 2 wk   2 wk   1 wk

Carbon Tetrachloride
Partial Hepatectomy

COMPENSATORY CELL
  PROLIFERATION

Fig.2.   Experimental protocol to study the effect of compensatory
         cell proliferation and mitogen-induced cell proliferation on
         the induction of GGT positive foci in liver of rats initiated
         with DENA, BP and MNU. Male Wistar rats (240-260 g) were
         given CCl$_4$ (2 ml/kg, i.g.), lead nitrate (100 μ mol/kg, i.v.),
         EDB (100 mg/kg, i.g.), CPA (100 mg/kg, i.g.) or nafenopin
         (200 mg/kg, i.g.). In some rats the proliferative stimulus
         was achieved through PH. During DNA synthesis, a non-necro-
         genic dose of DENA (20 mg/kg, i.p.), MNU (60 mg/kg, i.p.),
         or BP (200 mg/kg, i.g.) were administered at 20 hr after
         PH, 24 hr after EDB and CPA, 30 hr after lead nitrate and
         nafenopin, and 48 hr after CCl$_4$. After a 2-week recovery
         period, the initiated hepatocytes so formed were assayed
         as GGT positive foci using the resistant hepatocyte model
         (9).

coupled with 2 carcinogens, diethylnitrosamine (DENA) and benzo(a)pyrene
(BP) (Figure 3). The inability to achieve initiation by mitogen-
induced liver cell proliferation was not due to an inhibitory effect
of the chemicals used on the activity of GGT; in fact, biochemical
as well as histochemical determination of GGT following treatment
with lead nitrate revealed that the metal was able to significantly
induce GGT activity (data not shown).

    The possibility that the lack of formation of GGT-positive
foci in mitogen pretreated rats could be due to an insufficient
proliferative stimulus also appears to be unlikely because the
extent of cell proliferation at the time of carcinogenic treatment
is similar in animals pretreated with CCl$_4$, lead nitrate, and
EDB (Figure 4).

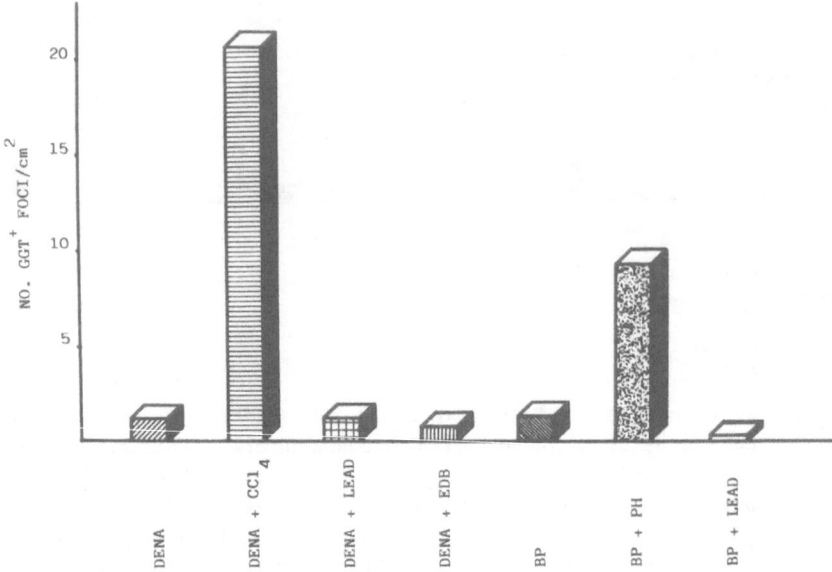

Fig.3.　Effect of different types of liver cell proliferative stimuli on the formation of GGT-positive foci induced by DENA and BP. The experimental protocol is given in Figure 2.

Since lead nitrate is known to inhibit the cytochrome P–450 system (28,29), it was possible that it could interfere with the metabolism of the carcinogens used, DENA and BP, both chemicals that require their metabolism in order to exert the carcinogenic effect. Thus, we further extended our studies on the effect of mitogen-induced cell proliferation on initiation of liver carcinogenesis by using i) 2 other hepatic mitogens, CPA (25) and nafenopin (29,30) which are not inhibitors of the cytochrome P–450 system, ii) another carcinogen, N-methyl-N-nitrosourea (MNU), which is a direct alkylating carcinogen and, iii) an additional phenotypic marker for the putative preneoplastic foci, the placental form of glutathione S-transferase (GST-P) (31–33).

As indicated in Figure 5, irrespectively of the carcinogen used, enzyme altered foci were seen only in rats whose liver cells were stimulated to divide by a regenerative stimulus, but not when the carcinogen was given during mitogen-induced cell proliferation.

The inability to achieve initiation by mitogen-induced cell proliferation is very intriguing for the following reasons: the extent of cell proliferation at the time of carcinogen treatment is almost identical in both types, i.e. compensatory and mitogen-induced liver cell proliferative systems, as shown by studies on labeled thymidine incorporation into DNA (Figure 4), and by autoradiography (data not shown), and b) the extent of DNA alkylation by

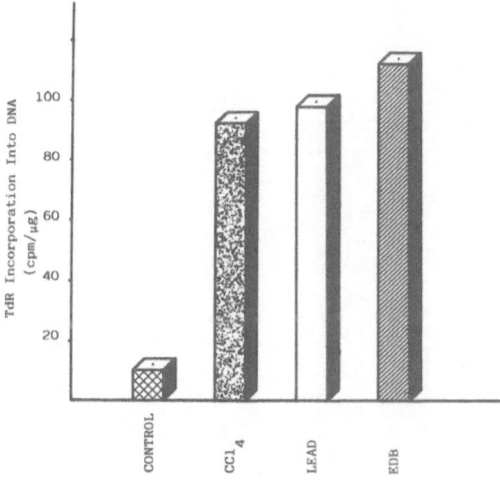

Fig.4.   Effect of different proliferative stimuli on TdR incorporation
          into liver DNA. Each animal received a single injection of
          TdR (20 μCi/100 g) at 23 hr (EDB pretreated rats), 29 hr
          (lead-pretreated rats) and 47 hr (CCl_4 pretreated rats). The
          animals were killed 1 hr after TdR administration.

MNU was not inhibited by pretreatment with lead nitrate (Table
1).

These results raise several questions pertaining to the role
of cell proliferation in the initiation process. Perhaps of greater
significance is the importance of these observations in understanding
the fundamentals of regulation of liver cell proliferation itself.

The absence of initiated hepatocytes when liver cell proliferative
stimulus was from mitogens could be because of such proliferative
stimulus was not conducive for achieving initiation. Alternatively,
such liver cell proliferation might have accomplish initiation,
but, the initiated hepatocytes are eliminated during the regression
phase following the cessation of the mitogenic stimulus (Figure
6). If the former hypothesis is valid, one wonders why one type
of cell proliferation (compensatory cell proliferation) achieves
initiation, but not the other type (mitogen-induced cell proliferation).
It is possible that during compensatory cell proliferation, certain
conformational changes in the genomic organization may occur such
that some genes, for example certain proto-oncogenes, may become
available for carcinogenic attack. Replication of these altered
genes may be the critical event in the initiation step. Whereas,
similar conformational changes may not occur during mitogen-induced
liver cell proliferation. An analysis of genes expressed during
these two types of liver cell proliferation may even lead to the

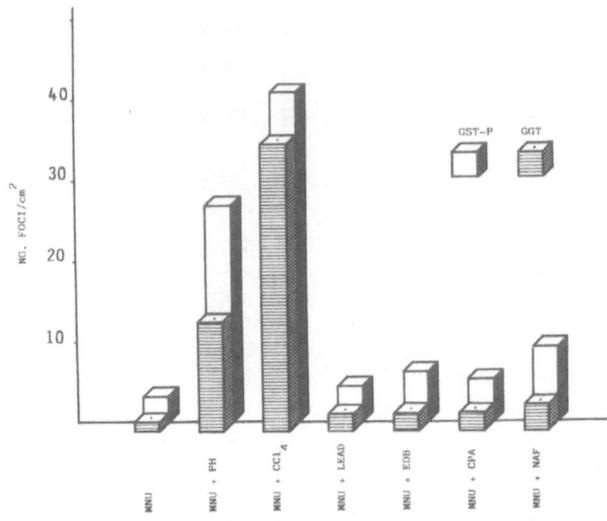

Fig.5.   Effect of different types of liver cell proliferative stimuli
on the formation of GGT and GST-P positive foci induced by
MNU. The experimental protocol is given in Figure 2.

identification of the genes that may be involved in the initiation
process.

    If the latter hypothesis is valid, i.e. the mitogen-induced
cell proliferation did achieve initiation but the initiated hepatocytes
are lost during the regression phase of liver hyperplasia, then
it has to be concluded that initiated hepatocytes are more proned
to apoptosis. This conclusion is based on the observation that
initiated hepatocytes (monitored as GGT positive foci) are randomly
distributed, that virtually no foci are seen when initiation was

Table 1. Presence of (^{14}C)-MNU Induced Methylated Purines in Rat Liver
         DNA Following Pretreatment with Lead Nitrate

Treatment	N-7-Methylguanine (cpm/mg DNA)	O^6-Methylguanine (cpm/mg DNA)
H_2O + (^{14}C)-MNU	484 ± 95	51 ± 8
Lead Nitrate + (^{14}C)-MNU	637 ± 95	66 ± 11

Rats were treated with either lead nitrate (100 μ mol/kg, i.v.) or H_2O. 30
hours later, the rats were given (^{14}C)-MNU (6 mg/40 μCi/100 g). Two hr
thereafter the rats were killed and N-7-MeG, and O^6-MeG were determined
in liver DNA (21) Values are the mean ± S.E.

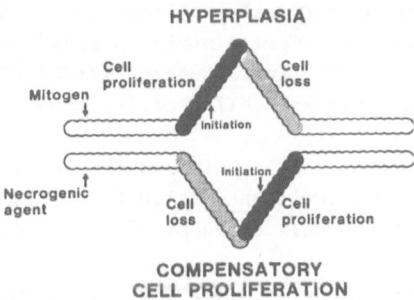

HYPERPLASIA

Fig.6. Schematic representation of the possible different fate of initiated cells depending upon the nature of the proliferative stimulus.

attempted with mitogen-induced cell proliferation, and that not all hepatocytes are lost during the regression phase of the mitogen-induced liver hyperplasia, only the excess cells being lost. If initiated hepatocytes are more prone to apoptosis it is tempting to speculate that the administration of compounds that induce the occurrence of this type of cell death may also influence the promotion phase of liver carcinogenesis. On this respect, it is interesting to note that hepatocytes of nodules generated by different models exhibit a higher incidence of apoptosis (25,34); in addition, our recent finding that repeated treatment with lead nitrate to rats previously exposed to an initiating dose of DENA did not promote the growth of GGT positive foci, eventhough a mitogenic wave occurred everytime the metal was injected (35), suggests that the foci cells stimulated to proliferate by lead may be eliminated during the apoptotic wave that follows the initial hyperplasia.

Further work in this area should provide interesting insights into the nature of the role of cell proliferation in the carcinogenic process and may open up new dimension in our understanding the basics of cell proliferation.

References

1. C.Boreck, and L.Sachs, The number of cell generations required to fix the transformed state in X-ray involved transformation. Proc.Natl.Acad.Sci.U.S.A., 57:1522 (1967).
2. V.M.Craddock, Cell proliferation and experimental liver cancer, in: "Liver Cell Cancer", H.M.Cameron, D.A.Linsel, G.P.Warwick, eds., Elsevier/North Holland Biomedical Press, Amsterdam, (1976).
3. A.D.Glinos, N.L.R.Bucher, and J.C.Aub, The effect of liver regeneration on tumour formation in rats fed 4-dimethylaminoazobenzene. J.Exp.Med., 93:313 (1951).

4. T.Kakunaga, Requirement for cell proliferation in the fixation and expression of the transformed state in mouse cells treated with 4-nitroquinoline-oxide, Int.J.Cancer, 14:736 (1974).

5. A.W.Pound, Carcinogenesis and cell proliferation, N.Z.Med.J., 67:88 (1968).

6. G.J.Todaro, and H.Green, Cell growth and the initiation of transformation by SV40. Proc.Natl.Acad.Sci.U.S.A., 55:302 (1966)

7. E.Warwick, Effect of the cell cycle on carcinogenesis, Fed.Proc., 30:1760 (1971)

8. A.W.Pound, Influence of carbon tetrachloride on induction of tumours of the liver and kidneys in mice by nitrosamines. Br.J.Cancer, 37:67 (1978).

9. E.Cayama, H.Tsuda, D.S.R.Sarma, and E.Farber, Initiation of chemical carcinogenesis requires cell proliferation, Nature, 275:60 (1978)

10. T.S.Ying, D.S.R.Sarma, and E.Farber, Induction of presumptive preneoplastic lesions in rat liver by a single dose of 1,2-dimethylhydrazine, Chem-Biol.Interact., 28:363 (1979).

11. A.Columbano, S.Rajalakshmi, and D.S.R.Sarma, Requirement of cell proliferation for the initiation of liver carcinogenesis as assayed by three different procedures, Cancer Res., 41:2079 (1981)

12. A.Loveless, Possible relevance of O^6 alkylation of deoxyguanosine to the mutagenicity and carcinogenicity of nitrosamines and nitrosamides, Nature, 223:206 (1969).

13. R.Goth, and M.F.Rajewsky, Persistence of O^6-ethylguanine in rat-brain DNA: Correlation with nervous system-specific carcinogenesis by ethylnitrosourea, Proc.Natl.Acad.Sci.U.S.A., 71:639 (1974).

14. J.W.Nicoll, P.F.Swann, and A.E.Pegg, The accumulation of O^6-methylguanine in the liver and kidney DNA of rats treated with dimethylnitrosamine for a short or long period, Chem-Biol.Interact., 16:301 (1977).

15. B.D.Preston, B.Singer, and L.A.Loeb, Mutagenic potential of O^4-methylthymine in vivo determined by an enzymatic approach to site specific mutagenesis, Proc.Natl.Acad.Sci.U.S.A., 83:8501 (1986).

16. J.A.Swendberg, M.C.Dyroff, M.A.Bedell, J.A.Popp, N.Huh, U.Kirstein, and M.F.Rajewsky, O^4-ethyldeoxythymidine, but not O^6-ethydeoxyguanosine, accumulates in hepatocyte DNA of rats exposed continuosly to diethylnitrosamine. Proc.Natl.Acad.Sci.U.S.A., 81:16 92 (1984).

17. B.Singer, and J.T.Kusmierek. Chemical mutagenesis, Ann.Rev.Biochem., 51:655 (1982).

18. S.Rajalakshmi, and D.S.R.Sarma, Replication of hepatic DNA in rats treated with dimethylnitrosamine. Chem-Biol.Interact., 11:245 (1975).

19. C.W.Shearman, and L.A.Loeb, Effects of depurination on the fidelity of DNA synthesis, J.Mol.Biol., 128:197 (1979).

20. S.E.Abanobi, A.Columbano, R.A.Mulivor, S.Rajalakshmi, and D.S.R.Sarma, In vivo replication of hepatic deoxyribonucleic acid of rats treated with dimethylnitrosamine: Presence of dimethylnitrosamine induced O^6-methylguanine, N-7-methylguanine and N-3-methyladenine in the replicated hybrid deoxyribonucleic acid, Biochemistry, 19:1382 (1980).

21. A.Columbano, G.M.Ledda-Columbano, P.M.Rao, S.Rajalakshmi, and D.S.R. Sarma, In vivo replication of carcinogen-modified DNA: Presence of dimethylnitrosamine-induced N-7-methylguanine and O^6-methylguanine in the parental and daughter strands of the in vivo replicated, hybrid DNA, Biochem.Arch., 1:121 (1985).

22. A.Columbano, G.M.Ledda, P.Sirigu, T.Perra, and P.Pani, Liver cell proliferation induced by a single dose of lead nitrate, Am.J. Pathol., 110:83 (1983).

23. A.Columbano, G.M.Ledda-Columbano, P.Coni, G.Faa, C.Liguori, G.Santacruz, and P.Pani, Occurrence of cell death (apoptosis) during the involution of liver hyperplasia, Lab.Invest., 52:670 (1985).

24. J.F.R.Kerr, A.H.Whyllie, and A.R.Currie, Cell death: The significance of apoptosis, Int.Rev.Cytol., 68:251 (1980).

25. W.Bursch, B.Lauer, I.Timmermann-Trosiener, G.Barthel, J.Schuppler, and R.Schulte-Hermann, Controlled cell death (apoptosis) of normal and putative preneoplastic cells in rat liver following withdrawal of tumor promoters, Carcinogenesis, 5:453 (1984).

26. E.Nachtomi, and E.Farber, Ethylene dibromide as a mitogen for liver, Lab.Invest., 38:279 (1978).

27. P.Scoppa, M.Roumengous, and W.Penning, Hepatic drug metabolizing activity in lead poisoned rats, Experientia, 29:970 (1973).

28. A.P.Alvares, S.Leigh, J.Cohn, and J.Kappas, Lead and methyl mercury: Effects of acute exposure on cytochrome P-450 and the mixed function oxidase system in the liver, J.Exp.Med., 135:1406 (1972).

29. W.G.Levine, M.G.Ord, and L.A.Stocken, Some biochemical changes associated with nafenopin-induced liver growth in the rat, Biochem. Pharmacol., 26:939 (1977).

30. R.B.Beckett, R.Weiss, R.E.Stitzel, and R.J.Cenedella, Studies on the hepatomegaly caused by the hypolipidemic drugs nafenopin and clofibrate, Toxicol.Appl.Pharmacol., 23:42 (1972).

31. L.C.Eriksson, R.N.Sharma, M.W.Roomi, R.K.Ho, E.Farber, and R.K. Murray, A characteristic electrophoretic pattern of cytosolic polypeptide from hepatocyte nodules generated during liver carcinogenesis in several models, Biochem.Biophys.Res.Commun., 117:740 (1983).

32. A.Kitahara, K.Satoh, and K.Sato, Properties of the increased glutathione S-transferase A form in rat preneoplastic hepatic lesions induced by chemical carcinogens, Biochem.Biophys.Res. Commun., 112:20 (1983).

33. K.Sato, A.Kitahara, K.Satoh, T.Ishikawa, M.Tatematsu, and N.Ito, The placental form of glutathione S-transferase as a new marker protein for preneoplasia in rat chemical hepatocarcinogenesis, Gann, 75:199 (1984).

34. A.Columbano, G.M.Ledda-Columbano, P.M.Rao, S.Rajalakshmi, and D.S. R.Sarma, Occurrence of cell death (apoptosis) in preneoplastic and neoplastic liver cells: A sequential study, Am.J.Pathol., 116:441 (1984).

35. G.M.Ledda-Columbano, A.Columbano, P.Coni, C.Liguori, and P.Pani, Repeated treatment with the mitogen lead nitrate fails to promote the growth of GGT-positive foci, Proc.Am.Assoc.Cancer Res., 28:663 (1987).

CELL DEATH (APOPTOSIS) IN NORMAL AND PRENEOPLASTIC LIVER TISSUE

W. Bursch and R. Schulte-Hermann

Institut für Tumorbiologie-Krebsforschung

Abtl. Onkologische Toxikologie

Borschkegasse 8a, A-1090 Wien

INTRODUCTION

Numerous compounds of "xenobiotic" origin such as the environmental pollutant α-hexachlorocyclohexane, the synthetic sex steroid cyproterone acetate (CPA), phenobarbital (PB) or various other lipophilic compounds have been found to produce liver tumors in long-term animal experiments, although they do not exhibit detectable genotoxic activity. Studies on the mechanisms of action of such nongenotoxic hepatocarcinogens revealed that these with respect to their chemical structure and general biological or pharmacological effects very heterogenous chemicals share the ability to increase activities of hepatic enzymes involved in the metabolism of lipophilic substrates and to increase the size (hypertrophy) and the number (hyperplasia) of hepatocytes. These changes are thought to reflect an adaptive program in the liver that is switched on consequently to the increased functional demands on the organ (Conney et al. 1960; Argyris and Magnus 1968; Schlicht et al. 1967, 1968; Koransky et al. 1969; Schulte-Hermann 1974; Schulte-Hermann et al. 1980a,b).

Furthermore, increase of drug-metabolism and liver enlargement were found to be largely reversible when the functional load is reduced after withdrawal of the growth stimulus. At least with some of the inducers, liver involution includes regression of hyperplasia (Levine et al. 1977, Schulte-Hermann et al. 1980 b). Recently, we suggested that cell death by apoptosis may be responsible for the regression of liver hyperplasia. It is important to note, that the occurrence of cell death in the liver after withdrawal of the growth inducer appears not to reflect toxic injury of hepatocytes. Rather, cell death by apoptosis appears to be a programmed process involved in the regulation of liver cell number, similar to the role of apoptosis in endocrine dependent

organs after hormone withdawal or during embryologic development (Kerr et al. 1972, Wyllie et al. 1980, Ferguson and
Anderson 1981; Bursch et al. 1984, 1985, 1986). In putative
preneoplastic (ppn) lesions of rat liver, however, mechanisms
controlling homeostasis of cell number appear to fail during
long term treatment with these agents. Thereby, nongenotoxic
hepatocarcinogens stimulate selective and excessive growth of
ppn lesions and promote the development of liver tumors.

In this paper, we will briefly describe the role of
apoptosis for the elimination of excessive cells in normal
liver. Subsequently, we compare cell death by apoptosis in
normal liver with apoptosis in ppn lesions and discuss the
role of cell death by apoptosis for growth and regression of
putative preneoplastic lesions in rat liver.

RESULTS AND DISCUSSION

Cell death (apoptosis) in normal liver tissue

The role of cell death by apoptosis for the regulation
of cell number in the normal liver has been studied using the
sex-steroid cyproterone acetate (CPA) as a model compound to
stimulate liver growth and the relation between CPA levels,
DNA content and incidence of apoptosis was closely followed
(fig.1).

Repeated treatment of rats with high doses of CPA
(100 and 130 mg/kg/d) caused an increase of liver DNA content
by about 60% and a doubling of liver size (not shown). The
increase of liver DNA content reflects liver hyperplasia
since hepatocellular DNA replication was found to be followed
by mitosis while no changes of hepatocellular ploidy were
detected (Schulte-Hermann et al. 1980 b,c). The increase of
liver DNA content (hyperplasia) was found to perist as long
as CPA treatment was performed. However, when the CPA treatment was stopped the liver DNA content declined rapidly:
within 3 to 5 days after cessation of treatment about 25% of
DNA present at maximal liver enlargement disappeared. On the
other hand, this decline in liver DNA content could be prevented by continued treatment with CPA (fig. 1).

These findings suggest that elimination of DNA is due to
elimination of CPA. Therefore, we measured the CPA concentration in the liver during a treatment of 7 days and thereafter
(fig. 1). There was a steep increase of CPA level in rat
liver within the first hours after treatment, followed by a
decrease. The increase in the CPA dose on day 3 did not cause
further enhancement of CPA levels. Rather, liver CPA levels
tended to decrease towards the end of the treatment period.
After cessation of treatment, CPA was found to be eliminated
almost completely within 48 hrs. Analysis of the elimination
kinetics of CPA revealed a relatively short biological half-
life of about 11 hours between 2 and 48 h post administration
(Bursch et al. 1986). These results strongly suggest that
involution of liver DNA occurs consequently to the elimination of the growth inducer rather than to cell damage.

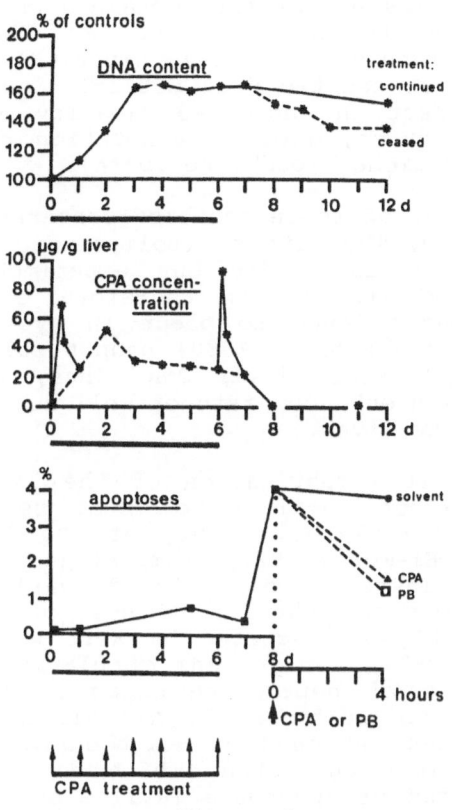

Figure 1.

Effect of CPA treatment and CPA withdrawal on DNA content, CPA concentration and of incidence of apoptoses in rat liver.

References: Bursch et al.(1985, 1986). Female Wistar rats were treated with cyproterone acetate (CPA) as indicated at the bottom of the figure; small arrows: 100 mg/kg/day, large arrows: 130 mg/kg/day. Liver DNA content (mg DNA/100g rat) is expressed as percentage of solvent-treated controls. Solid line: rats killed 24 hrs after the last treatment; treatment continued: initial CPA treatment as indicated below the abscissa followed by further treatment with 130 mg CPA/kg/day until day 11; treatment ceased (dashed line): rats killed between 2 and 5 days after the last (7th) treatment. CPA concentrations (µg/g liver) were determined 24 hrs after each dose (dashed line) and at closer intervals after the first and seventh dose (solid line). The CPA determinations were performed by B. Düsterberg, Schering,Berlin, FRG. Apoptoses: the number of apoptotic bodies (ABs, intra- and extra-hepatocellular ABs, with and without chromatin, cf. figure 2) found in histological sections is expressed as percentage of intact hepatocytes. For studies on inhibtion of apoptosis rats were initially treated with 7 doses of CPA. 2 Days after the last treatment, CPA or PB were administered in aqueous supensions at a dose of 130 mg/kg body weight and the rats were killed 4 hours thereafter. Note the different scales of the abscissa.

Furthermore, the CPA levels in rat liver revealed another important aspect of hepatic responses to this compound. It is of interest to compare the areas under the curves obtained after the first and seventh treatment. In the liver, the latter was 67% of that obtained on day 1. Furthermore, in the serum the peak area on day 7 was only 36% of that of day 1 (Bursch et al. 1986). Since CPA was found to be a potent inducer of hepatic drug metabolizing enzymes, these findings may reflect an increased capacity of the liver to metabolize the inducer, i.e. an adaptation of the liver to its increased functional load (see above).

The next question to be answered concerned the mechanism of DNA elimination. The rate of proliferation of hepatocytes is about 0,5% per day under our experimental conditions (Schulte-Hermann et al. 1980 b); therefore, a decrease of DNA synthesis previously found to occur in hyperplastic livers (Schulte-Hermann and Schmitz 1980) cannot solely explain the rapid decrease of excess liver DNA. Thus, we searched for signs indicating an enhanced rate of cell death in histological sections of the liver.

Histological investigation of the liver revealed no signs of diffuse or focal necrosis as seen after toxic, inflammatory or circulatory injury of the liver (Recknagel 1967; Farber and El-Mofty 1975; Trump et al. 1981; Popper and Keppler 1986). Instead we observed various cytological alterations indicating the occurrence of cell death by apoptosis (fig. 2) as described by Kerr et al. (1972) and Wyllie et al. (1980). For reasons of clarity, a schematical diagram of stages of hepatocyte death as found after CPA withdrawal is shown in figure 3. A small number of hepatocytes exhibited separation from neighbouring cells and condensation of nuclear chromatin, which reflect the earliest morphological signs of apoptosis (Wyllie et al. 1980; Bursch et al. 1985). Furthermore, in H&E stained liver sections many eosinophilic membrane bound bodies were found in the intercellular space (fig. 2). Such bodies are considered to be fragments of cells undergoing death by apoptosis and therefore are called apoptotic bodies (ABs). Histochemically, the extracellular ABs contained no or very few lysosomes with detectable acid DNAse, RNAse and phosphatase activity, indicating the lack of autolytic activity within ABs at this stage (Bursch et al. 1985). The histochemical findings were supported by measurements of the activity of glutamate-pyruvate transaminase (GPT) in serum, which was found to be at control level at the time of maximal increase of cell death (Bursch et al. 1986). The majority (about 80%) of the ABs, however, was found within apparently normal hepatocytes (intra-hepatocellular ABs, fig. 2), indicating that normal hepatocytes rapidly phagocytize the ABs. Evidence for phagocytosis of ABs by intact hepatocytes was provided by the divergent ^{3}H-TdR labelling of most ABs and nuclei within individual hepatocytes as shown in figure 4: in hepatocytes with labelled nuclei at least 66% of the ABs were not labelled. Since in binucleated hepatocytes both nuclei are always labelled (Schlicht et al. 1968; Schulte-Hermann et al. 1980 b), this result shows that the chromatin of these ABs must be derived from other cells than those in which they were found. Thus at least the majority of intracellular ABs with chromatin appears to be phagocytized by hepatocytes. In addition, phagocytosis of ABs by RES cells also occurs as shown by electron microscopy (Bursch, Aumüller, Schulte-Hermann, unpubl. observation). Furthermore, this experiment

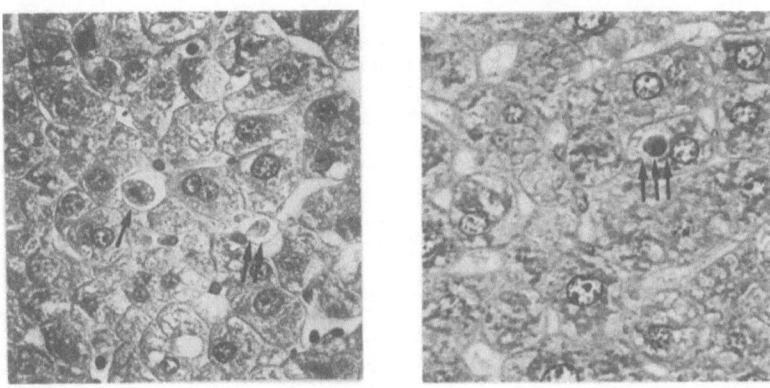

Figure 2.

Morphological signs of cell death by apoptosis in rat liver.

Extra-hepatoccelular AB with (↑) or without(↑ ↑) chromatin; intra-hepatocellular AB with chromatin (↑ ↑ ↑). Hematoxylin-eosin, x 500

CELL DEATH (APOPTOSIS)

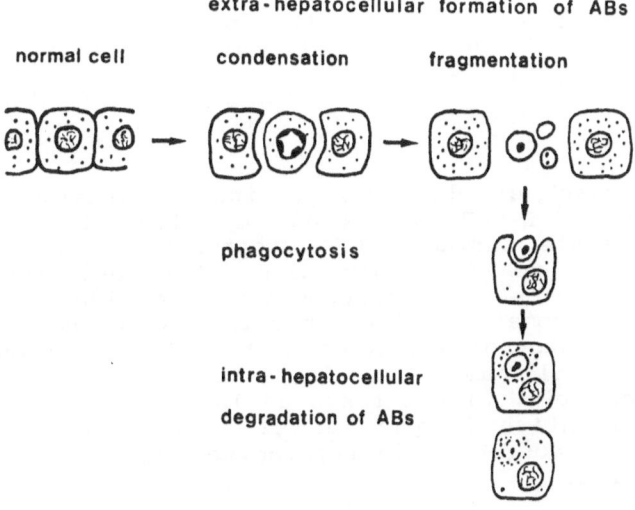

Figure 3.

Hypothetical diagram of the process of apoptosis during regression of liver hyperplasia. The figure is explained in the text.

revealed another interesting result: since most of the ABs (86%) were unlabelled, nonreplicating hepatocytes seem to be eliminated preferentially. This result confirmed the conclusion previously drawn from experiments with biochemical determination of the labelling of hepatocytes (Schulte-Hermann et al. 1980b).

Once the ABs have been phagocytized, they appear to be degraded by intra-hepatocellular lysosomes, whereas intra-apoptotic lysosomes seem to be inactive until the late stages of this degradation (Bursch et al. 1985).

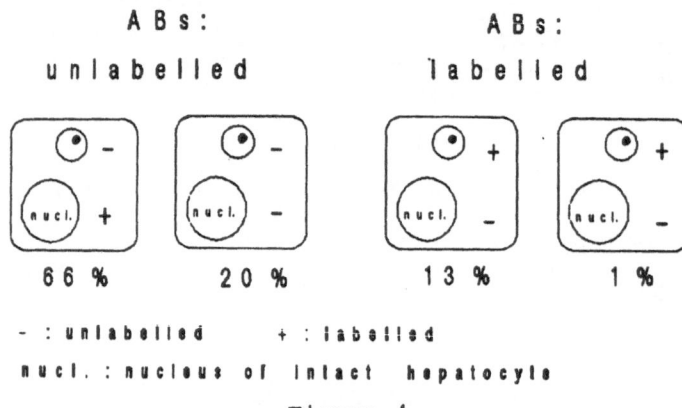

Figure 4.

Occurrence of labelled DNA in nuclei and ABs of the same hepatocytes

Reference: Bursch et al. 1985. Continuous infusion of ^{3}H-methyl-thymidine (^{3}H-TdR) was used to label all hepatocytes which proliferate during a CPA treatment for 7 days (see. fig. 1). Rats were killed two days after cessation of CPA, (at the peak incidence of apoptosis in the liver) and ^{3}H-TdR labelling of chromatin in hepatocytic nuclei and in ABs was determined by autoradiography of histological sections of the liver. The total number of intra-hepatocellular ABs with chromatin (cf. fig. 2) was taken as 100%; the data shown indicate the relative frequencies of ^{3}H-labelling of ABs as well as their occurrence in hepatocytes with or without ^{3}H-labelled nuclei.

In conclusion, the process of cell death by apoptosis observed in our studies revealed some important differences from necrosis as seen after toxic, inflammatory or circulatory injury of the liver (Recknagel 1967; Farber and El-Mofty 1975; Trump et al. 1981; Popper and Keppler 1986). What does the occurrence of cell death by apoptosis mean? Kerr et al. (1972) and Wyllie et al. (1980) suggested that apoptosis is a programmed form of cell death occurring during embryologic development and metamorphosis or after hormone withdrawal in endocrine-dependent organs. However, signs of cell death observed in the course of human viral hepatitis (councilman bodies) or alcoholic hepatitis (Meybehm et al. 1986) or after galactosamine administration exhibit some of the cytological alterations described for apoptosis. Therefore, it would appear unreasonable to denote the type of cell death observed in rat liver after CPA withdrawal as a programmed event (or apoptosis) purely on morphological grounds. However, analysis of the incidence cell death in rat liver as related to liver DNA content (hyperplasia) and CPA concentration should be taken into account for evaluation of the function of hepatic cell death after CPA withdrawal.

As shown in figure 1, the incidence of apoptoses increased coincident with CPA elimination. The highest incidence of apoptoses was found from 2 to 5 days after cessation of CPA treatment (Bursch et al. 1984, 1986). On the other hand, when CPA administration was resumed, the incidence of apoptoses was found to decrease by about 60% within 4 hours after a single dose of the inducer. A similar decrease of the incidence of apoptoses was found after treatment with other liver growth stimuli such as phenobarbital.

The decrease in the number of ABs after CPA suggested that the growth inducer inhibits the formation of ABs. Thus, following the time course of elimination of ABs should provide a means to determine the duration of apoptosis and of the stages of apoptosis as visible at light microscopy. As shown in figure 5 a, the AB incidence was lowered already two hours after CPA retreatment, the minimum was found 4 hours after dosing. The half-lives of the extra- and the intra-hepatocellular ABs (T/2 about 30 and 70 min., respectively) were determined separately, using the apparently linear segments of a semilogarithmic plot of the data for regression analysis (Fig. 5 b). The short duration of the visible apoptosis as found in these experiments supports the view that even a low number of ABs may reflect a high rate of cell turnover (Wyllie at al. 1980, Searle et al. 1987). In our experiments, the low AB incidence is consistent with the relatively extensive loss of DNA from the liver within a few days (Bursch et al. 1984, 1986). The longer half-life of intra-hepatocellular ABs as compared to extra-cellular ABs found in this experiment is in accordance with the higher relative frequency of intra-hepatocellular ABs found in previous experiments (Bursch et al. 1985).

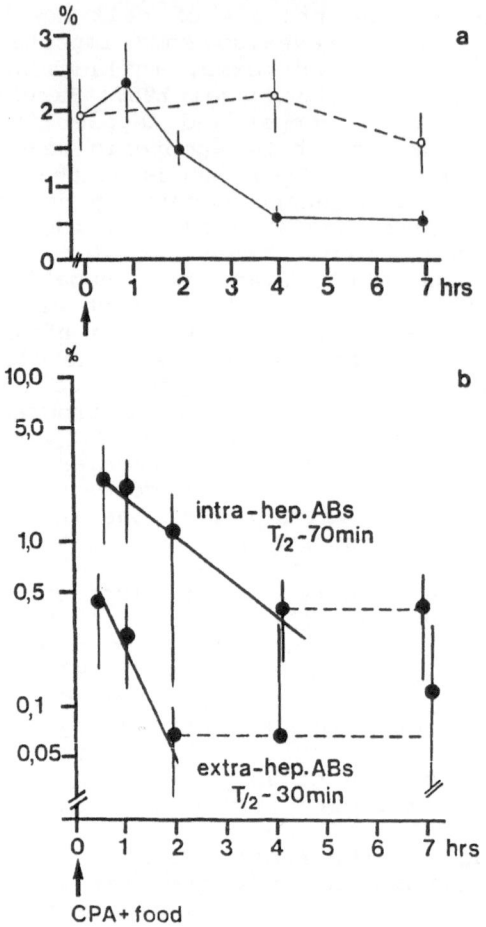

Figure 5.

Time course of decrease of AB incidence after CPA and food administration.

Rats received CPA for 7 days as described in figure 1. Two days after the last CPA dosing (i.e. at the peak incidence of ABs), rats were retreated with a single dose of CPA (130 mg/kg). Additionally, rats received food according to the feeding schedule (see Bursch et al. 1986); food uptake was found to decrease the AB incidence (Bursch, Lauer, Schulte-Hermann, unpubl. observation). In a) the incidence of the total number of ABs (intra-, extra hepatocellular ABs, ABs with and without chromatin) is given , in b) we differentiated between extra- or intra-hepatocellular localization of the ABs. ●——●: CPA and food at "0";○---○: no food and no CPA at "0". 7000 - 8000 hepatocytes were scored per liver for determination of the AB incidence. Each point represents the mean (±) SD of 5-6 animals.

In summary, the following arguments support the view that cell death by apoptosis is the major factor responsible for the rapid regression of DNA:
1. the short duration of apoptosis explains why low numbers of apoptotic bodies can account for the loss of about 25% of DNA within 3 - 5 days
2. the peak incidence of ABs coincides with the period of DNA regression
3. Apoptosis and DNA regression can be inhibited by continued treatment with CPA

Furthermore, these findings also suggest that the occurrence of cell death in CPA-treated livers does not reflect toxic injury to the liver, but is a programmed event serving to eliminate the excess of cells in hyperplastic livers:

1. the incidence of apoptosis correlates negatively with the concentration of CPA in the liver
2. a single dose of CPA obviously inhibits apoptosis. Phenobarbital and other inducers of liver growth (α-hexachlorocyclohexane, nafenopin; Bursch et al. 1985, 1986) also inhibit apoptosis, indicating that inhibition of apoptosis is not specific for CPA, but may be related to the growth stimulating potential of these compounds.

In conclusion, apoptosis appears to be an important regulator of cell number in adult liver. According to our hypothesis cells in a resting liver (G_0) have two options to leave G_0: replication or death. Application of a growth stimulus (e.g. CPA) will stimulate cell replication and inhibit cell death (apoptosis) and thereby create and maintain liver hyperplasia. The reverse will occur when the growth stimulus is removed. According to this hypothesis the occurrence of apoptosis after CPA withdrawal reflects an active process of de-adaptation which is switched on when the functional demands on the liver decrease. It is of interest to note that there exists evidence for the presence of gene(s) in a mammalian thymoma cell line that code for a cell suicide program resembling apoptosis (Ucker 1987).

Cell death (apoptosis) in putative preneoplastic liver tissue

Elucidation of the interaction of CPA or PB with cell death by apoptosis was of particular interest because CPA, PB and other inducers of liver growth promote the development of liver tumors in experimental animals (Peraino et al. 1975, Watanabe and Williams 1978, Schulte-Hermann 1985). The promoters have been found to accelerate growth of foci of altered cells which occur in the liver after exposure to initiating carcinogens; these foci (or some of them) seem to be precursors of hepatomas. Two observations caused us to investigate cell death (apoptosis) in ppn foci in rat liver:

1. In rats without promoting treatment a large discrepancy between the rate of cell proliferation in ppn liver foci and their actual growth rate was found. Even without promotion, the doubling time of foci growth was expected to be about 45 days. However, the actual growth rate of the average focus found was almost zero for several months and

then increased gradually (Schulte-Hermann et al. 1983). Thus, it seemed that ppn cells have a shorter life-span than normal hepatocytes, which is several hundred days (Epstein 1967; Kennedy et al. 1958, Schulte-Hermann et al. 1971,1977). Alternatively, the expression of the phenotype may be unstable, i.e. foci may remodel to a phenotype indiscriminable from normal hepatocytes.

2. It is widely assumed that tumor promotion, at least in the skin, may be reversible during early stages (Weinstein et al. 1978, Pitot and Sirica, 1980). We have noted that after cessation of a promoting treatment with phenobarbital or -hexachlorocyclohexane the majority of foci of altered cells disappeared (Schulte-Hermann et al. 1983). Therefore, we wondered whether those mechanisms responsible for the involution of hyperplasia in normal liver could be also involved in the disappearance of foci after promoter withdrawal.

Putative preneoplastic liver foci were initiated by administration of a single dose of N-nitrosomorpholine (NNM). Subsequent promoting treatment with phenobarbital (PB) served to stimulate foci growth. The incidence of cell death by apoptosis in normal as well as focal tissue of the same livers are shown in figure 6. As indicated the incidence of ABs is severalfold higher than in normal resting liver (without PB treatment). Pb treatment resulted in a moderate decrease, withdrawal of PB resulted in an excessive increase and readministration of PB again resulted in a decrease of ABs. It should be noted that under all experimental conditions foci exhibited a higher AB-incidence than the surrounding phenotypically normal tissue. Preliminary results indicate that the duration of visible stages of apoptosis in foci seems not to be longer than in normal tissue. These observations suggest that the increased AB-incidence in foci (as compared to normal tissue) reflect a high rate of cell turnover and not merely a prolonged degradation of ABs in phenotypically altered cells.

In summary, these findings suggest that (1) cell death (apoptosis) in foci is of a similar regulatory nature as in normal liver, (2) cell death is much more frequent in foci than in normal liver, and (3) PB treatment seems to prolong the life span of hepatocytes. With respect to the growth deficit noted in foci without promotion, we assume that a relatively high rate of cell death at least partially counterbalances the enhanced proliferative activity. An increased frequency of apoptosis in foci and in nodules was also observed by Columbano et al. (1984) using another model for studies on hepatocarcinogensis. In addition, remodeling of focal cells to the normal phenotype may also be a (negative) determinant of focal growth. As shown previously, without promoter treatment foci express their program to phenotypic alterations only incompletely (Schulte-Hermann et al. 1983). Incomplete expression is also found after withdrawal of the promotors (fig. 7), and this phenomenon is known as remodeling. It was suggested (Schulte-Hermann 1985) that the induction of the altered phenotype by a promotor like PB reflects an overexpression of the adaptive program. Consequently, remodeling after PB withdrawal should be regarded as a de-adaptation and involution as described above for noninitiated

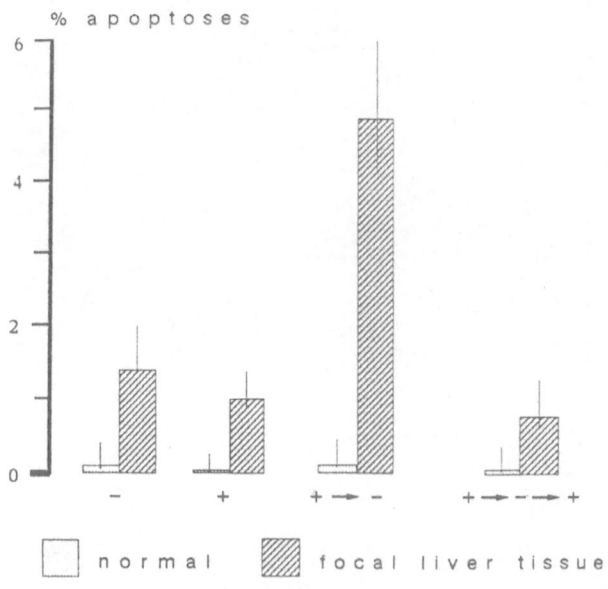

% a p o p t o s e s

normal ▨ focal liver tissue

Figure 6.

Effect of PB treatment and PB withdrawal on the incidence of ABs in normal liver and in liver foci.

Reference: Bursch et al. (1984). Briefly, rats were treated with a single dose of NNM (250 mg/kg). One subgroup received no further treatment (-). The other NNM treated rats received PB (50 mg/kg/d via the food) for 7 months and then were subjected to one of the following protocols: (1) continuous treatment until necropsy (+); (2) PB withdrawal until necropsy (+ → -); (3) PB withdrawal for 39 days, followed by PB treatment (50 mg/kg/d via the food) for 3 days (+ → - → +). The total number of ABs found in normal or in focal liver tissue is given, vertical bars indicate the 95% confidence limits.

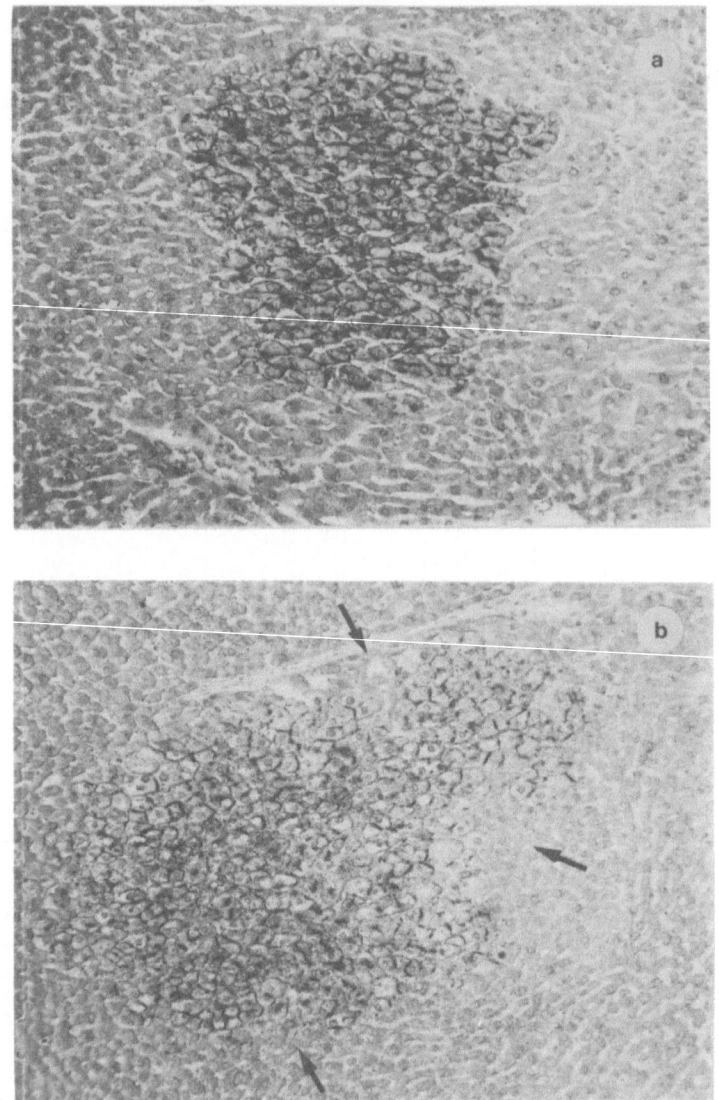

Figure 7.

Morphological appearance of GGT positive liver foci.

(a) liver focus with distinct border as found during PB administration; (b) focus with non distinct borders (area of
phenotypic remodelling, arrows) as it occurs 4 days after PB
withdrawal.

liver. We have therefore checked whether apoptosis would be associated with remodeling phenomena, and this appears to be the case (Schulte-Herman et al. 1986). Although no difference in cell proliferation was apparent, ABs were clearly more abundant in foci with indistinct borders than in their sharply demarcated counterparts. Thus, apoptosis in foci, to some extent, seems to be associated with incomplete phenotypic expression or remodeling and may reflect an involution phenomenon similar to that in normal liver when the functional load resulting in expression of certain gene programs is reduced.

Another important question may be raised in view of the increased rate of cell death by apoptosis in foci after PB withdrawal: Is the rate of cell death (apoptosis) sufficient for eradication of liver foci, i.e. is growth promotion of ppn liver foci reversible?

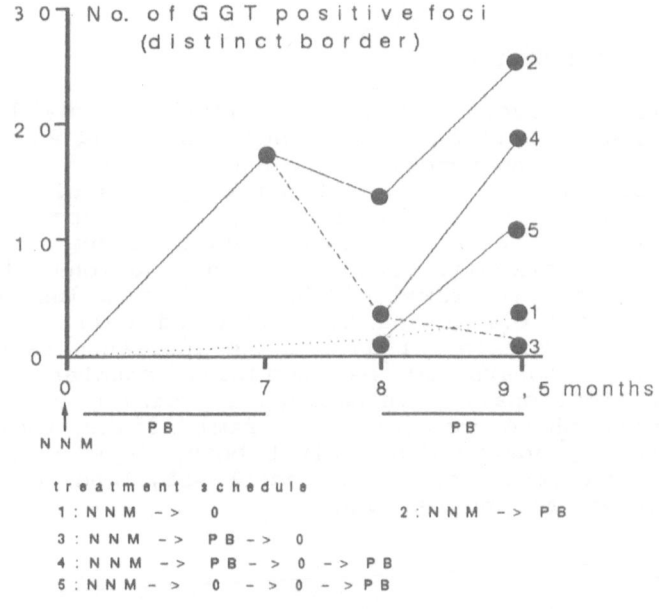

Figure 8.

Effect of withdrawal and retreatment with PB on number of GGT positive liver foci with distinct borders.

Reference: Schulte-Hermann et al. (1986). Treatment: rats were treated with a single dose of NNM (250 mg/kg). One subgroup received no further treatment (1). Another subgroup of NNM treated rats received PB (50 mg/kg/d via the food) for 7 months and then was subjected to one of the following protocols: (2) continuous treatment until necropsy; (3) PB withdrawal until necropsy; (4) PB withdrawal for 1 month followed by PB treatment for 1,5 months. Furthermore, NNM treated rats that had received no PB during the first 7 months were treated with PB from 8 months until necropsy (5). Foci numbers are given per square centimeter of section area.

A preliminary answer to this question is given in figure 8. In this experiment, NNM treatment was followed by PB treatment for 7 months. Then PB was withdrawn and as a result, the number of foci exhibiting a distinct border (cf. Fig.7) decreased rapidly. After 4 weeks on basal diet, PB treatment was reinitiated. It could be observed that the number of foci increased rapidly. Their number was clearly higher than in rats that had received no PB during the first 7 months. This finding indicates, that the foci are not completely eradicated after PB withdrawal. Thus, the question whether promotion is reversible gets two answers at present:

1. induction of phenotypic expression of ppn cells (adaptive program) seems to be readily reversible.

2. induction of cell multiplication seems not to be reversible i.e. the rate of cell death is not sufficient to eliminate ppn foci, at least not during a period of 5 weeks.

CONCLUSION AND SUMMARY

Homeostasis of liver cell number involves control of cell proliferation as well as of cell death by apoptosis. In normal rat liver, nongenotoxic hepatocarcinogens were found to induce proliferation and to inhibit apoptosis of parenchymal cells, and thereby create and maintain liver hyperplasia. The enhanced cell number is thought to reflect a new steady state of liver size (metabolic capacity) with functional demands on the liver. After withdrawal of the growth stimulus, excessive hepatocytes are eliminated by programmed cell death (apoptosis). In ppn foci in rat liver, the increased rate of cell proliferation appears to be partially counterbalanced by apoptosis. Additionally, incomplete expression or remodeling of the focal phenotype (gene program) limits foci growth. Tumor promoting agents can inhibit both, loss of phenotypic expression and cell death by apoptosis, and thereby accelerate growth of ppn lesions.

REFERENCES

Argyris T.S. and Magnus D.R. (1968) The stimulation of liver growth and demethylase activity following phenobarbital treatment. Dev Biol 17: 187-201

Bursch W., Düsterberg B and Schulte-Hermann R. (1986) Growth, regression and cell death in rat liver as related to tissue levels of the hepatomitogen cyproterone acetate. Arch Toxicol 59: 221-227

Bursch W., Lauer B., Timmermann-Trosiener T., Barthel G., Schuppler J, Schulte-Hermann R.,(1984) Controlled cell death (apoptosis) of normal and putative preneoplastic cells in rat liver following withdrawal of tumor promoters. Carcinogenesis 5: 453-458

Bursch W., Taper H.S., Lauer B., Schulte-Hermann R.,(1985)
Quantitative histological and histochemical studies on the
occurrence and stages of controlled cell death (apoptosis)
during regression of rat liver hyperplasia.
Virch Arch Cell Pathol 50: 153-166

Columbano A., Ledda-Columbano G.M., Rao, P.M., Rajalakshmi,
S. and Sarma, D.S.R. (1984) Occurrence of cell death
(apoptosis) in preneoplastic and neoplastic liver cells.
Am J Pathol 116: 441-446

Conney A.H., Davison C. Gastel R., Burns J.J. (1960) Adaptive
increases in drug-metabolizing enzymes induced by phenobarbital and other drugs. J Pharmacol Exp Ther 130:1-8

Epstein C.J., Moses H.L. Epstein L.B. and Garrison M.M.
(1967) A structural analysis of hepatomegaly induced by a
hormone-secreting tumor. Exp Mol Pathol 7: 304-326

Farber J.A. and El-Mofty S.K. (1975) The biochemical pathology of liver cell necrosis. Am J Pathol 81: 237-250

Ferguson D.J.P. and Anderson T.J. (1981) Morphological
evaluation of cell turnover in relation to the menstrual
cycle in the "resting" human breast. Br J Cancer 44: 177-181

Kennedy J.C., Pearce W.M., and Parrot D.M.V. (1958) Liver
growth in the lactating rat. J Endocrinol 17: 158-160

Kerr J.F.R., Wyllie A.H., Currie A.R. (1972) Apoptosis: a
basic biological phenomen with wide-ranging implications in
tissue kinetics. Br J Cancer 26: 239-257

Koransky W., Magour S., Noack G. and Schulte-Hermann (1969)
Über den Einfluß induzierender Substanzen auf Fremdstoff-
Oxydasen und andere Redoxenzyme der Leber.
Naunyn-Schmiedebergs Arch Pharmacol 263: 281-296

Levine W.G., Ord M.G. and Stocken L.A. (1977) Some
biochemical changes associated with nafenopin induced liver
growth in the rat. Biochem Pharmacol 26: 939-942

Meybehm M., Stiens R. and Gedigk P. (1986) Die Apoptose-
Mitosehäufigkeit in der Leber bei verschiedenen Lebererkran-
kungen. Verh Dtsch Ges Path 70: 562

Peraino C. ,Fry R.J.M., Staffeldt E. and Christopher J.P.
(1975) Comparative enhancing effects of phenobarbital,
amobarbital, diphenylhydantoin, and dichlorodiphenyltri-
chloroethane on 2-acethylaminofluorene-induced hepatic
tumorigenesis in the rat. Cancer Res 35: 2884-2890

Pitot H.C. and Sirica A.E., (1980) The stages of initiation
and promotion in hepatocarcinogenesis.
Biochem Biophys Acta 605: 191-215

Popper H. and Keppler D. (1986) Networks of interacting
mechanisms of hepatocellular degeneration and death.
Progress in liver disease, Vol VIII, pp. 209-235

Recknagel R.O. (1967) Carbon tetrachloride hepatotoxicity.
Pharmacol Rev 19: 145-149

Schlicht J., Koransky W. Magour S. Schulte-Hermann R. (1968)
Größe und DNS-Synthese der Leber unter dem Einfluß körper-
fremder Stoffe.
Naunyn-Schmiedebergs Arch Pharmacol 261: 26-41

Schlicht J., Koransky W.,Schulte-Hermann R.,(1967) Zur
Lebervergrößerung unter dem Einfluß von Pharmaka.
Verh Dtsch Ges Inn Med 73:251-255

Schulte-Hermann R. (1974) Induction of liver growth by
xenobiotic compounds and other stimuli. Crit Rev Toxicol 3:
97-158

Schulte-Hermann R. (1985) Tumor promotion in the liver.
Arch Toxicol 57: 147-158

Schulte-Hermann R. and Schmitz E (1980) Feedback inhibiton of
hepatic DNA synthesis. Cell Tiss Kinet 13: 371-380

Schulte-Hermann R., Hoffmann V., Parzefall W., Kallenbach M.,
Gerhardt A. and Schuppler J. (1980b) Adaptive responses of
rat liver to the gestagen and anti-androgen cyproterone
acetate and other inducers. II Induction of growth.
Chem Biol Interact 31: 287-300

Schulte-Hermann R., Koransky W., Leberl C. and Noack G.
(1971) Hyperplasia and hypertrophy of rat liver induced by
α-hexachlorocyclohexane and butylhydroxytoluene. Retention
the hyperplasia during involution of the enlarged organ.
Vir Arch Abt B, Zellpath 9:125-134

Schulte-Hermann R., Landgraf H. and Koransky W. (1977) Effect
of hypophysectomy on the stimulation of liver growth by
α-hexachlorocyclohexane, phenobarbital and partial
hepatectomy in the rat.
Naunyn-Schmiedebergs Arch Pharmacol 298: 137-142

Schulte-Hermann R., Parzefall W. and Bursch W. (1986) Role of
stimulation of liver growth by chemicals in hepatocarcinogensis. Banbury Report 25: Nongenotoxic Mechanisms in
Carcinogensis, in press

Schulte-Hermann R., Schuppler J., Timmermann-Trosiener I.,
Ohde G., Bursch W. and Berger H (1983) The role of growth of
normal and preneoplastic cell populations for tumor promotion
in rat liver. Enironmental Health Perspect. Vol 50,pp 185-194

Schulte-Hermann R. Hoffmann V., Landgraf H. (1980c) Adaptive
response of rat liver to the gestagen and anti-androgen cyproterone acetate and other inducers. III. Cytological changes. Chem Biol Interact 31: 301-311

Schulte-Hermann R., Parzefall W. (1980a) Adaptive response or rat liver to the gestagen and anti-androgen cyproterone acetate and other inducers. I. Induction of drug-metabolizing enzymes.
Chem Biol Interact 31: 279-286

Searle J., Harmon B.V., Bishop C.J. and Kerr J.F.R. (1987) The significance of cell death by apoptosis in hepatobiliary disease. J Gastroent and Heptol 2: 77-96

Trump B.F., Berezesky I.K. and Osornio-Vargas A.R. (1981) Cell death and disease process. The role of calcium. In: Bowen I.D., Lockshin R.A. (eds) Cell death in biology and pathology. Chapman and Hall, London, New York

Ucker D.S. (1987) Cytotoxic T lymphocytes and glucocorticoids acitvate an endogenous suicide process in target cells.
Nature 327: 62-64

Watanabe K., Williams G.M. (1978) Enhancement of rat hepatocellular-altered foci by the liver tumor promoter phenobarbital: evidence that foci are precursors of neoplasms and that the promoter acts on carcinogen-induced lesions.
J Natl Cancer Inst 61: 1311

Weinstein B., Wigler M., Fisher P.B. Sisskin E. and Pietrapaolo C. (1978) Cell culture studies on the biologic effects of tumor promoters. In: Slaga T.J., Sivak A. and Boutwell R.K. (eds) Carcinogensis Vol 2, Raven Press, New York pp. 313-333

Wyllie A.H., Kerr J.F.R., Currie A.R. (1980) Cell death: the significance of apoptosis. Int Rev Cytol 68: 251-306

BIOCHEMICAL ALTERATIONS DURING LIVER CARCINOGENESIS

A STUDY OF THE ACTIVITIES OF CARBOHYDRATE-METABOLIZING ENZYMES AND THE
LEVELS OF CARBOHYDRATE METABOLITES AND AMINO ACIDS IN NORMAL LIVER AND IN
HEPATOCELLULAR CARCINOMA

U. Gerbracht[1], E. Roth[2], K. Becker[3], M. Reinacher[4]
and E. Eigenbrodt[1]

[1]Institut für Biochemie und Endokrino-
logie, Giessen; [2]Chirurgische Universitätsklinik, Wien;
[3]Institut für Veterinär-Physiologie, Giessen; [4]Institut für
Veterinär-Pathologie, Giessen

ABSTRACT

    Primary hepatocellular carcinoma was induced by treatment with the
initiator N'nitrosomorpholine followed by the promoting agents phenobarbital or clofibrate. In those tumors, the activities of pyruvate kinase,
fructose 1,6-bisphosphatase and lactate dehydrogenase were reduced. A
reduction in the activities of pyruvate kinase and fructose 1,6-bisphos-
phatase along with an increase in malic enzyme activity were observed in
the host livers of tumor-bearing rats and in livers of rats pretreated
with the promoter alone, suggesting that these changes may be a general
effect of the xenobiotic which serves as the tumor promoter in chemical-
induced hepatocarcinogenesis. Such changes were independent of the promoter used, whereas alterations in the enzymes gamma-glutamyltransferase
and glucose 6-phosphate dehydrogenase were dependent on the promoter
type. Enolase activity was not affected by any treatment. In a second
experiment, relevant carbohydrate metabolites, amino acid levels and
selected carbohydrate metabolizing enzyme activities were determined in
hepatic tumors from rats which had received phenobarbital as the promoting drug. Serine dehydratase and glucose 6-phosphatase were strongly
depressed when compared to host livers and livers from rats treated only
with N'nitrosomorpholine. On the other hand, glucokinase activity was
reduced in tumors as well as in host livers of tumor-bearing rats, while
phosphofructokinase and 6-phosphogluconate dehydrogenase activities were
unaltered in all livers. The decrease in pyruvate kinase, fructose 1,6-
bisphosphatase, serine dehydratase and the subsequent decrease in pyruvate and alanine in hepatocellular carcinoma were positively correlated
with an increase in fructose 1,6-bisphosphate and glycine.

INTRODUCTION

    Alterations in carbohydrate metabolizing enzymes have been commonly
observed during the carcinogenic process in different tissues. A decrease
in differentiation and an increase in growth rate has been shown to be
paralleled by an increase in the activities of key glycolytic enzymes,
e.g. hexokinase and pyruvate kinase[1-5], while the activities of the
gluconeogenic enzymes, glucose 6-phosphatase and fructose 1,6-bisphos-
phatase, decreased[1,6-9]. However in some tissues, the activities of
phosphofructokinase and pyruvate kinase have also been shown to decrease

163

during the carcinogenic process[6-12]. These effects may be related to changes in the isozyme pattern or alternatively the isozyme pattern may be more important in tumor development than total enzyme activity[4,5,10,13]. Indeed all tumors with exception of chemical-induced primary hepatocellular carcinoma contain high levels of a specific form of pyruvate kinase, the type M_2[10-13]. We have shown that the increase in pyruvate kinase type M_2 found in homogenates of hepatocellular carcinomas results from an increase of type M_2 in stromal cells, but not in hepatocellular carcinoma cells[14]. On the other hand pyruvate kinase type L distribution is similar to those in normal liver.

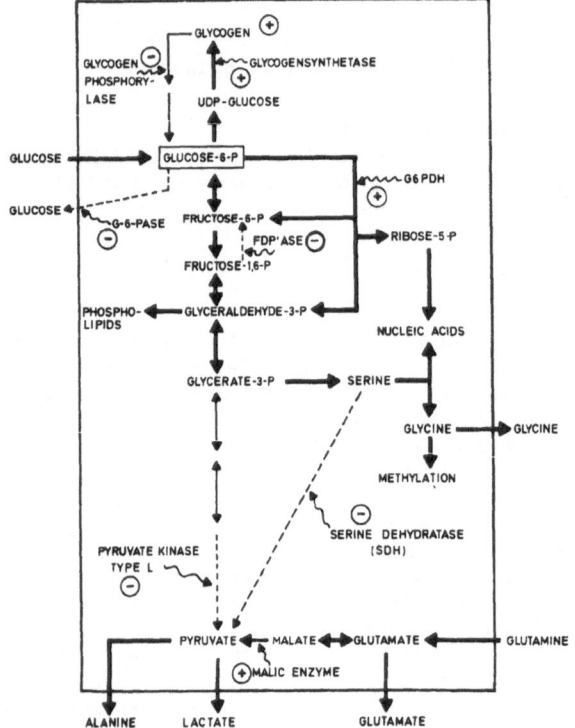

Fig. 1.
Diagrammatic carbohydrate enzyme activities and levels of metabolites in putative preneoplastic hepatocytes and in liver tumors. Alterations of enzyme activities and metabolite levels compared to normal cells, signs represent
o: unchanged,
-: decrease,
+: increase,
—>: minor pathway,
→: major pathway,
~>: enzyme activity.

The aim of these study was to investigate, whether the decrease in the glycolytic enzyme pyruvate kinase is compensated for an increase in the key glutaminolytic enzyme, malic enzyme, and whether these and other enzyme alterations are influenced by the promoter type. Two types of promoters have been identified namely, the classical cytochrome P-450 inducers such as phenobarbital or the peroxisome proliferators like clofibrate, with different mode of actions[19]. Alterations in carbohydrate enzyme activities may be a result in distinct changes of carbohydrate metabolites and amino acid levels[5]. Therefore the carbohydrate and amino acid levels have been investigated in the hepatocellular carcinomas of N'nitrosomorpholine and phenobarbital treated animals and non-tumorous liver tissues from animals pretreated only with N'nitrosomorpholine.

MATERIALS AND METHODS

Induction of hepatocarcinogenesis

Female Wistar rats 4 weeks of age, weighing 40-60 g were obtained from Zentralinstitut für Versuchstierzucht, Hannover, FRG. Two weeks

later the animals received a single dose of 250 mg/kg b.w. N'nitrosomorpholine, dissolved in water, by stomach tube. This was followed by application of phenobarbital or clofibrate in the feed beginning 8 weeks after
N'nitrosomorpholine treatment. Food was provided ad libitum, but the
dietary concentration of phenobarbital or clofibrate was adjusted during
the course of these experiments such that the daily intake of phenobarbital or clofibrate equalled 50 or 125 mg/kg b.w., respectively. Control
groups were either untreated or treated with a single dose of either
N'nitrosomorpholine alone or the promoting agent alone. Rats were killed
between 20 and 25 months after N'nitrosomorpholine treatment.

Abbreviations of treatment schedules: (0 → 0) control group,
(0 → PB) rats treated with phenobarbital, (0 → CF) rats treated with
clofibrate, (NNM → 0) rats treated with single dose of N'nitrosomorpholine, (NNM → PB) rats treated with N'nitrosomorpholine and phenobarbital, (NNM → CF) rats treated with N'nitrosomorpholine and clofibrate.

Determinations of enzyme activities

The rats were killed by decapitation. The livers were removed immediately, cut into small pieces and were stored at -90°C. For metabolite
assays, tissues were quickly frozen by using a freeze clamp technique and
stored at -90°C. Tumors from tumor-bearing rats were handed by the same
procedure. The tissues were then homogenized with a teflon pestle in a
buffer containing Tris-Cl (50 mM), mercaptoethanol (10 mM), 5-aminohexa-
nic acid (2 mM), phenylmethylsulfonylfluoride (0.2 mM) and EDTA (1 mM),
pH. 7.2. The homogenates were centrifuged at 50,000 x g for 20 minutes at
4°C and the supernatants were used for enzyme assays with exception of
those to be used for glucose 6-phosphatase activity determination. In
latter case, the homogenates were centrifuged at 11,000 x g for 30 minutes at 4°C. The supernatants were then sedimented by 100,000 x g for 60
minutes at 4°C and the pellets resuspended in ice-cold buffer.

The following enzyme activities were measured as described:
Glucokinase (EC 2.7.1.1), the final concentrations of the reagents in the
cuvette were: triethanolamine (42 mM), glucose (222 mM), MgCl₂ (67 mM),
NADPH (0.73 mM), glucose 6-phosphate dehydrogenase (0.5 U/ml), ATP
(2.7 mM) and the reaction was started with 50 µl of liver extract[20]; 6-
phosphogluconate dehydrogenase (EC 1.1.1.44), the concentrations in the
test solution were: glycylglycine (50 mM), MgCl₂ (20 mM), cysteine hydro-
chloride (6.5 mM), NADP (1.5 mM). The reaction was started with 50 µl
liver extract[21]; glucose 6-phosphatase (EC 3.1.3.9)[22]; pyruvate kinase
(EC 2.7.1.40)[23]; fructose 1,6-bisphosphatase (EC 3.1.3.11)[24]; phosphofructokinase (EC 2.7.1.11) was determined according to Brand and Söling[25]
with the following modifications: instead of triethanolamine, Tris-Cl was
used and the concentrations of fructose 6-phosphate and AMP were 4.9 and
1 mM, respectively; serine dehydratase (EC 4.2.1.13)[26]; NADP malic enzyme
(EC 1.1.1.40)[27]; glucose 6-phosphate dehydrogenase (EC 1.1.1.49)[28]; L-
gamma-glutamyltransferase (EC 2.3.2.2)[29]; lactate dehydrogenase (EC
1.1.1.27)[30] and enolase (EC 4.2.1.11)[31]. The activities of the enzmyes
are expressed as units/g or mU/g liver tissue. Specific activities of
enzymes are given as mU/mg soluble protein (nmoles per min per milligram
protein).

Abbreviations of enzymes: lactate dehydrogenase (LDH), gamma-glutamyltransferase (γ-GT), glucose 6-phosphate dehydrogenase (G6PDH),
fructose 1,6-bisphosphatase (FBPase).

Metabolite assays

1 g of liver tissue was immediately homogenized in 10 ml volume of
0.6 N ice-cold HClO₄. After homogenization the homogenizer was rinsed
with 1 ml HClO₄ and the washings were added to the homogenates. The
samples were placed in ice for 30 minutes and centrifuged at 20,000 x g

for 10 minutes at 4°C. The supernatants were collected and the pellets resuspended in 1 ml HClO₄ and than centrifuged again. The supernatants were pooled and then adjusted to pH 3.5 by addition of 5 m K₂CO₃. The samples were placed on ice for 30 minutes and sedimented for 10 minutes at 50,000 x g. The supernatants were used for metabolite assays. D-fructose 6-bisphosphate and D-glycerinaldehyde 3-phosphate[32], pyruvate, phosphoenolpyruvate[33], D-glucose 6-phosphate[34] were measured as indicated.

Determination of free amino acid concentrations

For determination of free amino acids the supernatants were lyophilized. The lyophilisates were weighed on a Chan 25 electrobalance and homogenized with 0.5 ml of a 40 g/1 solution of sulfosalicylic acid with 100 µM β-thienylalanine added as an internal standard. After centrifugation, the pH was adjusted to 2.2 with 0.2 M LiOH. The supernatants were stored at -80°C. The free amino acid concentrations were measured with an automated amino acid analyzer (Liquimat 3, Kontron, Zürich, Switzerland) equipped with an automating computing intergrator. A column packed with Durrum resin (Durrum-6A, Pierce, Rockford, IL) and a lithium buffer system (Durram-pico buffers, Pierce) with five buffers were used.

The soluble protein content was measured by the method of Bradford[35].

Statistics

Standard deviations were calculated in this study and significant differences were calculated using the Student's t-test.

RESULTS

Liver tumors were isolated from rats treated with N'nitrosomorpholine followed by continuous feeding with phenobarbital or clofibrate. The tumor tissue and surrounding liver were analyzed for their activity of carbohydrate-metabolizing enzymes. The glycolytic enzyme pyruvate kinase

2a)   Pyruvate Kinase activity

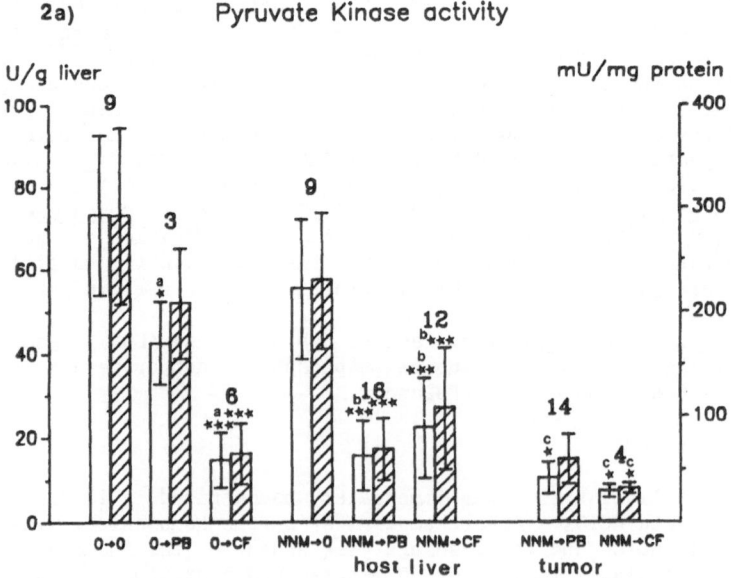

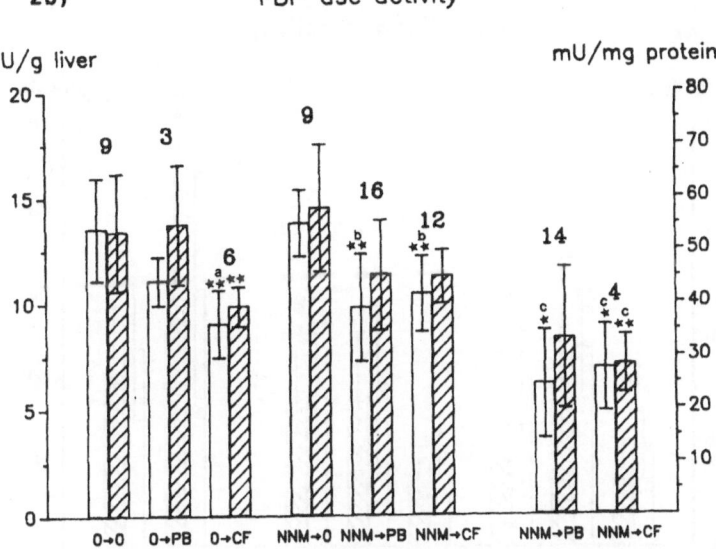

2b) FBP 'ase activity

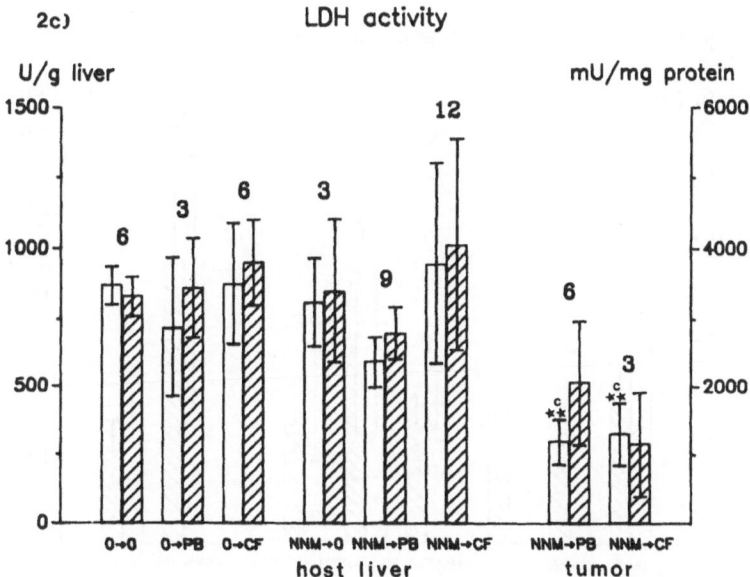

2c) LDH activity

(fig. 2a), the gluconeogenic enzyme fructose 1,6-bisphosphatase (fig. 2b) and lactate dehydrogenase (fig. 2c) were reduced in tumors as compared to the surrounding tissue. In contrast to the decrease in those enzymes, the glutaminolytic enzyme, malic enzyme, was increased (fig. 2d). The data suggest that these alterations seem to be a common effect in the development of hepatocellular carcinoma and further reveal that the variations are independent of the different treatment schedules at least in phenobarbital- and clofibrate-treated rats.

However certain alterations in enzyme activity were dependent on the promoting agent used in this experiment. Glucose 6-phosphate dehydro-

2d) Malic Enzyme activity

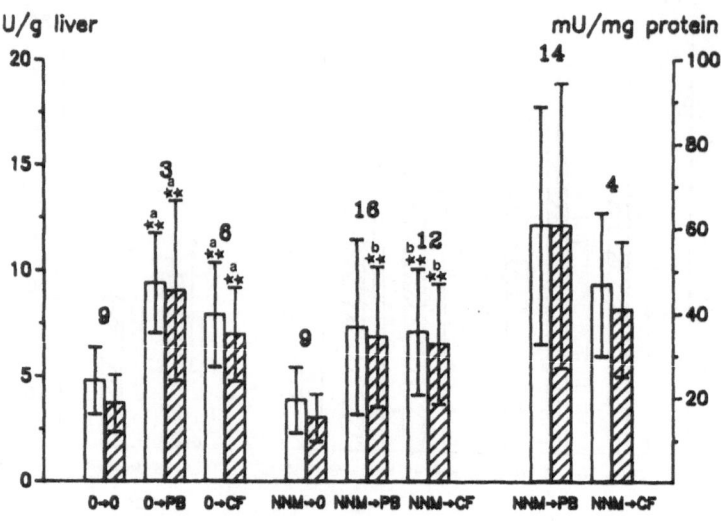

2e) G6PDH activity

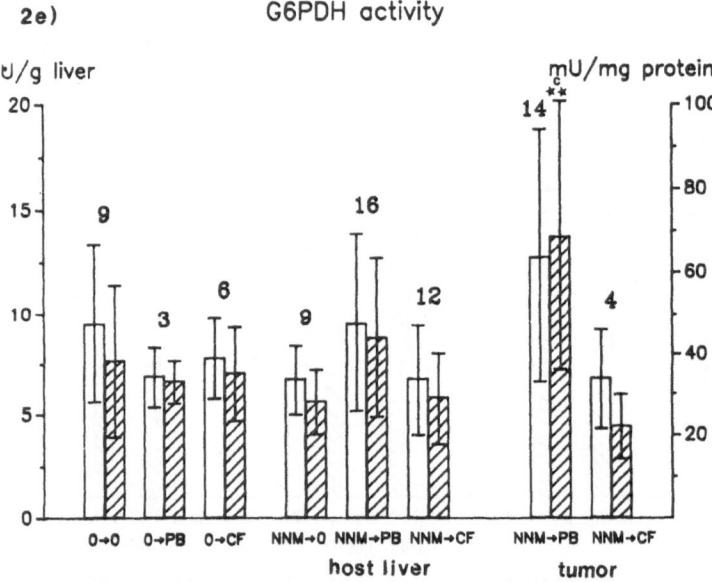

genase (fig. 2e), an enzyme of the pentose phosphate pathway, and gluta-myltransferase, a clinical tumor marker, were increased only in tumors of phenobarbital-treated rats (fig. 2e, 2g). The enolase activity was not affected by clofibrate or phenobarbital feeding (fig. 2f).

Of particular interest is the fact that some changes in enzyme activities were also found in host livers of tumor-bearing rats and in animals treated with the promoter alone. Alterations of this nature were found in pyruvate kinase, malic enzyme, fructose 1,6-bisphosphatase and gamma-glutamyltransferase activities.

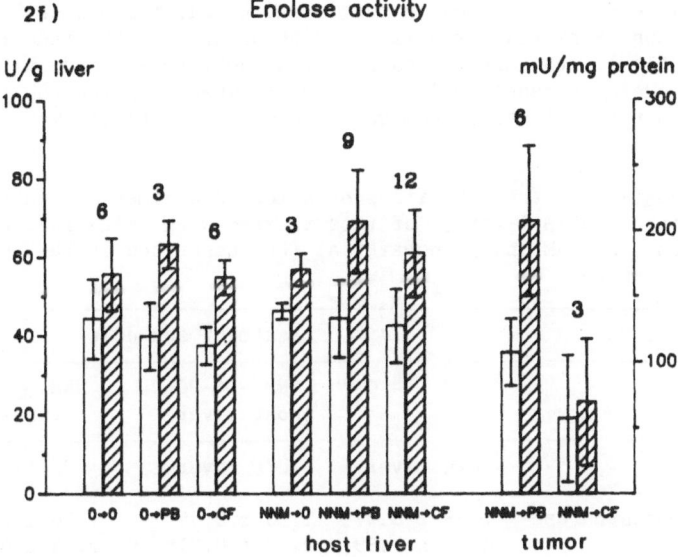

2f)

Enolase activity

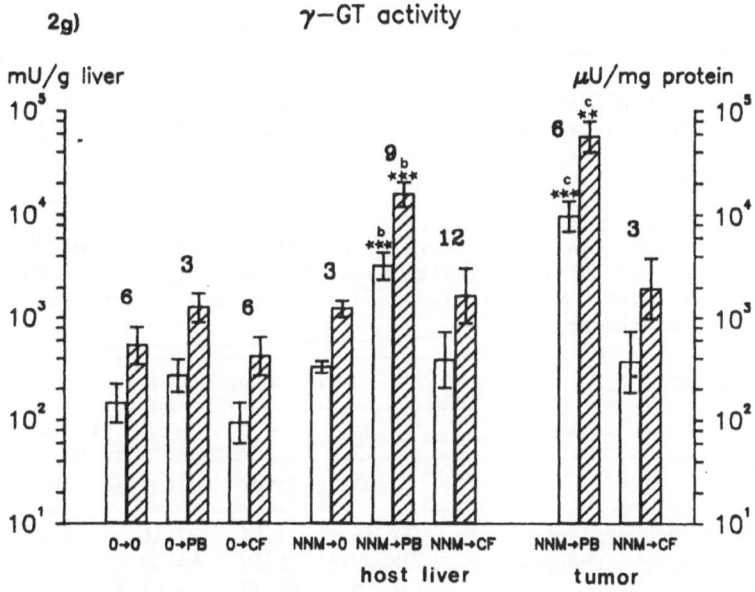

2g)

γ–GT activity

Fig. 2. Activities of enzymes are presented in U/g liver (left) and mU/mg protein (right columns). All values are means ± standard deviations. Significance of difference was checked by means of Student's t-test, a) significantly different from 0 → 0 group, b) significantly different from N'nitrosomorpholine (NNM) → 0 treated group, c) significantly different from host livers. Numbers of animals are given above the columns.

To gain more insight into metabolism of hepatic tumors, additional carbohydrate metabolizing enzymes, relevant carbohydrate metabolites and amino acid levels were studied in tumors and normal tissues of N'nitrosomorpholine and N'nitrosomorpholine and phenobarbital treated rats. As shown in table 1, the activities of serine dehydratase and glucose 6-phosphatase were strongly reduced in tumors when compared to the host livers and to normal livers. However, glucokinase activity was decreased

Table 1. Changes in the activities of selected enzymes of carbohydrate metabolism in livers, of rats treated with N'nitrosomorpholine (NNM) or NNM and phenobarbital (PB) described in the Materials and Methods.

enzymes	treatment schedule		
	NNM —> 0	NNM —> PB (host liver)	NNM —> PB (tumor)
	U/g liver	U/g liver	U/g liver
Glucose 6-phosphatase	2.36 ± 0.47	1.90 ± 0.55	1.26 ± 0.32[b)]**
Glucokinase	4.01 ± 0.99	2.23 ± 0.81[a)]**	2.23 ± 0.73
6-Phosphogluconate dehydrogenase	15.50 ± 3.54	13.66 ± 4.13	14.76 ± 6.27
Phosphofructokinase	5.20 ± 1.35	4.08 ± 1.32	4.37 ± 1.32
Serine dehydratase	2.63 ± 1.01	2.67 ± 1.92	0.70 ± 0.57

All values are means ± standard deviations. Significant difference was checked by means of Student's t-test.
* = $p < 0.05$, ** = $p < 0.01$, *** = $p < 0.001$,
a) significantly different from NNM —> 0 treated rats,
b) significantly different from NNM —> PB (host liver).

Table 2. Changes in the concentrations of selected metabolites in livers, of rats treated with N'nitrosomorpholine (NNM) or NNM and phenobarbital (PB) as described in the Materials and Methods.

metabolites	treatment schedule	
	NNM —> 0	NNM —> PB (tumor)
	nmol/g liver	nmol/g liver
Glycerinaldehyde 3-phosphate	37.26 ± 21.61	22.10 ± 2.82
Fructose 1,6-bisphosphate	22.89 ± 8.10	44.40 ± 14.38**
Pyruvate	137.29 ± 48.12	58.01 ± 29.71*
Phosphoenolpyruvate	54.39 ± 5.83	45.44 ± 23.99
Glucose 6-phosphate	166.26 ± 129.02	141.44 ± 183.37

in both tumors and host livers. With phosphofructokinase and 6-phosphogluconate dehydrogenase no alterations were found. The relevant carbohydrate metabolites and amino acid levels are summarized in tables 2 and 3. A marked increase in the levels of fructose 1,6-bisphosphate, glutamate and glycine have been demonstrated in tumor tissues in addition with a reduction of pyruvate and alanine.

DISCUSSION

The data presented show that in primary hepatocellular carcinomas from animals treated with N'nitrosomorpholine followed by phenobarbital or clofibrate, simultaneous changes in the activities of different enzymes in the carbohydrate metabolism occur. Our results are in general accordance with data from several investigations with the following exception: other investigators have reported an increase in pyruvate kinase and phosphofructokinase[1,6,7,2-4] whereas we found that pyruvate kinase activity was strongly decreased and phosphofructokinase activity was unchanged (table 1, fig. 2a). Yet other investigators, using chemical-induced primary hepatocellular carcinomas, reported a strong decrease in pyruvate kinase activity[8]. In liver cell homogenates two isoenzymes of pyruvate kinase were found, the type L and M_2. A decrease in type L and an increase in type M_2 have been reported in cell homogenates during hepatocarcinogenesis[6-8]. Immunohistological and cell separation studies by our group revealed that the type of pyruvate kinase found in liver cells and in hepatocellular carcinoma cells is the type L[14]. Additionally we showed that the pyruvate kinase type M_2 is increased in stromal cells but not in hepatocellular carcinoma cells[14]. Investigations of several different rat tumors revealed that those tumors derived from tissues containing pyruvate kinase type M_1 and type M_2 (e.g. brain, lung and breast) displayed a strong increase in pyruvate kinase activity, type M_2[10-13].

Besides pyruvate kinase, it has been reported that the other key glycolytic enzymes, hexokinase and phosphofructokinase, were increased[2-5,10-13]. In contrast, we found that tumors derived from tissues (e.g. liver) containing pyruvate kinase type L showed a strong decrease in pyruvate kinase activity, whereas there was no change in phosphofructokinase activity (table 2, fig. 2a). Tumor cells generate energy mainly by two pathways: the glycolytic and the glutaminolytic one. Therefore it is evident that the decrease in the key glycolytic enzyme, pyruvate kinase, may be compensated for a strong increase in malic enzyme, the key glutaminolytic enzyme (fig. 2a, 2d)[15-18]. It is interesting to note that one other enzyme, the serine dehydratase, is able to by-pass the pyruvate kinase reaction (fig. 1). We have therefore investigated the activity of this enzyme in tumors which exhibited a decrease in the activity of pyruvate kinase. Our data show a decrease in serine dehydratase activity from 2.6 units/g liver in tissues of control rats to 0.7 units/g in hepatocellular carcinomas (table 1). This decrease in the lower glycolytic pathway (pyruvate kinase, serine dehydratase) should lead to an accumulation in the metabolites like fructose 1,6-bisphosphate, serine and glycine[5] (fig. 1). In normal liver cells these amino acids are converted to fructose 1,6-bisphosphate and then to fructose 6-phosphate by the fructose 1,6-bisphosphatase reaction. The decrease in fructose 1,6-bisphosphatase should cause an increase in fructose 1,6-bisphosphate, glycine or serine (fig. 1). Indeed we found a 2-fold increase of fructose 1,6-bisphosphate and glycine levels in hepatocellular carcinomas (table 2, 3). This increase in fructose 1,6-bisphosphate has also been reported by other investigators[5]. The reduction of serine dehydratase and pyruvate kinase is able to reduce the formation of pyruvate and alanine from glucose. On the other hand the decrease in lactate dehydrogenase may enhance pyruvate level (fig. 1). Indeed this alteration were found in our investigation. A possible explanation for the reduced pyruvate level is a fact that the glutaminolytic pathway is unable to compensate for the reduction in pyruvate formation from glycolytic substrates. The increase in glutamate within hepatocellular carcinomas indicates that the flux from glutamate to pyruvate is rate limiting (fig. 1, table 2, 3). To draw any further conclusions, investigations of all enzymes and metabolites, located in the glutaminolytic pathway, had to be done. Alterations in pyruvate, alanine and glycine levels as reported here have been described in tumors and other proliferating tissues[5].

Table 3. Amino acid contents in normal livers from N'nitrosomorpholine treated rats and in hepatocellular carcinomas induced by N'nitrosomorpholine and phenobarbital. The amino acid levels are given in nmol/g liver ± standard deviations.

amino acid	normal liver (n = 10)	tumor liver (n = 5)
P-Serine	191.2 ± 73.2	184.3 ± 50.1
Taurine	3597.4 ± 1742.5	3272.1 ± 582.5
Aspartate	695.0 ± 323.4	1238.1 ± 621.2
Threonine	308.9 ± 86.3	418.8 ± 121.2*
Serine	477.3 ± 127.4	396.3 ± 96.3
Glutamate	1248.5 ± 283.4	1795.7 ± 291.2**
Glutamine	3755.1 ± 1308.8	3819.5 ± 621.1
Proline	129.5 ± 49.3	140.4 ± 64.2
Glycine	1956.6 ± 489.9	3396.8 ± 827.7***
Alanine	1829.6 ± 510.3	874.6 ± 144.4***
Citrulline	195.8 ± 107.8	346.2 ± 60.5
Valine	126.4 ± 29.5	140.7 ± 20.4
Methionine	34.8 ± 11.6	30.9 ± 7.9
Isoleucine	65.7 ± 18.9	68.6 ± 15.5
Leucine	153.5 ± 46.6	146.5 ± 24.9
Tyrosine	40.4 ± 32.1	47.4 ± 40.8
Phenylalanine	73.9 ± 28.5	80.2 ± 34.1
Ornithine	147.7 ± 34.4	183.3 ± 50.6
Lysine	469.3 ± 121.9	386.3 ± 64.8
Histidine	382.3 ± 117.5	407.3 ± 120.1
Arginine	11.1 ± 10.2	9.3 ± 9.5
Total AA	15823.0 ± 3575.5	17611.6 ± 2313.5

These studies indicate mayor changes in carbohydrate metabolism following xenobiotic treatment in normal liver tissue and in tumor cells. Interesting new data are presented for first time, namely a simultaneous decrease in pyruvate kinase and serine dehydratase activities and in the levels of the reaction products of those enzymes, pyruvate and alanine, and an increase in fructose 1,6-phosphate and glycine. These changes are important both from the point of view that pyruvate is a regulator of cell growth[37,38] and that glycine, as a precursor of glutathione, plays a crucial role in detoxification. The observed metabolic alterations support the assumption that in the carcinogenic process, the metabolic pattern changes from toxification to detoxification and from gluconeogenesis to nucleogenesis.

Acknowledgements: The authors wish to thank Dr. Schulte-Hermann for providing the animal facilities used during the course of these experiments and Dr. L.W. Robertson for critically reviewing the manuscript. We would also like to thank the Umweltbundesamt (FU 106.03.060) and BMFT (CMT 32A) for financial support.

REFERENCES

1. G. Weber, Enzymology of cancer cells. N. Engl. J. Med. 3:486 (1977).
2. D. Balinski, C.E. Platz, and J.W. Lewis, Enzyme activities in normal, dyplastic and cancerous human breast tissue. JNCI 72:217 (1984).
3. S.H. Gregory and S.K. Bose, Density gradient changes in hexose transport, glycolytic enzyme levels and glycolytic rates in uninfected and murine sarcoma virus-transformed rat kidney cells. Exp. Cell Res. 110:387 (1977).
4. K.D. Hammond and D. Balinsky, Isoenzyme studies of several enzymes of carbohydrate metabolism in human adult and fetal tissues, tumor tissues and cell cultures. Cancer Res. 38:1323 (1976).
5. E. Eigenbrodt, P. Fister, and M. Reinacher, New perspectives on carbohydrate metabolism in tumor cells (review), in: "Regulation of carbohydrate metabolism," R. Breitner, ed., CRC Press Inc., Boca Raton (1984).
6. K. Sato, I. Hatayama, K. Hoshino, F. Imai, S. Tsuchida, T. Sato, K. Nishimura, M. Tatematsu, and N. Ito, Enzyme deviation patterns in primary rat hepatomas induced by sequential administration of two chemically different carcinogens. Cancer Res. 41:4147 (1981).
7. P.R. Walker and R. van Potter, Isozymes studies on adult, regenerating, precancerous and developing liver in relation to findings in hepatomas. Advances in Enzyme Regulation 10:339 (1972).
8. D. Silber, E. Checinska, J. Rabczynski, A.A. Kasprzak, and M. Kochman, Isozyme pattern of pyruvate kinase during hepatocarcino genesis induced by 2-acetylaminofluorene in rat liver. Eur. J. Cancer 14:729 (1977).
9. S. Yanagi, S. Makiura, M. Arai, K. Matsumura, K. Hirao, N. Ito, and T. Tanaka, Isozyme pattern of pyruvate kinase in various primary liver tumors induced during the process of hepatocarcinogenesis. Cancer Res. 34:2283 (1974).
10. F.A. Breemer, A.M.C. Vlug, M.F. Rousseau-Merck, C.W.M. Veelen, G. Rijksen, and G.E.J. Staal, Glycolytic enzymes from human neuroectodermal tumors of childhood. Eur. J. Cancer Clin. Oncol. 20:253 (1984).
11. F.H. Breemer, A.M.C. Vlug, G. Rijksen, H. Hamburg, and G.E.J. Staal, Characterisation of some glycolytic enzymes from human retina and retinoblastoma. Cancer Res. 42:4228 (1982).
12. R. Oskam, G. Rijksen, G.E.J. Staal, and S. Vora, Isozymic composition and regulatory properties of phosphofructokinase from well differentiated and anaplastic medullar thyroid carcinomas of the rat. Cancer Res. 45:135 (1985).
13. M. Reinacher and E. Eigenbrodt, Immunohistological demonstration of the same type of pyruvate kinase isoenzyme (M_2-PK) in tumors of chicken and rat. Virchows Arch. (Cell Pathol.) 37:79 (1981).
14. M. Reinacher, E. Eigenbrodt, U. Gerbracht, G. Zenk, I. Timmermann-Trosiener, P. Bentley, F. Waechter, and R. Schulte-Hermann, Pyruvate kinase isozymes in altered foci and carcinoma of rat liver. Carcinogenesis 7:1351 (1986).
15. R.W. Moreadith and A.L. Lehniger, The pathway of glutamate and glutamine oxidation by tumor cell mitochondria. J. Biol. Chem. 259:6215 (1984).
16. L.A. Sauer, R.T. Dauchy, W.O. Nagel, and H.P. Morris, Mitochondrial malic enzymes. Mitochondrial $NADP^+$-dependent malic enzyme activity and malate dependent pyruvate formation are progression-linked in Morris hepatomas. J. Biol. Chem. 255:3844 (1980).
17. W.L. McKeehan, Glycolysis, glutaminolysis and cell proliferation. Cell. Biol. int. Rep. 6:635 (1982).
18. L.J. Reitzer, B.M. Wice, and D. Kennell, Evidence that glutamine, not sugar, is the major energy source for cultured HeLa-cells. J. biol. Chem. 254:2667 (1979).

19. K. Furukawa, S. Numoto, K. Furuya, N.T. Furukawa, and G.M. Williams, Effects of hepatocarcinogen nafenopin, a peroxisome proliferator, on the activities of rat liver glutathione-requiring enzymes and catalase in comparison to the action of phenobarbital. Cancer Res. 45:5011 (1985).

20. H. Bergmeyer, Glucokinase, in: "Methoden der enzymatischen Analyse," I:502, H. Bergmeyer, ed., Verlag Chemie, Weinheim (1974).

21. H. Bergmeyer, 6-phosphogluconat-Dehydrogenase, in: "Methoden der enzymatischen Analyse," I:533, H. Bergmeyer, ed., Verlag Chemie, Weinheim (1984).

22. E.S. Baginski, P.P. Fao, und B. Zak, Glucose-6-Phosphatase, in: "Methoden der enzymatischen Analyse," I:909, H. Bergmeyer, ed., Verlag Chemie, Weinheim (1974).

23. E. Eigenbrodt and W. Schoner, Purification and properties of the pyruvate kinase isoenzymes type L and M_2 from chicken liver. Hoppe-Seyler's Z. Physiol. Chem. 358:1033 (1977).

24. A. McPherson, D. Burkey, and P. Stankiewicz, Crystalline alkaline from fructose-1,6-diphosphatase. J. Biol. Chem. 252:7031 (1977).

25. I.A. Brand and H.D. Söling, Rat liver phosphofructokinase. J. Biol. Chem. 249:7824 (1974).

26. M. Suda and H. Nakagawa, L-serine dehydratase, in: "Methods in Enzymology," Part B, 17:346, S.P. Colowick and N.O. Kaplan, eds., Academic Press, New York and London (1971).

27. M. Zelewski and J. Swierczynski, The effect of clofibrate feeding on the NADP-linked dehydrogenase activity in rat tissue. Biochim. Biophys. Acta 758:152 (1983).

28. G.W. Löhr und H.D. Waller, Glucose-6-phosphat-Dehydrogenase, in: "Methoden der enzymatischen Analyse," I:673, H. Bergmeyer, ed., Verlag Chemie, Weinheim (1974).

29. J. P. Persijn and W. van der Silk, L-γ-Glutamyltransferase. J. Clin. Chem. Clin. Biochem. 14:421 (1976).

30. U. Bergmeyer, K. Grawehn, und M. Graßl, Lactat-Dehydrogenase, in: "Methoden der enzymatischen Analyse," I:513, H. Bergmeyer, ed., Verlag Chemie, Weinheim (1974).

31. U.Bergmeyer, K. Grawehn, und M. Graßl, Enolase, in: "Methoden der enzymatischen Analyse," I:476, H. Bergmeyer, ed., Verlag Chemie, Weinheim (1974).

32. G. Michal und H.O. Beutler, D-Fructose-1,6-diphosphat, Dihydroxyaceton-phosphat und D-Glycerinaldehyd-3-phosphat, in: "Methoden der enzymatischen Analyse," II:1359, H. Bergmeyer, ed., Verlag Chemie, Weinheim (1974).

33. R. Czok und W. Lamprecht, Phosphoenolpyruvat und D-Glycerat-2-phosphat, in: "Methoden der enzymatischen Analyse," II:1491, H. Bergmeyer, ed., Verlag Chemie, Weinheim (1974).

34. H. Bergmeyer und G. Michal, D-Glucose-6-phosphat, in: "Methoden der enzymatischen Analyse," II:1279, H. Bergmeyer, ed., Verlag Chemie, Weinheim (1974).

35. Bio-Rad Laboratories, Bio-Rad protein assay instruction manual. Bio-Rad Laboratories GmbH, München (1983).

36. T. Kitagawa and H.C. Pitot, The regulation of serine dehydratase and glucose-6-phosphatase in rat liver during diethylnitrosamine and N-2-fluorenylacetamide feeding: a histochemical study. Cancer Res. 35:1075 (1975).

37. W.J. Wasilenko and A.C. Marchok, Pyruvate regulation of growth and differentiation in primary cultures of rat tracheal epithelial cells. Exper. Cell Res. 155:507 (1984).

38. J. Groelke and H. Amos, Transaminase inhibitors block glycolysis and G_1 to S phase progression in chick embryo fibroblasts. Reversal by α-Keto acids. J. Cell Phys. 119:133 (1984).

39. E. Eigenbrodt and M. Reinacher, Carbohydrate metabolism in neoplastic tissue. Infusionstherapie 13:85 (1986).

THE EXPRESSION OF CELL SURFACE RECEPTORS IN

REGENERATING AND NEOPLASTIC LIVER TISSUE

Lennart C Eriksson(1), Pehr Rissler(1), Niclas Andersson(1), Christer Möller (2), Gunnar Norstedt(2), and Göran Andersson(1,3)

Departments of Pathology(1), Medical Nutrition(2) and Oral Pathology(3), Huddinge hospital, S-141 86 Huddinge, Sweden

ABSTRACT

In this work we have investigated the expression of different cell surface receptors, representing different cell functions and different mechanisms for receptor regulation in persistant liver nodules, regenerating and normal liver. Results are presented from work on the transferrin receptor, the asialo-glycoprotein receptor and the epidermal growth factor receptor. In addition, the expression of insulin-like growth factor I and II in fetal, regenerating, and nodular liver tissue as well as in hepatomas is presented.

Transferrin is necessary for normal cell growth and for optimal cell proliferation. The receptor is recycled with the apotransferrin still bound after iron has been released in the cell. Asialo-glycoprotein receptor, on the other hand, recirculates after ligand dissociation and the ligand is degraded in the lysosomes. Epidermal growth factor receptor is endocytosed with its ligand and shunted to the lysosomes where both the receptor and its ligand appears to be degraded. A minor fraction of the ligand is secreted to the bile. The main findings of the present study are that:

- Cells forming liver nodules contain 60-fold higher number of transferrin bindings sites, but only 80% of the number of asialo-glycoprotein binding sites and epidermal growth factor binding sites, compared to normal cells. The receptor affinities in liver nodules are, however, not markedly different from those of the normal receptors.
-Subcellular distribution of binding sites, for these three receptor systems, show a pronounced enrichment in a low density membrane fraction enriched in Golgi derived membranes and endocytic vesicles. In nodules Golgi/endosome enrichment is less accentuated.
-The increased ferrotransferrin receptor density, found in nodular cells, is not associated with increased cellular uptake of iron.
-Inability to acidify endosome compartments, with the subsequent failure to dissociate the receptor-ligand complex, is

suggested to explain receptor relocalization and the deficient iron accumulation seen in liver nodules. Incapacity of the proton pump, involved in acidification, may also explain the increase in the number of transferrin receptors.
-Liver nodules are resistant to downregulation of a low-affinity form of the epidermal growth factor receptor by 2-acetylaminofluorene. This may contribute to their ability to grow in the presence of the compound during promotion/selection.

Insulin-like growth factors (IGF-I and IGF-II) are required for normal fetal and post-pubertal growth. Fetal liver express a high rate of IGF-II production, measured as IGF-II mRNA, and a low rate of IGF-I synthesis. In adult liver the opposite situation occurs, i.e a high level of IGF-I mRNA and a low level of IGF-II mRNA.
The expression of IGF-I is lower than normal in nodules and carcinomas. IGF-II appears in the majority of hepatomas, suggesting the possibility of autocrine, or paracrine growth regulation in malignancy.

INTRODUCTION

In our work on mechanisms of chemical carcinogenesis using the liver model we have become increasingly interested in regulation of cellular behaviour by agonist-receptor interaction, receptor internalization, signal transduction and second messengers.

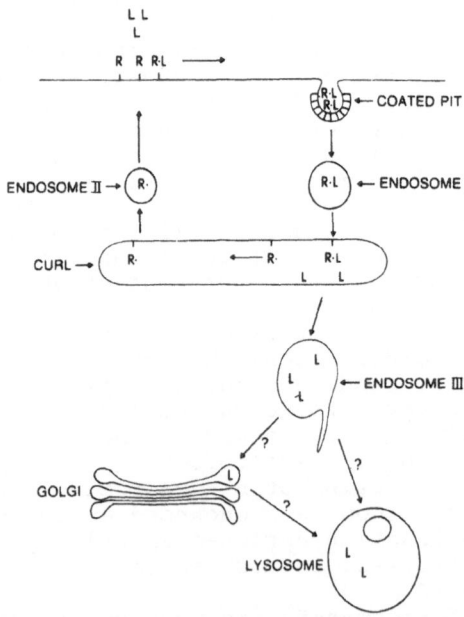

Fig 1.   Schematic presentation of receptor-ligand internalization. L=ligand, R=receptor, CURL=compartment for receptor-ligand dissociation. (From Andersson, GN and Glaumann H. In Lysosomes: their role in protein breakdown. Academic Press, 1987.)

In this presentation we will present data on three different cell surface receptors, which represent three different cell functions and which are internalized and transported intracellularly in three different ways. The receptors are transferrin receptor, taking up nutritional iron, asialoglycoprotein receptor, taking up galactose or N-acetylgalactosamine terminated glycoproteins for degradation, and epidermal growth factor receptor, presumably mediating growth regulating signals ιo the cell. In the second part of the presentation we summarize work performed on the expression of insulin-like growth factors I and II in fetal, regenerating and preneoplastic liver tissue as well as in experimentally produced hepatomas.

Liver nodules exhibit an iron storage deficiency upon exposure to excess of iron (1), and are low in microsomal heme (2). These data suggest that the nodules have some defect in iron uptake/storage and metabolism. The expression of asialo-glycoprotein binding sites on the surface of cells from liver nodules is very low (3), although the cellular content of receptor mRNA is not different from normal (4). These data point in the direction of receptor relocalization in nodular cells, the mechanism of which is still obscure. A lower than normal density of epidermal growth factor binding sites on the surface of cells isolated from liver nodules has been reported (5). Despite this reduction nodular hepatocytes respond to mitogenic signals as efficient as normal cells (6). The described changes of receptor density on nodular cells encouraged us to perform this study with the aim to elucidate the mechanisms of receptor density regulation and the functional aspects of changes in receptor expression.

EXPERIMENTAL PROCEDURES

Liver nodules and carcinomas were produced in male Wistar rats by intermittent feeding with 2-acetylaminofluorene (7). Partial hepatectomy was performed as described by Higgins and Anderson (8). Receptor binding was quantitated in a total membrane fraction (TPF) to estimate the total cell content of accessible binding sites. We also prepared a microsomal fraction and a fraction enriched in Golgi-derived membranes as well as endocytic vesicles (low density membrane fraction, LDF). The fractionation procedures are described in detail in (9). Radio-iodinated ligands were used for the binding studies. Binding of ferrotransferrin was measured as in (9). Asialoglycoprotein receptors were measured by binding of asialo-orosomucoid (ASOR) as described by (10) and epidermal growth factor (EGF) receptor was measured as binding to high and low affinity binding sites (1 and 10 nM concentration of ligand, respectively). Insulin-like growth factor mRNA was measured as described in (11).

RESULTS

The binding of ferrotransferrin to different subfractions in normal liver, regenerating liver (48h after partial hepatectomy) and liver nodules, produced by intermittent feeding of 2-acetylaminofluorene is illustrated in Fig 2a. The ligand binding to the total particulate fraction (TPF), containing the total complement of cellular membranes, were

177

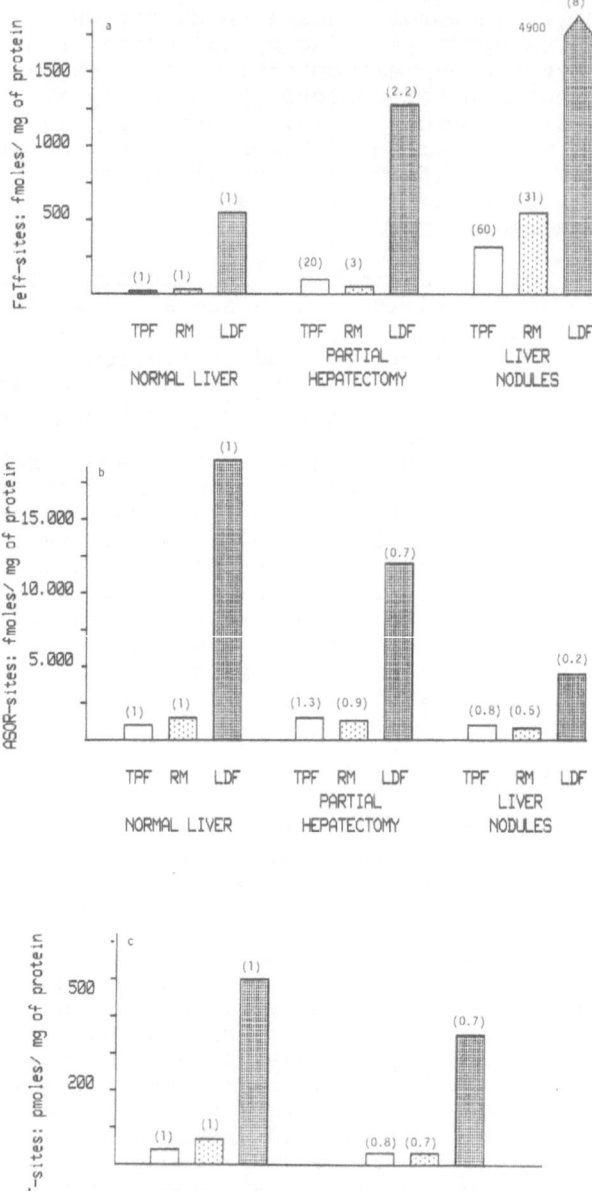

Fig 2.   Binding of FeTf, ASOR and EGF to different subfractions prepared from normal liver, liver nodules and regenerating liver. TPF=Total particulate fraction. RM=residual microsomes, LDF=low density membrane fraction. Numbers in parenthesis on top of the bars represent relative induction ratios. The specific receptor content in membrane fractions from normal rats is normalized to 1.

increased above normal in regenerating liver and even more so in liver nodules, which expressed a 60-fold increase in ferrotransferrin ᛉ binding. The binding sites were heterogeneously distributed amoung different subcellular compartments. The highest specific content was found in the Golgi/endosome-enriched fraction. Regenerating liver and persistent liver nodules showed a similar intracellular distribution pattern although the degree of enrichment in the low density fraction was considerably less pronounced, indicating a relocalization of binding sites in these two tissues.

Binding characteristics, as jugdged by Scatchard analysis indicated the presence of a homogeneous receptor population. Only the number of binding sites varied in the three tissues, no significant differencies were detected in binding affinities. Table I lists the K_D values in LDF. In spite of the increased number of binding sites in liver nodules, the uptake of iron was slower than normal after intraportal injection of 59-Fe-labelled transferrin. (Fig. 3.)

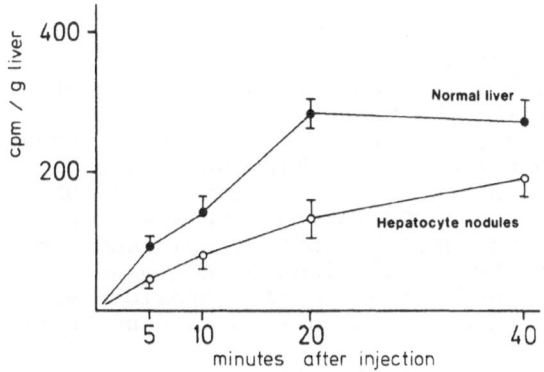

Fig 3. Uptake of 59-Fe into normal liver and liver nodules following intraportal injection of 59-Fe-transferrin. Data from (9).

Regarding the asialo-glycoprotein receptor, measured as asialo-orosomucoid (ASOR) binding sites, the highest specific binding was found in the Golgi/endosome-enriched fraction, LDF (Fig2b). No significant change could be seen in ASOR binding to TPF of regenerating liver tissue and only a slight reduction of ASOR binding to the membranes of nodular liver tissue compared to normal liver was noted. However, a considerable relocalization of binding sites within the cell was appearant, with a relative reduction of LDF binding sites in nodules, to 25% of normal binding. Also in the case of ASOR binding, affinity constants and ligand specificities were not altered and only a single, homogeneous receptor population was detected. For K_D see Table I.

Table I. Dissociation constants (K_D) for ferrotransferrin receptor, ASOR-receptor and EGF-receptor in LDF from different liver tissues (nM).

	FeTf	ASOR	EGF High affinity	EGF Low affinity
Normal liver	0.53	0.38	0.82	8.2
Partial hepatectomy	0.51	0.39	nd	nd
Liver nodules	0.41	0.34	1.2	11.2
2-AAF treatment	nd	nd	2.8	18.6

2-AAF treatment was performed by feeding 0.05% 2-AAF for 2 weeks (nd= not determined).

The number of binding sites for EGF on the surface of nodular liver cells have been reported to be markedly lower than normal (5,13). The binding of EGF to the total membrane fraction (TPF) was, however, only slightly reduced in nodules, retaining 80% of normal binding (Fig 2c). The specific content of EGF binding sites was highest in LDF and similar to transferrin and ASOR binding. This enrichment was less pronounced in nodules. In both normal and nodular liver tissue there are two populations of EGF binding sites, one high affinity binder with a K_D of approximatively 1 nM, and one low affinity binder, with a K_D of around 10 nM (Table I).

The number of EGF binding sites on the cell surface can be downregulated by ligand interaction (EGF or TGF-alpha). Intriguing is also the decrease in receptor number noted upon 2-acetylaminofluorene treatment (13). As is evident from our data presented in Fig 4a and 4b, 2-AAF treatment affects the low and high affinity sites differently in nodular liver cells, compared to normal liver cells. In untreated cells the high affinity binder decreases immediately after 2-AAF exposure (Fig 4a), while in nodules, this binder decreases following a transient increase. The number of low affinity binding sites in normal cells also decreases upon exposure to 2-AAF (Fig 4b). In liver nodules the EGF binding increases to a level 2.5 fold the normal in 4 days. A plateau is reached at a level of 1.5-fold the normal.

Insulin-like growth factor (IGF) expression was measured by determining the mRNA levels for IGF-I and IGF-II in livers of fetal, neonatal, adolescent and adult rats as well as in regenerating liver, liver nodules and hepatomas. IGF-II mRNA was expressed in fetal and neonatal liver, but decreased soon after birth. IGF-I, however, was low in fetal liver and increased after birth to be maintained at a constant high level throughout the adult life (11). During regeneration no change in this balance was noted (11).

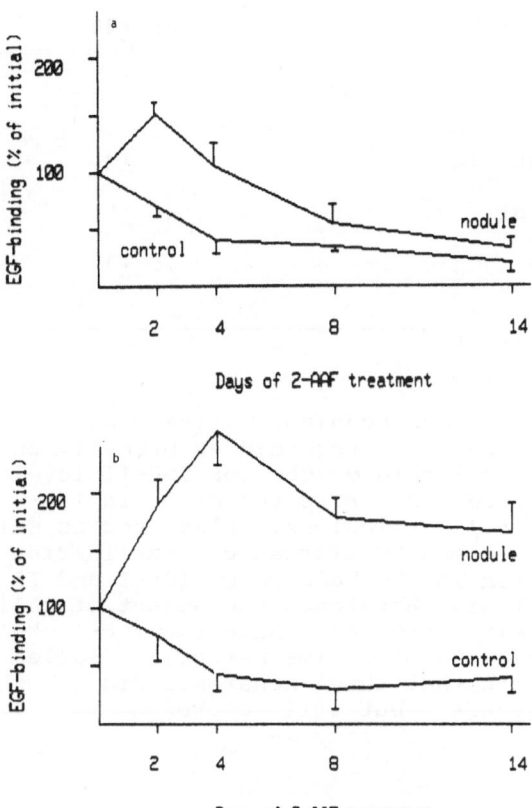

Fig 4.   Binding of EGF to membrane fractions prepared from
          normal and nodular rats fed 0.05% 2-AAF diet for
          the time indicated. Data are the mean of three
          experiments ± SD.

Table II. Levels of IGF-I and IGF-II mRNA in normal liver, liver nodules and in hepatomas.

Experimental group (n)	IGF-I mRNA	IGF-II mRNA
	molecules/cell	
Normal liver (7)	222 +12	< dl
Liver nodules (8)	125 +23	< dl
Hepatomas		
Moderate-poor (3)	7 +3	125 +26
Moderate (3)	20 +6	20 +9
Moderate (3)	15 +3	< dl

dl=detection limit.

Persistant liver nodules, developing in the process of hepatocarcinogenesis and regarded as premalignant precursors to hepatomas, maintained the low IGF-II levels of normal liver, but showed a moderate reduction in IGF-I mRNA content (Table II). In liver lesions, diagnosed as malignant hepatocellular carcinomas by microscopic examination considerable changes were seen in the balance of IGF-I and II expression. In six out of nine hepatomas the amount of cellular IGF-II mRNA was markedly increased, while the IGF-I mRNA was reduced to levels below 20 molecules per cell (Table II). It is important to note that three hepatomas did not show increased IGF-II mRNA levels, but still expressed very low values of IGF-I mRNA.

DISCUSSION

The mechanisms of receptor regulation is complex and involves receptor synthesis and transport, availability of ligand, receptor-ligand binding, endocytosis, dissociation of receptor-ligand complex, degradation of receptor or receptor recycling. In the case of nodular cells, the receptor expression is apparently different from that of normal liver cells. It is possible that normal and nodular cells, in vivo, might be exposed to different ligand concentrations, for instance due to differencies in blood supply. Future tissue culture experiments will separate the part of the nodular phenotype that is genetically controlled from the part that is regulated via humoral differential factors.

Regarding the recycling receptors, ferrotransferrin receptor and asialo-glycoprotein receptor, our data can be interpreted to suggest a defect acidification of the endosome compartment in nodules as a common mechanism explaining the nodular receptor profile. A reduced proton pump activity would result in an insufficient pH reduction in endosomes and lysosomes to allow ligand dissociation from the receptors. Ferrotransferrin-receptor complexes would then not release the iron but the entire complexes would recirculate back to the cell surface. The resulting low uptake of iron, could then induce, by feed-back regulatory mechanisms, an increased receptor synthesis. In the case of ASOR receptor, a defect protonpump could inhibit receptor-ligand dissociation and recirculation, thus shunting the entire complex to the lysosomes. In fact, treatment with weak bases like chloroquine, well known for its inhibitory effect on the acidification of the lysosomal compartment, and phenobarbital increase the amount of transferrin receptors in rat liver (unpublished data).

The mechanisms or the consequences of EGF receptor changes in persistant liver nodules is not known. It is, however, intriguing to speculate that maintained high levels of EGF low affinity receptor in nodular cells in the presence of 2-AAF may explain the resistance of the initiated cells to the mitoinhibitory effect of 2-AAF and as a result promote their ability to grow in presence of the compound. This differential response to toxic substances have been suggested to be fundamental in 2-AAF selection/promotion (14).

Our data on IGF expression in the process of hepatocarcinogenesis suggest an association of IGF-I decrease with premalignant growth behavior. Cell growth can still be controlled, although the basal rate of proliferation is higher than normal in this tissue. The malignant transformation and autonomous growth properties is correlated to the appearance of high levels of IGF-II mRNA. Rechler et al. (15) have shown that IGF-II receptors are present in both normal and transformed liver cells. It is therefore tempting to suggest that the late appearance of IGF-II might result in a growth advantage of neoplastic cells by an autocrine or paracrine mechanism. The fact that three lesions, characterized as hepatomas, did not show increased levels of IGF-II mRNA may be explained, for instace, by mRNA degradation or overdiagnosis in the microscopic classification of malignancy. It is also possible that the results reflect a true heterogeniety among different cancers suggesting that there are alternative pathways by which the state of malignant growth is reached.

During the process of chemical hepatocarcinogenesis many different cellular alterations appear, the relevance of which for the development of cancer remains to be clarified. It is, however, intriguing to speculate that in a multistep process a series of cellular changes, including up and down regulation of growth factors and growth factor receptors, may result in a growth advantage. The establishment of autocrine and/or paracrine growth regulation might explain the autonomy in tumor cell behavior.

AKNOWLEDGEMENTS

This work was supported by the Swedish Medical Research Council.

REFERENCES

1. G. M. Williams and R. S. Yamamoto, Absence of stainable iron from preneoplastic and neoplastic rat liver with 8-hydroxyquinoline-induced siderosis. J. Natl. Cancer Inst. 49:685 (1972).

2. D. L. Stout and F. F. Becker, Heme enzyme pattern in rat liver nodules and tumours. Cancer Res. 47:963 (1987).

3. R. P. Evarts, E. R. Marsden, P. Hanna, P. J. Wirth, and S. S. Thorgeirsson, Isolation of preneoplastic rat liver cells by centrifugal elutriation and binding to asialofetuin. Cancer Res, 44:5718 (1984).

4. B. E. Huber, I. B. Glowinski and S. S. Thorgeirsson, Transcriptional and post-transcriptional regulation of the asialoglycoprotein receptor in normal and neoplastic rat liver. J. Biol. Chem. 261:12400 (1986).

5. L. Harris, V. Preat and E. Farber, Decreased epidermal growth factor (EGF), asialoorosomucoid (ASOR) and apoprotein-E (APO-EL) binding during rat hepatocarcinogenesis. Proc. Amer. Assoc. Cancer Res. 27:842 (1986).

6. J. Rotstein, D. S. R. Sarma and E. Farber, Sequential alterations in growth control and cell dynamics of rat hepatocytes in earley precancerous steps in hepatocarcinogenesis. Cancer Res, 46:2377 (1986).

7. L. C. Eriksson, U-B. Torndal and G. N. Andersson, Isolation and characterization of endoplasmic reticulum and Golgi apparatus from hepatocyte nodules in male Wistar rats. Cancer Res, 43: 3335 (1983).

8. G. M. Higgins and R. M. Andersson, Experimental pathology of the liver. I. Restoration of the liver of the white rat following partial surgical removal. Arch. Pathol 12: 186 (1931).

9. L. C. Eriksson, U-B. Torndal and G. N. Andersson, The transferrin receptor in hepatocyte nodules: binding properties, subcellular distribution and endocytosis. Carcinogenesis, 7:1467 (1986).

10. R. L. Hudgin, W. E. Pricer, G. Ashwell Jr., R. J. Stockert, A. G. Morell, J. Biol. Chem., 249: 5536 (1974).

11. G. Norstedt, C. Möller, L. C. Eriksson and G.N. Andersson, Expression of insulin-like growth factor (IGF-I) and IGF-II during hepatic development, proliferationa and carcinogenesis in the rat. Carcinogenesis, In press.

12. L. Harris, V. Preat and E. Farber, Patterns of ligand binding to normal, regenerating, preneoplastic and neoplastic rat hepatocytes. Cancer Res.In Press (1987).

13. Z. Josefsberg, B. I. Carr, D. Hwang, G. Barseghian, C. Tomkinson and A. Lev-Ran, Effect of 2-acetylaminofluorene on the binding of epidermal growth factor to microsomal and Golgi fractions of rat liver. Cancer Res, 44:2754 (1984).

14. E. Farber, Cellular biochemistry of the stepwise development of cancer with chemicals: G.H.A. Clowes Memorial Lecture. Cancer Res, 44: 5463 (1984).

15. M. W. Rechler, J. Zapf, S. P. Nissely, E. R. Froesch, A. C. Moses, J. M. Podskalny, J. E. Shilling and R. E. Humbel, Interactions of insulin-like growth factors I and II and multiplication-stimulating activity with receptors and serum carrier proteins. Endocrinology, 107:1451 (1980).

CHOLESTEROL METABOLISM DURING CELL PROLIFERATION

P.Pani, S.Dessì and B.Batetta

Istituto di Farmacologia e Patologia Biochimica, Università di Cagliari, Cagliari, Italy

Cholesterol metabolism has been extensively studied for its role in cell replication and growth (1). Besides the fact that cholesterol is a constitutive physiological compound of plasma membranes, it is believed that intermediate molecules of its metabolism are directly implied with DNA synthesis (2). Several experimental reports support these assumptions. The following general considerations can be recalled:

1. A "continuous" flow of cholesterol synthesis is needed during cell proliferation in order to supply the cholesterol required for biogenesis of new membranes that must accompany cell growth (3).

2. The pioneering work of Siperstein showed the loss of feedback inhibition by cholesterol on hydroxy-methyl-glutaryl coenzyme A (HMGCoA) reductase in tumoral tissue (4).

3. In the last decade different Authors have repeatedly given "in vitro" experimental evidence that isoprenoid units are directly correlated with DNA synthesis (5-7).

4. Cholesterol synthesis and correlated metabolic pathways (hexose monophosphate (HMP) shunt, cholesterol esterification, lipoprotein metabolism) are synchronized with DNA synthesis and with the extent of parenchymal cell proliferation (8-12).

The occurence of parenchymal proliferation in the whole organism implies the cooperation of different organs and metabolic systems in order to keep a physiological omeostasis between parenchymal masses and body weight. An impairment in any step of this network may unbalance the capacity of different tissues to mantain their own physiological proliferative state or to respond to mitogenic stimuli. On the other hand, an ouburst of parenchymal proliferation may alter the general asset of the same biochemical pathways associated with cell replication and growth. It is then conceivable that alterations of cholesterol metabolism during cell proliferation may take place may take place not only in the organ site of this biological process, but also in systems that control or are affected by intracellular cholesterol metabolism (lipoproteins in the plasma compartment). It can be also expected that an impairment in the overall cholesterol metabolism and related metabolic pathways may restrain the capacity of tissue to proliferate.

The proliferative state of a tissue can be modified by different stimuli, both endogenous or exogenous. A question arises: do metabolic changes, occurring during cell proliferation, follow a general trend irrespectively of the mitogenic stimulus? In order to verify if this occur, hepatic cell proliferation was studied under different experimental conditions: a. Compensatory, in liver regeneration after partial surgical hepatectomy; b. Chemically, with the mitogen lead nitrate; c. Metabolically, in diabetic rats given insulin and in refed-fasted rats; d. In nodular liver hyperplasia during the course of chemical carcinogenesis. In addition kidney hyperplasia and pancreatic and human lung tumors were also studied.

An increase of cholesterol synthesis was observed as early as at 24 hours in liver regeneration after partial hepatectomy (8). In lead nitrate-treated rats, the increase in thymidine incorporation induced by the metal, was preceded and accompanied by an enhanced synthesis of cholesterol (9,10). Similar findings were also observed during hyperplasia induced by insulin in diabetic rats and by refeeding in fasted rats (11). In these models the peak of cholesterol synthesis clearly preceded the maximum incorporation of labeled thymidine into DNA (13).

A higher rate of glucose-6-phosphate dehydrogenase (G6PD) and 6-phosphogluconate dehydrogenase (6PGD), the key enzymes of HMP shunt pathway, was also found in all models of hepatic cell proliferation studied (8-13). HMP shunt provides NADPH for HMGCoA reductase and riboses for nucleic acid synthesis. The utilization of NADPH for lipid synthesis and the consequent fall of NADPH/NADP ratio is a possible mechanism by which HMP shunt enzymes are induced in proliferating cells.

The same trend of biochemical modifications was also seen in preneoplastic liver nodules. They were obtained according to the procedure of Cayama et al. (14). A concomitant increase of HMP shunt enzymes and cholesterol synthesis was observed in these nodular cells actively proliferating as shown by thymidine incorporation (15). It was not possible, as it has been observed in other models of cellular proliferation, to demonstrate a sequential timing of cholesterol synthesis, HMP shunt and DNA synthesis during the course of chemical carcinogenesis. However experimental evidences are accumulating on the significance of these metabolic pathways also during the progression of neoplastic growth toward malignancy (12), including the early report by Siperstein and Fagan concerning the loss of feedback inhibition of HMGCoA reductase by cholesterol in hepatic tumoral tissue (4).

Liver is the major organ to synthesize cholesterol. It is then likely that the cholesterol required by this organ for biological processes, such as cell proliferation, can be provided by endogenous synthesis. Alternatively for other organs, cholesterol could be made available through its moiety carried in plasma by lipoproteins. In this regard, kidney is devoid, under physiological conditions of any cholesterol synthesizing activity. Kidney, as liver, does not proliferate in adult rats, but it is able to respond to mitogenic stimuli, such as lead nitrate. The same biochemical modifications, seen during liver hyperplasia, were also observed in the renal tissue (16). The increase of cholesterol synthesis furtherly supports the fact that "de novo" cholesterol synthesis, and not simply cholesterol itself as an end-product, is also needed in a proliferating parenchyma otherwise devoid of any cholesterol synthesizing activity.

Our results not only point the fact that an endogenous source of newly synthesized cholesterol is immediately utilized for membrane biogenesis, but also that a pool of esterified cholesterol is needed during cell proliferation. An accumulation of cholesterol esters was found in most models studied (8-10). These data were furtherly confirmed by studies on the regulation of cholesterol esterification in two different pancreatic tumors, fast and slow growing tumors transplanted in nude mice (17). Both tumors showed the rate of cholesterol synthesis positively related to the degree of growth. In addition an increase in the acyl-CoA: cholesterol acyltransferase (ACAT), the intracellular esterifying enzyme of free cholesterol during the active tumoral growth phase was also observed. The enzymatic activity was significantly higher in fast than in slow growing tumors. In the same study a decrease of circulating lecithin:cholesterol acyltransferase (LCAT), the esterifying enzyme of free cholesterol in the plasma, was also found. A reduction of LCAT activity with a concomitant fall in HDL_2 lipoprotein fraction also occurs in liver regeneration after partial hepatectomy (8) as well as in liver hyperplasia induced by lead nitrate (10), suggesting that alteration of cholesterol metabolism are not only occurring in the proliferating organ but also in other related systems such as plasma compartment.

The possible role of cholesterol synthesis and correlated metabolic pathways (HMP shunt, cholesterol esterification and lipoprotein metabolism) during cell proliferation are summarized in Figure 1.

The increase in cholesterol synthesis serves at least two essential fuctions during processes of cellular proliferation. Firstly, it provides free cholesterol for the biogenesis of new membranes. Secondly, mevalonate or other related isoprenoid units may regulate cell proliferation by playing a direct role in DNA replication.

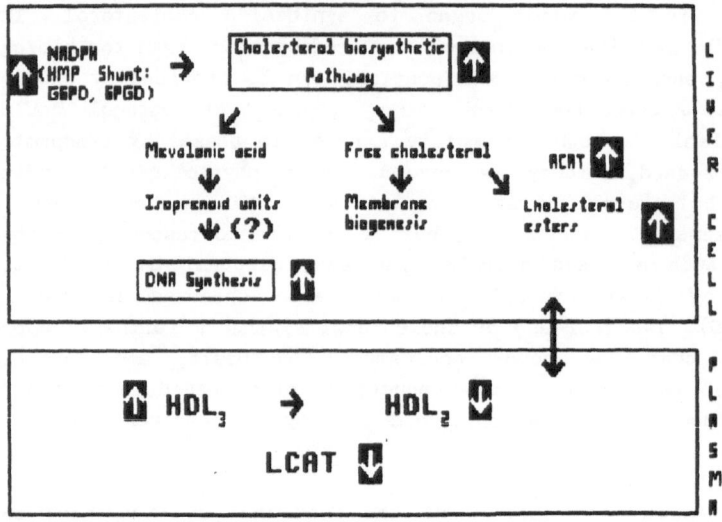

Fig. 1. Cholesterol synthesis and other correlated
metabolic pathways during cell proliferation.

The bulk of newly synthesized cholesterol causes a stimulation
of the rat of cholesterol esterification, catalyzed by ACAT, leading
to an accumulation of cholesterol esters. Being the HMP shunt pathway
regulated by the intracellular NADPH/NADP ratio, the utilization
of NADPH for cholesterol synthesis, may results in a fall of this
ratio with the consequent activation in the HMP shunt enzymes.

Finally, the increased utilization, and the storage of cholesterol
esters in the proliferating tissues, may also result in a less
availability of cholesterol in the plasma compartment with consequent
impairment of circulating cholesterol metabolism, as indicated by
the decrease in LCAT levels and by the fall of HDL_2 lipoprotein
fraction.

If the observed biochemical changes, seen during cell proliferation, have a physiological significance, one would expected that
inhibition of cholesterol synthesis and HMP shunt enzymes could
restrain the proliferative capacity of the organ following a mitogenic
stimulus. This has been repeatedly demonstrated "in vitro": Compactin,
and other inhibitors of cholesterol synthesis, are able to block
DNA synthesis in different cultured cell lines (18-20). In order
to test this possibility "in vivo", the liver mitogen lead nitrate
was administered during fasting. This metabolic condition causes
a fall in cholesterol synthesis and HMP shunt enzymes. In spite of
such inhibition, liver parenchyma of fasted rats still responds to
the mitogenic stimulus of lead in a similar fashion as in fed rats:
the peak of DNA synthesis is reached at 36 hours as in fed animals
(Figure 2,3). Lead also reverts the inhibition of cholesterol synthesis
(Figure 4), and HMP shunt enzymes (Figure 5). This suggests that

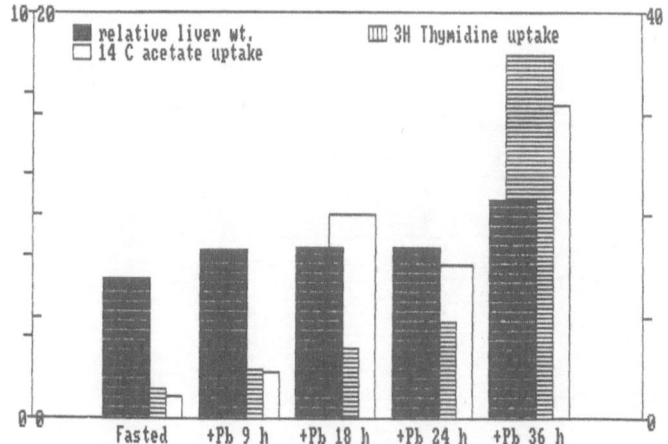

Fig. 2. Effect of a single dose of lead nitrate on
hepatic DNA and cholesterol synthesis in
fasted rats.
36 h fasted rats were injected intravenously
with lead nitrate (100 µ mol/kg body wt.).
During the experiment the rats received no
further food. The number of animals was 4
per group.

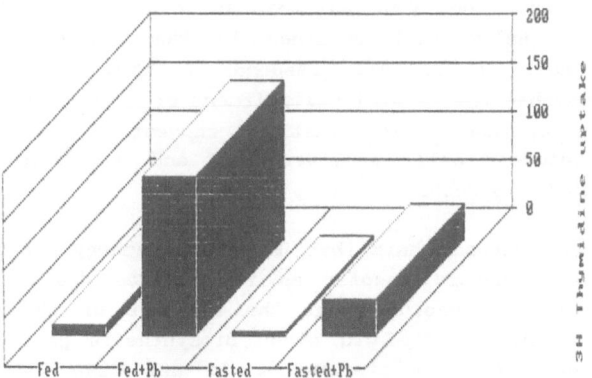

Fig. 3. Comparative effect of single dose
of lead nitrate on DNA synthesis
in fed and fasted rats.
Lead was injected intravenously
at a dose of 100 µ mol/kg body wt.
The number of animals was 5 per
group.

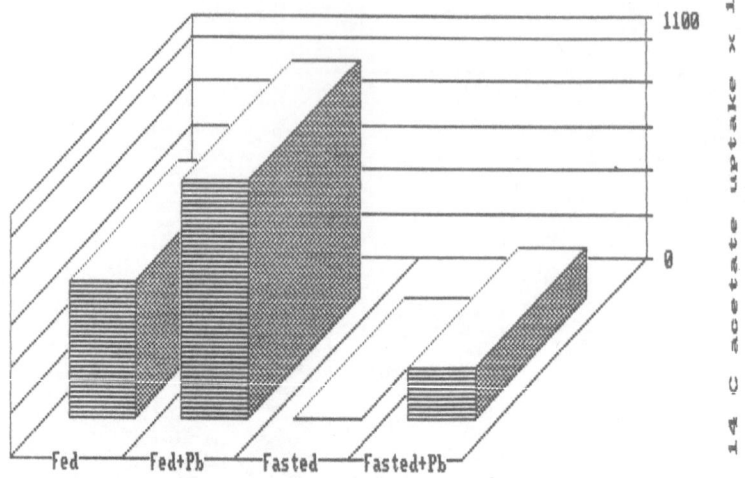

Fig. 4. Comparative effect of single dose of lead nitrate
on cholesterol synthesis in fed and fasted rats.
Lead was injected intravenously at a dose of 100
µmol/kg body wt. The number of animals was 5 per
group.

cell proliferation is able to overcome   strong metabolic inhibitions.
However, the degree of DNA and cholesterol synthesis, and of the
activities of G6PD and 6PGD enzymes in lead-treated rats during
fasting remains below that obtained in the fed state (Figures
3,4,5). Such restrain to fully respond to the mitogenic stimulus
of lead well matches the metabolic impairment of cholesterol synthesis
and HMP shunt enzymes during fasting, suggesting again a strict
correlation between cell proliferation and metabolic pathways
associated with the process itself.

It has been already said that HMP shunt pathway can be related
to cholesterol synthesis insofar as it provides NADPH for HMGCoA
reductase. We do not exclude that the increase of this metabolic
pathway may be also related to other biosynthetic processes (e.g.
riboses for nucleic acid synthesis). In any case, its increase
is a constant finding of cell proliferation, and it has often
taken as a marker of tumoral progression, in preneoplastic lesions
as well as in malignant cells (21-23). G6PD, the first enzyme
of HMP shunt, is lacking in the inherited disease, G6PD-deficiency.
The physiological relevance of this enzymatic activity strikes
with the fact that a G6PD-deficient cell population can meet the
requirement of NADPH, even if alternative biochemical pathways
can provide this reducing cofactor. We have studied the levels
of this enzymatic activity in tumoral and surrounding normal lung

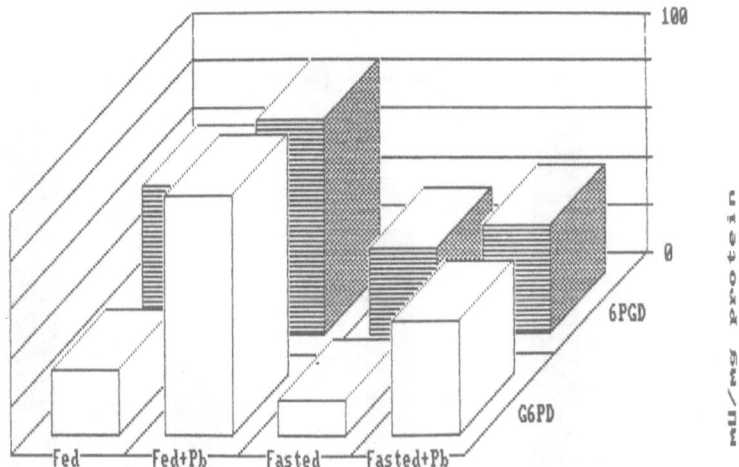

Fig. 5. Comparative effect of a single dose of lead nitrate
on G6PD and 6PGD enzymatic activities in fed and
fasted rats.
Lead was injected intravenously at a dose of 100
μ mol/kg body wt. The number of animals was 5 per
group.

tissue, taken from normal and G6PD-deficient subjects. In G6PD
normal patients an increase of the enzymatic activity was constantly
observed in tumoral tissues (Figure 6). In spite of a barely measurable
G6PD activity in the surrounding lung parenchyma of G6PD-deficient
patients (in some cases no activity was detected), the lung tumoral
tissue always revealed significant levels of the enzyme, at least
comparable to those found in the surrounding normal lung tissue
of G6PD-normal patients (Figure 6). Even if a cause-effect relationship
between G6PD and cell proliferation can not be definitely stated,
these observations provide further insights on the possibility
that G6PD is a necessary requisite for cell proliferation.

In our opinion, the observed biochemical changes in proliferating
tissues and in the correlated systems, namely in plasma, not only
could represent suitable markers to identify the progression of
a proliferative or tumoral process, but also control points for
the biological process of cell proliferation, neoplastic and non.

ACKNOWLEDGEMENTS. This work was supported by CNR (No. 86.00510.44),
by Ministero Pubblica Istruzione (40%, 60%), Rome, Italy, by Assesso-
rato Igiene e Sanità, Regione Autonoma della Sardegna, Cagliari, Italy.
The authors thank Mrs. Bruna Melis and Mr. Paolo Deidda for technical
assistance.

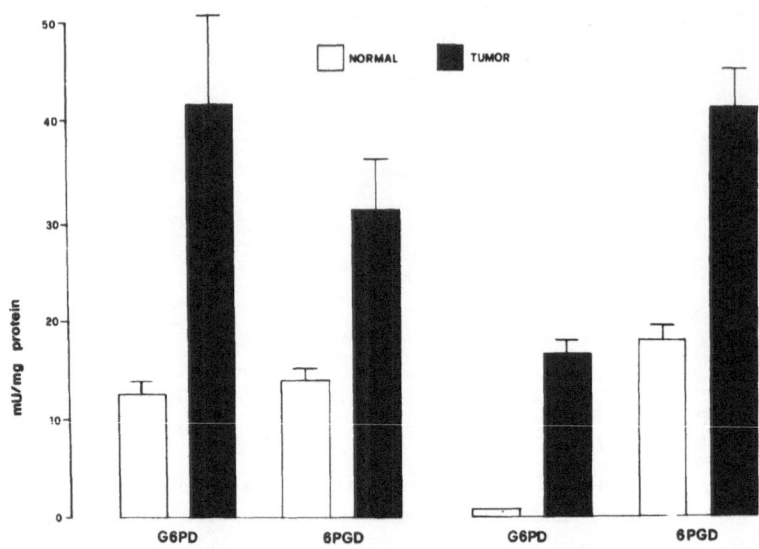

Fig. 6. G6PD and 6PGD activities in normal and tumoral lung tissues of erythrocyte G6PD normal and deficient subjects.

References

1. P.S. Coleman and B.B. Lavietes, Membrane cholesterol and tumori-genesis, C.R.C. Critical Rev. Biochem. 11:341 (1981).
2. M.D. Siperstein, Role of cholesterogenesis and isoprenoid synthesis in DNA replication and cell growth, J.Lipid Res. 5:3 (1964).
3. R.B. Clayton, The utilization of sterols by insects, J.Lipid Res. 5:3 (1964).
4. M.D. Siperstein and M.V. Fagan, Deletion of the cholesterol negative feedback system in liver tumors, Cancer Res. 24:1108 (1964).
5. M.S. Brown and J.L. Goldstein, Multivalent feedback regulation of HMGCoA reductase, a control mechanism coordinating isoprenoid synthesis and cell growth, J.Lipid Res. 21:505 (1980).
6. A.J.R. Habenicht, J.A. Glomset, and R. Ross, Relation of cholesterol and mevalonic acid to the cell cycle in smooth muscle and Swiss 3T3 cells stimulated to divide by platelet growth factor, J.Biol. Chem. 255:5134 (1980).
7. V. Quesney-Huneeus, M.A. Galik, M.D. Siperstein, S.K. Erickson, T.A. Spencer, and J.A. Nelson, The dual role of mevalonate in the cell cycle, J.Biol.Chem. 258:378 (1983).
8. S.Dessì, C.Chiodino, B.Batetta, A.M.Fadda, C.Anchisi, and P.Pani, Hepatic glucose-6-phosphate dehydrogenase, cholesterogenesis, and serum lipoproteins in liver regeneration after partial hepatectomy, Exp.Mol.Pathol. 44:169 (1986).
9. S.Dessì, B.Batetta, E.Laconi, C.Ennas, and P.Pani, Hepatic choles-terol in lead nitrate induced liver hyperplasia, Chem.Biol. Interact. 48:271 (1984).

10. P.Pani, S.Dessì, K.N.Rao, B.Batetta, and E.Laconi, Changes in serum and hepatic cholesterol in lead induced liver hyperplasia, Toxicol.Pathol. 12:162 (1984).

11. S.Dessì, C.Chiodino, B.Batetta, E.Laconi, C.Ennas, and P.Pani, Hexose monophosphate shunt and cholesterol synthesis in the diabetic and fasting states, Exp.Mol.Pathol. 43:177 (1985).

12. K.N.Rao, S.Kottapally, and H.Shinozuka, Acinar cell carcinoma of rat pancreas: mechanisms of deregulation of cholesterol metabolism, Toxicol.Pathol. 12:62 (1984).

13. S.Dessì, C.Chiodino, B.Batetta, M.Armeni, M.F.Mulas, and P.Pani, Comparative effects of insulin and refeeding on DNA synthesis, HMP shunt and cholesterogenesis in diabetic and fasted rats, Pathology submitted for publication.

14. E.Cayama, H.Tsuda, D.S.R.Sarma, and E.Farber, Initiation of chemical carcinogenesis requires cell proliferation, Nature 275:60 (1978).

15. G.M.Ledda-Columbano, A.Columbano, S.Dessì, P.Coni, C.Chiodino, and P.Pani, Enhancement of cholesterol synthesis and pentose phosphate pathway activity in proliferating hepatocyte nodules, Carcinogenesis 6:1371 (1985).

16. G.M.Ledda-Columbano, A.Columbano, S.Dessì, P.Coni, C.Chiodino, G.Faa, and P.Pani, Hexose monophosphate shunt and cholesterogenesis in lead-induced kidney hyperplasia, Chem.Biol.Interact. in press (1987).

17. K.N.Rao, S.Kottapally, E.D.Eskander, H.Shinozuka, S.Dessì, and P.Pani, Acinar cell carcinoma of rat pancreas: regulation of cholesterol esterification, Br.J.Cancer 54:305 (1986).

18. M.S.Brown, J.R.Faust, J.L.Goldstein, I.Kaneko, and A.Endo, Induction of 3-hydroxy-3-methylglutaryl coenzyme A reductase activity in human fibroblasts incubated with compactin (ML-236B), a competitive inhibitor of the reductase, J.Biol.Chem. 253:1171 (1978).

19. M.Astruc, M.Laporte, C.Tabacik, and A.Crastes de Paulet, Effect of oxygenated sterols on 3-hydroxy-3-methylglutaryl coenzyme A reductase and DNA synthesis in phytohemagglutinin-stimulated human lymphocytes, Biochem.Biophys.Res.Commun. 85:691 (1978).

20. S.Yachnin, Mevalonic acid as an initiator of cell growth. Studies using human lymphocytes and inhibitors of endogenous mevalonate biosynthesis, Oncodevelop.Biol.Med. 3:111 (1982).

21. W.R.Bezwoda, D.P.Derman, N.See, and N.Mansoor, Relative value of oestrogen receptor assay, lactoferrin content, and glucose-6-phosphate dehydrogenase activity as prognostic indicators in primary breast cancer, Oncology 42:7 (1985).

22. A.W.Evans, N.W.Johnson, and R.G. Butcher, A quantitative biochemical study of the glucose-6-phosphate dehydrogenase activity in premalignant and malignant lesions of human oral mucosa, Histochem.J. 15:483 (1983).

23. E.J.Zampella, E.L.Bradley, and T.G.Pretlow, Glucose-6-phosphate dehydrogenase: a possible clinical indicator for prostatic carcinoma, Cancer 49:384 (1982).

MECHANISM OF THE INHIBITION OF LIVER HEPATOCARCINOGENESIS PROMOTION BY

S-ADENOSYL-L-METHIONINE

Francesco Feo, Renato Garcea, Lucia Daino and Rosa Pascale

Istituto di Patologia generale dell'Università di Sassari

Via Padre Manzella 4, 07100 Sassari.Italy

INTRODUCTION

The identification and subsequent characterization of preneoplastic lesions in different tissues, in animals subjected to chemical carcinogens and in man, gives rise to a new and attractive outlook in the prevention of cancer development. It might be possible, by modulating the promotion and progression steps of carcinogenesis to inhibit the development of preneoplastic tissue as well as its progression to neoplasia. The disappearance of preneoplastic lesions has been recently obtained after treatment with certain antioxidants, hypolipidemic drugs, dehydroepiandrosterone and some other related hormones[1-5].

Choline-devoid, methionine-deficient diet is a weak initiator[5-7] and a strong promoter[5,7-9] of liver carcinogenesis. Recent observations have demonstrated that the treatment of normal rats with phenobarbital (PB), a known promoter, reduces the S-adenosyl-L-methionine (SAM) liver content[10]. This suggests that a fall in lipotrope content could be a general mechanism of the promotion process.

Lipotropes are involved in some methabolic pathways important in cell biochemistry and function (Fig. 1). SAM is synthesized from L-methionine through a reaction catalyzed by SAM-synthetase[11]. SAM is catabolized through three pathways in mammalian cells: (I) transformation to 5'-methylthioadenosine (5'-MTA) and 2-aminobutyrolactone; (II) decarboxylation followed by the synthesis of polyamines (PA) and, again, of 5'-MTA; (III) methylation reactions in which the SAM methyl group is transferred to various acceptors, such as, for instance, nucleic acids and phosphatidylethanolamine. The end products of this reaction are methylated compounds and S-adenosylhomocysteine (SAH). Interestingly, some metabolites synthesized in these pathways exhibit some opposite effects: PA are growth stimulators, while 5'-MTA is a growth inhibitor[12,13]. In addition, a high SAM/SAH ratio enhances methylation reactions while a low ratio inhibits them[14]. SAH is a homocysteine precursor and the latter is involved in the synthesis of methionine and GSH. A SAM load reconstitutes GSH level in GSH-depleted liver cells[15]. Thus, variations in the lipotrope liver level could influence some important mechanisms, such as growth, DNA methylation and GSH conjugation reactions which play a role in the carcinogenic process.

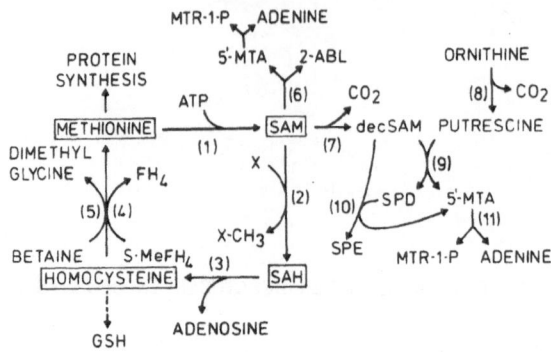

Fig. 1. Interconnections between the metabolism of lipotrope compounds, polyamine and 5'-MTA synthesis, and methylation reactions. (1) SAM synthetase; (2) methyltransferases; (3) SAH hydrolase; (4) N^5-methylFH$_4$: homocysteine methyltransferase; (5) betaine:homocysteine methyltransferase; (6) SAM lyase; (7) SAM decarboxylase; (8) ornithine decarboxylase; (9) spermidine synthetase; (10) spermine synthetase; (11) 5'-MTA phosphorylase. Abbreviations: 2-ABL, 2-aminobutyrolactone; decSAM, decarboxylated SAM; HF$_4$, tetrahydrofolate; S-MeHF$_4$, S-methyl-tetrahydrofolate; 5'-MTA, 5'-methylthioadenosine; MTR-1-P, methylthioribose-1-phosphate; SAM, S-adenosyl-L-methionine; SAH, S-adenosylhomocysteine; SPD, spermidine; SPE, spermine.

LIPOTROPE LEVEL DURING HEPATOCARCINOGENESIS PROMOTION

As a first approach in the study of the role of modifications in lipotrope liver content during carcinogenesis promotion, we verified if variations of lipotrope content occurred in experimental carcinogenesis models which are not based on the administration of a lipotrope-deficient diet.

We used the "resistant hepatocyte"[16] and the triphasic[17] models. In the first one, male Wistar rats were subjected to an initiating and a proliferative stimulus (a necrogenic dose of diethylnitrosamine, DENA) followed, two weeks later, by a selection step, during which initiated cells were stimulated to grow, by a partial hepatectomy (PH), and a second carcinogenic stimulus (2-acetylaminofluorene, 2-AAF), which inhibits normal cells growth, is given. In the triphasic model the selection step was followed by a PB treatment.

Our results are summarized in Fig. 2. SAM liver content decreases 24-35% in the animals subjected to DENA/2-AAF/PH, with respect to normal controls, between 2 and 6 weeks after starting 2-AAF feeding. No variations of SAM levels have been found in rats treated with 2-AAF alone, while a 42% decrease occurs in controls subjected to 2-AAF/PH (not shown). This, however, is followed by a recovery in SAM content up to the level found in normal liver, 3 weeks after starting 2-AAF feeding. This suggests that the reparative growth which follows PH is associated with a fall in SAM liver content which is recovered, in non-initiated rats, after completion of liver regeneration.

Chronic SAM treatment was started at the end of the selection step of carcinogenesis and continued for a maximum of 18 weeks (Fig. 2). SAM administration, in carcinogen-treated rats without PB, results in a complete recon-

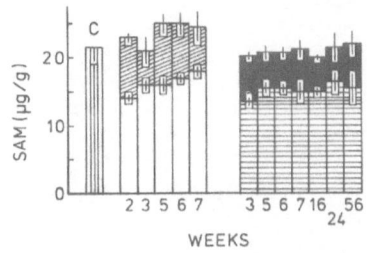

Fig. 2. SAM content in carcinogen-treated liver. Male
Wistar rats received a single i.p. dose (150 mg/
Kg) of DENA and, 2 weeks later, a diet containing 0.03% 2-AAF for 14 days, with PH on the 7th
day. PB (0.05% in the diet) and SAM (25 mg/Kg,
i.m., every 4 hr) treatments were started at the
end of 2-AAF feeding, and were continued for a
maximum of 18 weeks. The rats were killed between
9:0 and 10:0 a.m. and SAM determined in the acid
extract by HPLC analysis. The abscissa values
refer to the period of time after the start of
2-AAF feeding. Data are means ± SD of triplicate
determinations with 6-12 animals. Symbols: ▦,
untreated controls; ☐, DENA/2-AAF/PH; ▨, DENA/
2-AAF/PH/SAM; ▤, DENA/2-AAF/PH/PB; ■, DENA/
2-AAF/PH/PB/SAM. "t"-test: with SAM vs without
SAM: different for at least $P < 0.05$.

stitution of the SAM liver pool, 2 and 3 weeks after starting 2-AAF feeding.
Between the 5th and the 7th week a 11-14% increase in SAM content was found.
In PB-treated rats a complete recovery took place.

LIPOTROPE CONTENT AND DEVELOPMENT OF PRENEOPLASTIC AND NEOPLASTIC TISSUES

The enhancement of rat liver carcinogenesis by lipotrope-deficient
diet[5,7-9] indicates the possibility that the maintenance of a high lipotrope
liver content during hepatocarcinogenesis promotion, has an antipromotion
effect. Indeed, dietary methionine supply has been shown to partially prevent
ethionine-induced liver carcinomas[18] and benzo(a)pyrene-induced skin carcinomas[19]. However, this contrasts with the observation that long-term methionine administration, during promotion of DENA-initiated hepatocarcinogenesis,
does not influence tumor yield[20].

Our results (Fig. 3) indicate that SAM administration during hepatocarcinogenesis promotion largely prevents the development of putative preneoplastic foci (evidenced by the histochemical reaction of γ-glutamyltrans-
peptidase, GGT) in the rats subjected to DENA/2-AAF/PH ± PB. The decrease in
the percentage of GGT-positive liver, in SAM-treated rats, depends on a decrease in both the number and areas of GGT-positive foci (not shown). After
interruption of PB treatment (24th and 56th week) there is a marked decrease
in GGT-positive liver, whose development at this stage of the experiment, is
scarcely inhibited by SAM. However, in the 24th week hyperplastic nodules
(HN) are present in 92% of rats and represent about 32% of liver weight
(Table 1). On the 56th week relatively few HN are present in only 33% of
animals, while hepatocellular carcinomas (HC) have been found in 89% of rats.
SAM completely prevents the development of both HN and HC.

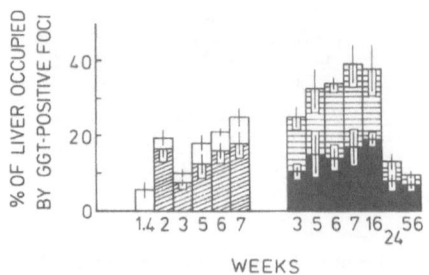

Fig. 3. Effect of SAM on the development of GGT-positive foci in the liver of carcinogen-treated rats. The same conditions of Fig. 2. Data are means ± SD of triplicate determinations with 4-12 animals. The abscissa values refer to the period of time after the start of 2-AAF feeding. Symbols: ☐, DENA/2-AAF/PH; ▨, DENA/2-AAF/PH/SAM; ▤, DENA/2-AAF/PH/PB; ■, DENA/2-AAF/PH/PB/SAM. "t"-test: with PB versus without PB, different for at least P < 0.05 between weeks 3 and 7. With SAM versus without SAM, different for at least P < 0.01 between weeks 2 and 7 in the rats not treated with PB; different for at least P < 0.01 between weeks 3 and 56 in PB-treated rats.

Table 1. The Development of GGT-positive Foci, Hyperplastic Nodules and Hepatocellular Carcinomas in the Liver of Carcinogen-treated rats.

Treatments	Time[a] (weeks)	Sur- viving rats	Body[c] wt.	RLW[c] (%)	No of rats bearing		Liver occupied by[c]		
					HN	HC	GGT+[d] foci	HN[e]	HC[e]
DENA/2-AAF/ PH/PB	24	12	413 ±44	6.6 ±0.6	11	0	12.8 ±2.6	32.2 ±2.5	
	56	9	487 ±29	6.9 ±0.9	3	8	10.2 ±1.3	4.2 ±0.8	44.8 ±3.0
DENA/2-AAF/ PH/PB/SAM	24	8	377 ±23	3.9 ±0.1	0	0	8.1 ±2.4		
	56	10	470 ±46	4.7 ±2.1	0	0	6.8 ±0.9		

[a]Period of time after the start of 2-AAF feeding.
[b]Data are means ± SD. The relative liver weight (RLW) includes the hyperplastic nodules (HN) and hepatocellular carcinomas (HC) weights.
[c]Calculated as a percentage of the surface-area of 5-7 liver sections.
[d]Calculated as a percentage of the total liver weight.
[e]Mean ± SD of 3 rats.
[f]Different from DENA/2-AAF/PH/PB for P < 0.001.

When the relative liver weight is determined after PH in carcinogen-treated rats (Fig. 4), it may be appreciated that liver regeneration proceeds relatively slowly, reaching completion 2 weeks after PH; PB has only a slight enhancing effect. Liver regeneration is almost complete in one week in rats no subjected to the initiation/selection treatment (not shown). The labelling index (LI) of surrounding liver, relatively high one week after PH, returns to normal values (0.18-0.25%; not included in Fig. 4) by the 2nd week. One week after PH, GGT-positive foci exhibit a high LI which is further stimulated by PB. Thereafter a progressive decrease occurs. However, after completion of liver regeneration DNA synthesis is still relatively high in GGT-positive foci. In the late stages of promotion (16-56 weeks after the start of 2-AAF feeding) GGT-positive foci grow slowly, even before PB withdrawal (16th week), when 38% of liver is still GGT-positive. After interruption of PB treatment LI is 4-6 times higher in the foci, in respect to surrounding liver, but it is 27-32 times higher in HN and HC. SAM treatment clearly results in a great inhibition of DNA synthesis in preneoplastic foci.

CELL LOSS DURING PROMOTION

Tissue growth results from a balance between cell growth and cell loss. Cell loss may depend on cell differentiation and cell death. After discontinuing a promotion treatment the majority of enzyme altered foci and nodules disappear[21]. This may depend on phenotypic reversion (remodelling), during which putative preneoplastic cells gradually lose the phenotypic markers and acquire the morphology, histochemical patterns, and levels of DNA synthesis identical to those of normal liver cells[21-23]. Cell death through apoptosis may also contribute to this process[24]. Our data indicate that no increase in size and number of foci occurs between the 7th and the 16th week of promotion, even though DNA synthesis in the foci is still 5-6 times higher than in surrounding liver. This could depend on cell loss by remodelling and apoptosis, a phenomenon which could be enhanced by SAM. Accordingly, we found that remodelling foci, relatively rare in the 3rd week after starting 2-AAF feeding, progressively increase from the 3rd to the 56th week in the rats subjected to the initiation/selection steps of carcinogenesis without PB. As expected (cfr. ref. 21), PB has an inhibitory effect. SAM greatly stimulates foci remodelling in the rats treated with PB and completely prevents the inhibition by PB (Fig. 5). As already known[21], non-uniform foci exhibit a LI lower than that of uniform foci (Fig. 6). SAM causes a significant LI decrease in both uniform and non-uniform foci.

As already observed[24], the percentage of apoptotic bodies (AB, including the intra- and extra-cellular bodies and those with and without chromatin) exhibits a fall in PB-treated rats. A sharp increase of AB occurs three days after the arrest of PB treatment. SAM treatment causes a significant increase in the foci AB either during or after PB treatment (Table 2).

POLYAMINE SYNTHESIS

Several observations have correlated PA synthesis with growth. PA content and activity of PA synthesizing enzymes are high in rapidly growing tissues, both normal and tumor[25-28]. Active DNA synthesis is preceeded by a burst of active PA synthesis[29]. Inhibition of PA synthesis by various compounds is coupled with growth inhibition[30].

Different reports have evidentiated an increased PA synthesis during the promotion of skin and liver carcinogenesis[31-35]. According to the results of recent work in our laboratory[35,36], liver PA content and the activity of ornithine decarboxylase (ODC), a key enzyme of PA synthesis, are clearly related to the extent of GGT-positive liver as well as to the DNA synthesis

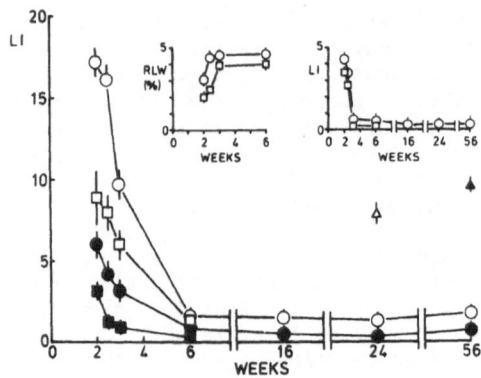

Fig. 4. Labelling indexes of GGT-positive foci, HN and HC.
The same conditions of Fig. 2. The rats were given
4 i.p. injections of [methyl-H^3]thymidine (0.5 μCi/
g body wt.) every 6 hr before killing. The LI was
determined by counting 6,000-8,000 hepatocytes per
liver in 100-160 GGT-positive foci and in 10-20 HN,
or 5,000-7,000 hepatocytes in HC and in surrounding
liver. Insert on the left: relative liver weight
(g/100 g body wt., RLW); insert on the right: LI
in surrounding liver. Data are means ± SD of 4-8
experiments. The abscissa values represent the
period of time from the start of 2-AAF feeding.
Symbols: squares: DENA/2-AAF/PH without (□), with
(■) SAM. Circles: DENA/2-AAF/PH/PB without (○),
with (●) SAM. "t"-test: PB vs without PB, different for P < 0.001 between weeks 2 and 3. SAM vs
without SAM, different for P < 0.001, without PB,
between weeks 2 and 3, and for at least P < 0.05,
with PB, between weeks 2 and 56.

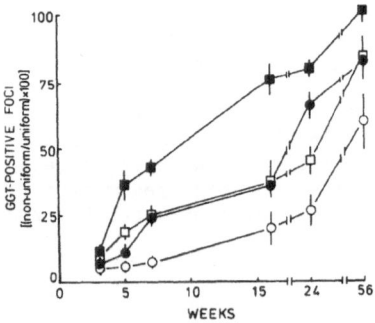

Fig. 5. Effect of SAM on the percentage of non-uniform foci
in carcinogen-treated rats. The same conditions of
Fig. 2. Data are means ± SD of 5-7 experiments. The
abscissa values represent the period of time from the
start of 2-AAF feeding. Symbols: squares: DENA/2-AAF/
PH without (□), with (■) SAM. Circles: DENA/2-AAF/
PH/PB without (○), with (●) SAM. "t"-test: PB vs
without PB, different for at least P < 0.05 between
weeks 5 and 56; SAM vs without SAM, different for
P < 0.001, without PB, and for at least P < 0.01,
with PB, between weeks 5 and 56.

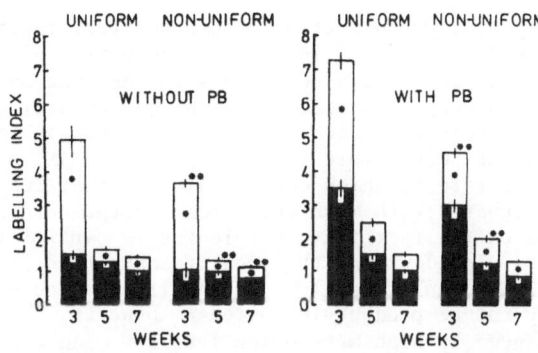

Fig. 6. Effect of SAM on DNA synthesis in uniform and
non-uniform foci. The same conditions of Fig. 5.
Data are means ± SD of 5 experiments. The abscissa
values represent the period of time after the
start of 2-AAF feeding. □ , without SAM; ■ , with
SAM. *With vs without SAM, different for at least
P < 0.05. **Non-uniform vs uniform, different for
P < 0.001.

Table 2. Effect of SAM on the incidence of apoptotic bodies in foci and
surrounding liver.

Treatment[a]	Time[b] (hours)	Foci[c]	Surrounding[c]
		(AB per 100 hepatocytes)	
DENA/2-AAF/PH		$0.89 \pm 0.24_d$	0.09 ± 0.02
DENA/2-AAF/PH/SAM		1.47 ± 0.15^d	0.09 ± 0.03
DENA/2-AAF/PH/PB	0	$0.34 \pm 0.13_d$	0.03 ± 0.00
DENA/2-AAF/PH/PB/SAM	0	0.83 ± 0.23^d	0.03 ± 0.00
DENA/2-AAF/PH/PB	72	$3.14 \pm 0.54_d$	0.09 ± 0.03
DENA/2-AAF/PH/PB/SAM	72	4.99 ± 0.32^d	0.08 ± 0.02

[a]The same conditions of Fig. 2. Fresh liver tissue was fixed with cold acetone.
5 μm thick sections were stained with H&E . Nuclear changes representing
apoptosis and apoptotic bodies (AB) were determined by scoring 2,500-
3,500 cells in surrounding liver . Clear cell and eosinophilic foci were
identified and a total of 350-5,000 focal cells were counted per liver.
[b]Period of time after the end of PB treatment.
[c]Data are means ± SD of 6 experiments.
[d]Different from DENA/2-AAF/PH PB for P < 0.001.

in preneoplastic tissue. This indicates the existence of a close relationship
between PA synthesis and growth of preneoplastic foci.

A decrease in the lipotrope liver content has been found to be associated with a high ODC activity[38] , which suggests that the reconstitution
of the liver SAM pool should inhibit PA synthesis. This has indeed been observed in rats during hepatocarcinogenesis promotion[36,37].

A study was effected in order to assess the mechanism of the inhibition of PA synthesis by SAM. Preincubation of hepatocytes, isolated from normal rats, with 0.1-1 mM SAM resulted in a great inhibition of ODC activity (Fig. 7). However, no inhibition occurred when the same SAM amounts were added directly to the reaction medium for the determination of ODC activity (not shown). It has been concluded that a SAM metabolite, formed during incubation with SAM was responsible for inhibition by SAM. Surprinsingly, 1 mM L-methionine had no effect, which could indicate that less SAM is available to hepatocytes incubated with methionine that to those incubated with SAM. This could depend on the fact that methionine is partially used for protein synthesis (Fig. 1). In addition, the product inhibition of SAM synthetase could limit the SAM cellular level[38]. In the liver there exists a SAM synthetase which may not be product-inhibited[39]. However, the product-inhibited enzyme may be induced by high methionine levels[38]. SAM also inhibits liver cell growth in vitro. Once again, 1 mM methionine has no effect (Fig. 7). We may conclude that the accumulation of relatively high amounts of an inhibitory metabolite, in the cells incubated with SAM, is responsible for the inhibition of PA synthesis and growth. 5'-MTA could be that metabolite. In fact, 5'-MTA inhibits spermine and spermidine synthetases[12,40], SAH hydrolase[41] (Fig. 1), cAMP phosphodiesterase[13] and DNA methylation[43]. We observed that it also inhibits ODC activity and that it does not need preincubation with intact liver cells to exhibit this inhibition (Fig. 7). Accordingly, adenine, which inhibits the phosphorolytic cleavage of 5'-MTA[43] (Fig. 1), enhances the inhibition of ODC activity and of in vitro hepatocyte growth by both SAM and 5'-MTA (Fig. 7).

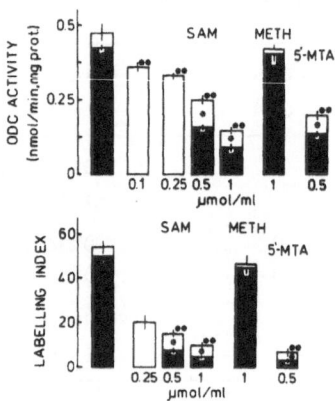

Fig. 7. Effect of SAM, methionine and 5'-MTA on DNA synthesis
and ODC activity of normal rat hepatocytes. Hepatocytes (8 x 10[6]/ml), suspended in Williams E medium
containing 20% rat serum, were incubated 1 hr at 37°C
and then centrifuged to isolate the cytosolic fraction
used as crude ODC. When indicated SAM, L-methionine,
and 2 mM adenine (■), were included in the medium.
5'-MTA was added directly to the reaction mixture for
ODC determination. For determination of LI, hepatocytes, suspended in the above medium enriched with hormones, were plated at 25,000/cm[2]. When indicated, SAM,
methionine, 5'-MTA and 2 mM adenine (■) were included
in the medium. 24 hr after plating EGF was added to the
medium, followed, 24 hr later, by 1 μCi/ml of [methyl-
H[3]]thymidine. After additional 96 hr LI was evaluated
by counting 3,000 cells per culture. Data are means ± SD
of 6 experiments. *Different for at least $P < 0.05$.
**Different from control for $P < 0.001$.

The above in vitro observations do not necessarily correspond to the in vivo conditions. Consequently, in vivo studies have been performed in order to compare DNA synthesis, ODC activity, and SAM and 5'-MTA content in preneoplastic foci, surrounding liver, HN and HC in the late stages of the promotion process (Fig. 8). The liver of rats subjected to the initiation/promotion treatment, according to the triphasic model, exhibit, 16 weeks after starting 2-AAF feeding, a decrease of around 37% in SAM and 5'-MTA contents. The decrease consists in 25-35% for the surrounding liver on the 24th and 56th week. This is coupled with a 45-80% increase in ODC activity and a 4-6-fold increase in LI. In HN, SAM and 5'-MTA contents decrease by 60-70%, ODC increases by 326% and LI increases by about 30 times. In HC these figures are 61, 66 and 352%. Therefore, a SAM decrease in preneoplastic tissue is associated with a decrease in 5'-MTA content and an enhancement in growth. A SAM load causes SAM and 5'-MTA accumulation and inhibition of ODC activity.

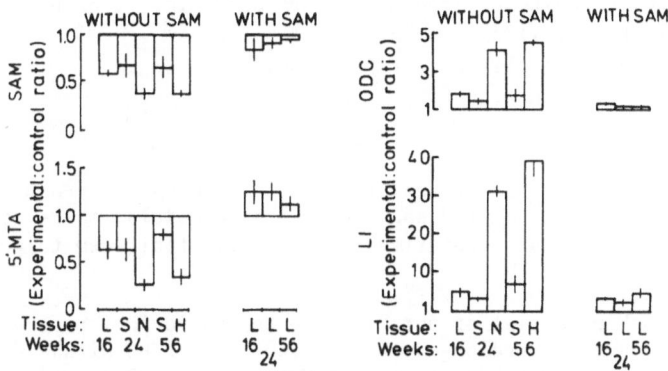

Fig. 8. Effect of SAM administration on the SAM and 5'-MTA contents, ODC activity and LI of liver, HN and HC in carcinogen-treated rats. The same conditions of Fig. 2. LI was determined in GGT-positive liver as described in the legend of Fig. 4. Data are means ± SD of triplicate determinations with 5-12 rats. Control: normal rats. Weeks: period of time after the start of 2-AAF feeding. Abbreviations: L, liver; S, surrounding; N, nodules; H, hepatocellular carcinoma.

The data in Fig. 8 also indicate that during active PA synthesis no 5'-MTA accumulation occurs in growing tissues. This could depend on an increased catabolism of 5'-MTA in these tissues. In accordance with this hypothesis, 5'-MTA phosphorylase (Table 3) is 61% and 123% higher in surrounding liver of carcinogen-treated rats, 24 and 56 weeks after starting 2-AAF feeding, in respect to normal liver. In HN and HC there occurs respectively a 396% and a 411% increase in phosphorylase activity.

CONCLUSIONS

Available evidence indicates that variations in the lipotrope content modulate liver carcinogenesis promotion[8-10,35,36]. There exist complex relationships between the SAM liver level and PA synthesis and growth. The following points have been established:

Table 3. 5'-MTA phosphorylase activity in hyperplastic nodules and hepatocellular carcinoma.

Treatments	Tissues	Time[a] (weeks)	Specific[b] activity
None	Normal liver		2.59 ± 0.63
DENA/2-AAF/PH/PB	Surrounding	24	4.19 ± 0.90
	Nodules	24	$10.26 \pm 2.21^{c,d}$
	Surrounding	56	5.85 ± 1.02^{c}
	Carcinoma	56	$13.26 \pm 4.65^{c,d}$
DENA/2-AAF/PH/PB/SAM	Liver	24	3.42 ± 0.99^{c}
	Liver	56	3.12 ± 0.95^{c}

[a]Period of time after the start of 2-AAF feeding.
[b]nmol of methylthioribose-1-phosphate formed/30 min, mg of protein. Data
are means ± SD of 7-11 experiments.
[c]Different from normal liver for $P < 0.001$.
[d]Different from surrounding for $P < 0.001$.

(1) During the early stages of hepatocarcinogenesis promotion, according
to the "resistant hepatocyte" and the triphasic models, there occurs a great
increase in PA synthesis. Putative preneoplastic foci seem to contribute to
this increase.

(2) Growth potential of putative preneoplastic foci progressively decreases even during a prolonged PB treatment. After PB withdrawal, GGT-positive foci undergo a great decrease but HN and HC develop. HN could derive
from a cell population that acquires the capacity to produce high PA amounts
and maintains this capacity permanently or at least for a long period of time.

(3) A decrease in liver SAM during hepatocarcinogenesis promotion may
be observed in an experimental model which is not based on the administration
of a lipotrope-deficient diet. Such a decrease is related to a high growth
potential, a prerequisite for promotion.

(4) SAM decrease is coupled with a high PA synthesis. This synthesis, as
well as a rise in total methylations, could explain the fall in SAM content
during growth. The fact that a high PA synthesis occurs together with a SAM
fall indicates that this fall is not due to impairment of SAM synthesis.

(5) Our data demonstrate an antipromoting effect of SAM and suggest
that this effect at least in part depends on inhibition of PA synthesis by
5'-MTA accumulation.

PB has been shown to promote carcinogenesis by increasing cell proliferation, stabilizating the altered phenotype and inhibiting cell death[44]. If we
consider these features as a general mechanism of the promotion, the antipromoting effect of SAM becomes evident. In fact, SAM inhibits growth of preneoplastic tissue, enhances the remodelling process and enhances the death of
putative preneoplastic cells.

The results of several groups have shown the existence of different
metabolic changes suggesting that some biochemical and functional alterations
occur in preneoplastic tissue. Among them the increment of detoxification

reaction[45,46], the decreased activation of some xenobiotics in HN[47], the variations of carbohydrate metabolism leading to an increased production of NADPH and ribose[46], appears to be particularly interesting. These changes have been interpreted as tne consequence of an "over-specialization" of preneoplastic cells for efficient performance of drug metabolism and cell proliferation[44]. If we consider our data in this context, the increase of the activities of ODC, PA synthetase[35], and 5'-MTA phosphorylase, could be interpreted as a part of an "adaptive program" which gives putative preneoplastic tissue a high growth potential and resistance to 5'-MTA toxicity. This program may represent a selective advantage for preneoplastic cells and may become a stable phenotypic characteristic only of relatively few cells.

ACKNOWLEDGEMENTS

This work was supported by grants from the "Progetto Finalizzato Oncologia" of CNR, and "Ministero della Pubblica Istruzione" (program 60%).

REFERENCES

1. A. B. Deangelo and C. T. Garrett, Inhibition of development of pre-neoplastic lesions in the livers of rats fed a weakly carcinogenic environmental contaminant, Cancer Lett. 20:199 (1983).
2. W. Stäuli, P. Bentley, F. Bieri, E. Frölich, and F. Waechter, Inhibitory effect of nafenopin upon the development of diethylnitrosamine-induced enzyme-altered foci within the rat liver, Carcinogenesis, 5:41 (1984).
3. M. A. Moore, W. Thamavit, H. Tsuda, K. Sato, A. Ichihara, and N. Ito, Modifying influence of dehydroepiandrosterone on the development of dihydroxy-d-n-propylnitrosamine-initiated lesions in the thyroid, lung and liver of F344 rats, Carcinogenesis 7:311 (1986).
4. R. Garcea, L. Daino, R. Pascale, S. Frassetto, P. Cozzolino, M. E. Ruggiu, and F. Feo, Inhibition by dehydroepiandrosterone of liver pre-neoplastic foci formation in rats after initiation-selection in experimental carcinogenesis, Toxicol. Pathol., in press.
5. Y. B. Mikol, K. L. Hoover, D. Creasia, and L. A. Poirier, Hepatocarcinogenesis in rats fed methyl-deficient amino acid-deficient diets, Carcinogenesis 4:1619 (1983).
6. A. K. Goshal and E. Farber, The induction of liver cancer by dietary deficiency of choline and methionine without added carcinogens, Carcinogenesis 5:1367 (1984).
7. S. Yokoyama, M. A. Sells, T. V. Reddy, and B. Lombardi, Hepatocarcinogenic and promoting action of a choline-devoid diet in the rat, Cancer Res. 45:2842 (1985).
8. B. Lombardi and H. Shinozuka, Enhancement of 2-acetylaminofluorene liver carcinogenesis in rats fed a choline-devoid diet, Int. J. Cancer 23: 565 (1979).
9. A. E. Rogers, G. Lehnart, and G. Morrison, Influence of dietary content of lipotropes and lipid on aflatoxin B1, N-2-fluorenylacetamide, 1,2-dimethylhydrazine carcinogenesis in rats, Cancer Res. 40:2802 (1980).
10. N. Shivapurkar and L. A. Poirier, Decreased levels of S-adenosylmethionine in the livers of rats fed phenobarbital and DDT, Carcinogenesis 5:589 (1982).
11. R. L. P. Adams and R. H. Burdon, "Molecular Biology of DNA Methylation" Springer-Verlag, New York (1985).
12. A. E. Pegg, R. T. Borchardt, and J. K. Coward, Effect of inhibitors of spermidine and spermine synthesis on polyamine concentrations and growth of mouse transformed fibroblasts, Biochem. J. 194:79 (1981).
13. M. K. Riscoe, P. A. Tower, and A. J. Ferro, Mechanism of action of 5'-methylthioadenosine in S49 cells, Biochem. Pharmacol. 33:3639 (1984).

14. G. L. Cantoni, The role of S-adenosylhomocysteine in the biological util-
    ization of S-adenosylmethionine, in: "Biochemistry and Biology of DNA
    Methylation", G. L. Cantoni and A. Razin, eds., p. 47, Alan R. Liss,
    Inc., New York (1985).

15. F. Feo, R. Pascale, R. Garcea, L. Daino, L. Pirisi, S. Frassetto, M. E.
    Ruggiu, D. Di Padova, and G. Stramentinoli, Effect of the variations
    of S-adenosyl-L-methionine liver content on fat accumulation and
    ethanol metabolism in ethanol-intoxicated rats, Toxicol. Appl.
    Pharmacol. 83:331 (1986).

16. D. B. Solt, A. Medline, and E. Farber, Rapid emergence of carcinogen-in-
    duced hyperplastic lesions in a new model for sequential analysis of
    liver carcinogenesis, Am. J. Pathol. 88:595 (1977).

17. M. Lans, J. de Gerlache, H. S. Taper, V. Préat, and M. B. Roberfroid,
    Phenobarbital as a promoter in the initiation-selection process of
    experimental rat hepatocarcinogenesis, Carcinogenesis 2:1283 (1983).

18. E. Farber and H. Ichinose, The prevention of ethionine-induced carcinoma
    of the liver in rats by methionine, Cancer Res. 18:1209 (1958).

19. Z. Brada, J. Hillova, M. Hill, N. H. Altman, and S. Bulba, Effect of
    methionine on development of benzopyrene (BP) induced sarcomas, Proc.
    of AACR, abstr. n° 478, Cancer Res. 27:121 (1986).

20. N. Shivapurkar, K. L. Hoover, and L. A. Poirier, Effect of methionine and
    choline on liver tumor promotion by phenobarbital and DDT in diethyl-
    nitrosamine-initiated rats, Carcinogenesis 5:547 (1986).

21. K. Enomoto and E. Farber, Kinetics of phenotypic maturation of remod-
    elling of hyperplastic nodules during liver carcinogenesis, Cancer Res.
    42:2330 (1982).

22. R. Schulte-Hermann, J. Schuppler, I. Timmermann-Trosiener, G. Ohde, W.
    Bursch, and H. Berger, The role of growth of normal and preneoplastic
    cell populations for tumor promotion in rat liver, Environ. Health
    Perspect. 50:185 (1983).

23. M. A. Moore, H-J. Hacker, and P. Bannasch, Phenotypic instability in
    focal and nodular lesions induced in a short term system in the rat
    liver, Carcinogenesis, 5:595 (1983).

24. W. Bursch, B. Lauer, I. Timmermann-Trosiener, G. Bartel, J. Schuppler,
    and R. Schulte-Hermann, Controlled death (Apoptosis) of normal and
    putative preneoplastic cell in rat liver following withdrawal of tumor
    promoters. Carcinogenesis 5:453 (1984).

25. J. Jänne, H. Pösö, and A. Raina, Polyamines in rapid growth and cancer,
    Biochim. Biophys. Acta 473:241 (1978).

26. O. Heby, Role of polyamines in the control of cell proliferation and dif-
    ferentiation, Differentiation 19:1 (1981).

27. G. Scalabrino and M. A. Ferioli, Polyamines in mammalian tumors. Part I,
    Adv. Cancer Res. 35:151 (182).

28. G. Scalabrino and M. A. Ferioli, Polyamines in mammalian tumors. Part II,
    Adv. Cancer Res. 36:1 (1982).

29. S. Thrower and M. G. Ord, Hormonal control of liver regeneration,
    Biochem. J. 144:361 (1974).

30. O. Heby, A. Anheus, M. Linden, and S. Oresson, Tumor cell proliferation
    as affected by changes in intracellular and extracellular polyamine
    levels, Adv. Poly am. Res 3:357 (1981).

31. T. G. O'Brien, R. C. Simsiman, and R. K. Boutwell, Induction of the poly-
    amine biosynthetic enzymes in mouse epidermis and their specificity
    for tumor promotion, Cancer Res. 35:2426 (1975).

32. G. Scalabrino, H. Pösö, E. Holttä, P. Hannonen, A. Kallio, and J. Jänne,
    Synthesis and accumulation of polyamines in rat liver during chemical
    carcinogenesis, Int. J. Cancer 21:239 (1978).

33. S. Yamagi, K. Sasaki, and N. Yamamoto, Induction by phenobarbital of
    ornithine decarboxylase activity in rat liver after initiation with
    diethylnitrosamine, Cancer Lett. 12:87 (1981).

34. J. W. Olson and D. H. Russell, Prolonged ornithine decarboxylase induction in regenerating carcinogen-treated liver, Cancer Res. 40:4373 (1980).

35. F. Feo, R. Garcea, L. Daino, R. Pascale, L. Pirisi, S. Frassetto, and M. E. Ruggiu, Early stimulation of polyamine biosynthesis during promotion of diethylnitrosamine-induced rat liver carcinogenesis. The effects of variations of the S-adenosyl-L-methionine cellular pool, Carcinogenesis, 6:1713 (1985).

36. R. Garcea, R. Pascale, L. Daino, S. Frassetto, P. Cozzolino, M. E. Ruggiu, M. G. Vannini, L. Gaspa, and F. Feo, Variations of ornithine decarboxylase activity and S-adenosyl-L-methionine and 5'-methylthio-adenosine contents during the development of diethylnitrosamine-induced liver hyperplastic nodules and hepatocellular carcinoma, Carcinogenesis, in press.

37. Y. B. Mikol and L. A. Poirier, An inverse relationship between hepatic ornithine decarboxylase and S-adenosylmethionine in the rats, Cancer Lett. 13:195 (1981).

38. K. Oden and S. Clarke, S-adenosyl-L-methionine synthetase from human erythrocytes: role in the regulation of cellular S-adenosylmethionine levels, Biochemistry 22:2978 (1983).

39. C. Matsumoto, Y. Suma, and K. Tsukada, Changes in the activities of S-adenosylmethionine synthetase isozymes from rat liver with dietary methionine, J. Biochem. 25:287 (1984).

40. R. L. Pajula and A. Raina, Methylthioadenosine, a potent inhibitor of spermine synthase from bovine brain, FEBS Lett. 99:343 (1979).

41. A. J. Ferro, A. A. Vandenbarki, and M. R. MacDonald, Inactivation of S-adenosylhomocysteine hydrolase by 5'-deoxy-5'-methylthioadenosine, Biochem. Biophys. Res. Commun. 100:523 (1981).

42. J. A. Lautenberg and S. Linn, The deoxyribonucleic acid modification and restriction enzymes of Escherichia coli B. I. Purification, subunit structure, and catalytic properties of the modification methylase, J. Biol. Chem. 247:6176 (1972).

43. H. G. Williams-Ashman, A. E. Pegg, and D. H. Lockwood, Mechanisms of the regulation of polyamine and putrescine biosynthesis in male genital glands and other tissues of mammals, Adv. Enzyme Regul. 7:292 (1972).

44. R. Schulte-Hermann, Tumor promotion in the liver, Arch. Toxicol. 57:147 (1985).

45. A. Aström, J. W. DePierre, and L. Eriksson, Characterization of drug-metabolizing systems in hyperplastic nodules from the livers of rats receiving 2-acetylaminofluorene in their diet, Carcinogenesis 4:577 (1983).

46. R. Schulte-Hermann, I. Timmermann-Trosiener, and J. Schuppler, Aberrant expression of adaptation to phenobarbital may cause selective growth of foci of altered cells in rat liver, in: "Models, Mechanisms and Etiology of Tumor Promotion", M. Börzsönyi, K. Lapis, N. E. Day and Y. Yamasaki, eds., IARC Scientific Publlication 56:67 (1984).

47. F. Feo, R. A. Canuto, R. Garcea, O. Brossa, and G. C. Caselli, Phenobarbital stimulation of cytochrome P-450 and aminopyrine N-demethylase in hyperplastic liver nodules during DL-ethionine carcinogenesis, Cancer Lett. 5:25 (1978).

NUCLEAR AND GENETIC ALTERATIONS DURING LIVER CARCINOGENESIS

LONG TERM EFFECT OF DIETHYLNITROSAMINE (DEN) ON THE PRODUCTION OF

MICRONUCLEI IN PRECANCEROUS RAT LIVER

H.Barbason, B.Bouzahzah, S.Massart, D. Brumioul,
B.Robaye and Ch.Herens
Pathology, University of Liège

Pathology, B 23, Sart Tilman, B-4000 Liège, Belgium

The mechanisms of hepatocarcinogenesis induced by nitrosamines have been mainly considered in relation to "initiation" processes. Alkylation of O^6-guanine associated with DNA synthesis has been frequently correlated with point mutations to explain the emergence of putative preneoplastic foci and this has been directly connected with various types of tumorigenesis[1-4].

However, O^6-alkylguanine has a short half life of about 1 day[5,6]. This does not seem a long enough effect to explain the multiple morphological and biochemical modifications obtained after the end of a single nitrosamine treatment. Moreover, these effects occur in precancerous cells as well as in the phenotypical normal surrounding tissue, during the long delay between the initiation and the occurence of detectable malignant transformation. The disturbances in the regulation of liver cell proliferation and specific functions, the selective growth of the precancerous cells, the roles played by non-carcinogenic promotors[7-12] (that must continue for many months after the end of the carcinogen administration) ... imply long term effects of nitrosamines.

In this respect, little attention has been focused to the evolution of other "nuclear lesions" different from O^6-guanine alkylation during the successive stages of the carcinogenic process. However, different experimental findings indicate the stability of other potentially important alkylation sites in DNA and also potentially persistent DNA breaks that can give rise to "chromosomal aberrations" in proliferative cells. These are detectable a long time after an acute exposure to the chemical carcinogen[4,6,13,14].

Alkylating agents including nitrosamines, and also X-irradiation can induce in the cell a number of nuclear lesions some of which may remain latent after the treatment and are revealed only by a subsequent mitosis[4,15,16]. These last cytogenetical damages are useful to study the development of malignancy since they could have some relation to the phenotypical expression of oncogens[17].

The present communication deals with the persistence of potential nuclear lesions following a first nitrosamine treatment and their possible relationship to mitotic aberrations and hepatocarcinogenesis.

The production of micronuclei has been chosen as a representative "indicator" of chromosome aberrations. It must be kept in mind that a micronucleus can be the result of a chromosome break. The acentric chromosome fragment is not included in the anaphase movements and becomes after telophase a small nuclear satellite of the main nucleus. To be mor- phologically expressed, micronucleus formation thus requires first a nuclear preclastogenic lesion and second a mitotic process. Because of their relatively short life estimated to be a few days (14) they also are, by themselves, a deletion of at least an important chromosome fragment which could be implicated in the oncogen activation as it is the case in the transforming retinoblastomas process[18,19]. The number of micronuclei produced by partial hepatectomy performed at various times after a nitro- samine treatment is thus a good mirror of the preclastogenic lesions evo- lution due to a first nitrosamine treatment.

We have previously compared, in this respect, the long term effect of a single dose of X-rays (450 R) or of a single injection of dimethylni- trosamine (DMN; 30 mg/kg). Both agents, combined with partial hepatectomy induce a production of morphologically similar micronuclei. But, partial hepatectomy performed at various times after the treatments shows very different evolution of the induced preclastogenic damages according to the type of first agent[4,15,16] (see fig. 1).

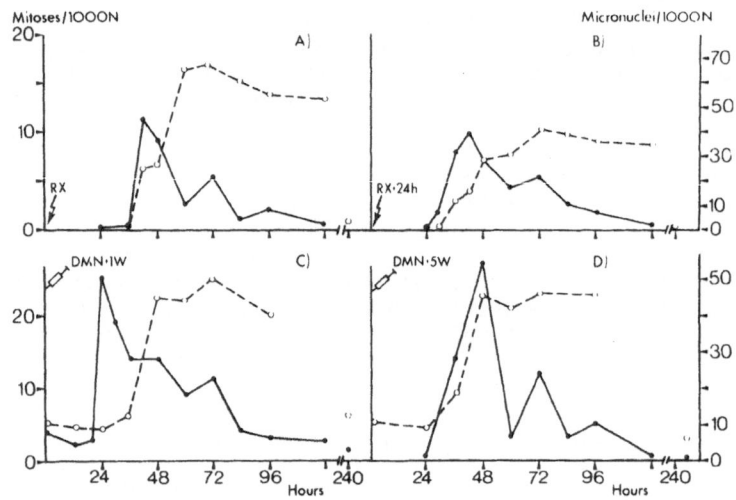

Fig.1. Mitotic activity (●) and micronuclei production(o) following the partial hepatectomy against the post- operative hours.
experimental groups : A. X-irradiation (450R) given 1 hour before the operation; B. X-irradiation (same dose) given 24 hours before the operation; C.DMN (30 mg/kg)given 1 week before the operation; D. DMN (same dose)given 5 weeks before the operation.

After X-rays (Fig.1A), partial hepatectomy performed 1 hour after the treatment induces a number of micronuclei occuring immediately after the mitotic activity. This peaks at about 3 days after the operation and decreases after the mitotic wave to reach low values at the 10th post- operative day. This confirms that the mean micronucleus life is only of a few days[14]. When a 24 hours delay is introduced between the irradiation and the partial hepatectomy (Fig. 1B), the micronuclei production is significantly reduced in spite of a quantitatively similar mitotic activity.

One week after a single DMN injection (Fig.1C), partial hepatectomy induces an important number of micronuclei occuring immediately after the mitotic wave. But, contrarily to X-rays, when the operation is performed up to 5 weeks later, about the same number of micronuclei are still revealed (Fig. 1D).

In order to obtain a general view about the persistence of preclasto-genic nuclear lesions, we have compared the maximum of micronuclei (obtained 72 hours after partial hepatectomy) when the operation is delayed up to 10 weeks, either after X-rays or after a single DMN injection (Fig.2).

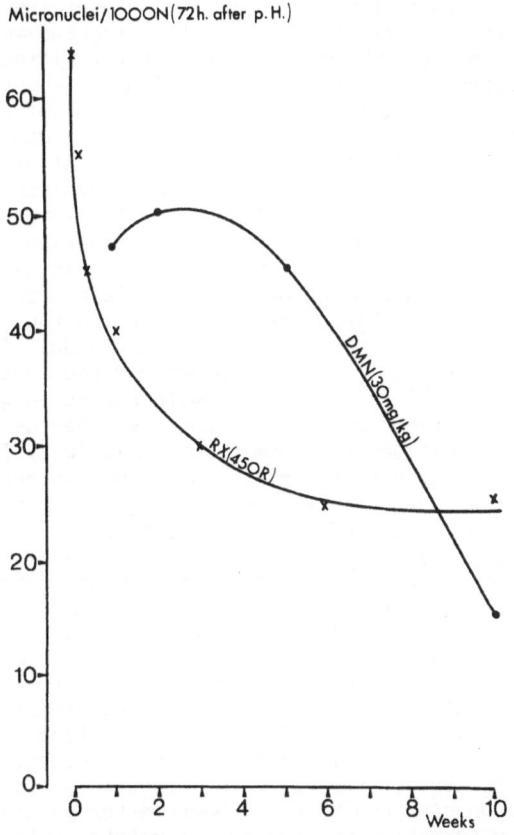

Fig.2. Micronuclei frequency revealed by partial hepatectomy against the delay after X-irradiation (X; 450R) or DMN (●; 30 mg/kg). In each case, micronuclei have been counted at the 72th post-operative hour corresponding to the maximum frequency.

The results clearly show a very different pattern of evolution according to the type of toxic agent. After X-rays, the production of micronuclei by the regenerating mitotic activity rapidly decreases to low values after a few days. On the contrary, after a single injection of DMN, the emergence of micronuclei by the same mitotic process is slightly increased in the first 2 weeks and begin to decrease significantly after the 5th week to reach low values after 10 weeks. These last results have been confirmed thereafter by Tates et al.[13,14].

In order to explain the differences observed in the long term effect of both genotoxic agents, we have suggested that micronuclei are in both case the expression of DNA breaks. It is well known that X-rays induce immediate DNA breaks. These can be rapidly repaired while, nitrosamines promotes a progressive occurence of DNA breaks so that they can be accumulate for a long time after the treatment without efficient repair. Thereafter, they could be expressed by a subsequent mitosis[4,15,16]. Supporting this interpretation is the fact that various experimental data indicate that DNA lesions such as bound adducts (principally O^2-thymine and alkylphosphotriesters) and potential DNA breaks, may persist for a long time after a single nitrosamine injection[6,13,14]. More precisely, alkylphosphotriesters may interfere with DNA-handling enzymes by bloking the polymerases, nucleases and other DNA-binding proteins[20,21,22]. These biochemical effects could be the cause of the progressive accumulation and of the persistence of DNA breaks after a first nitrosamine treatment. The above results are perfectly compatible with the interpretation of Tates et al.[6,13,14]. They declare[14] that "the extent of preclastogenic damage at a given time interval after injection will depend on a number of factors including 1. the formation and persistence of preclastogenic primary DNA modifications; 2. the formation and persistence of secondary preclastogenic lesions; 3. the rate liver cell turn-over".

The experimental procedure producing a combination between these 3 factors such that the micronuclei production is high imply an increased clastogenic risk and as a consequence, a possible cancer risk. That is the reason why we have tested this hypothesis, by using the same methods, in our previously described hepatocarcinogenesis model[7-12]. It uses diethylnitrosamine (DEN) which induces precisely the most persistent preclastogenic lesions[6,13,14], combined with subsequent experimental procedures inducing various mitotic control disturbances[7-12]. The different experimental conditions are summarized in Table 1. It compares a subcarcinogenic DEN administration of 2 weeks with a carcinogenic DEN treatment of 6 weeks. Both DEN treatments are given in drinking water (10 mg/kg/day) and are followed by 1 week without any treatment. This interruption intends to eliminate the acute toxic lesions due to the first drug administration. Thereafter, animals of each group (at minimum 25 rats per group) are submitted to 4 different regimes or treatments : none, partial hepatectomy, limited or continuous phenobarbital addition in the water (15 mg/rat/day). In each case, the evolution of precancerous lesions (PAS positive foci, neoplastic nodules, hepatomas) the median time of death and the hepatic tumor incidence observed at autopsy have been registered[12]. This allows us to estimate the "promoting effect" introduced after the DEN administration by the different subsequent treatments.

At various intervals, after different treatments, we have compared the number of micronuclei expressed 72 hours after partial hepatectomy. Since micronucleus formation depends on the mitotic activity and this varies in the different experimental conditions[12], we must correlate the number of micronuclei accumulated to the number of mitoses effectively computed as previously described[15]. The micronuclei index is thus defined as the ratio of the number of micronuclei containing cells 72 hours after the partial hepatectomy to the integrated number of mitoses occuring during this post-operative period. In the figure 3, this pôst-operative micronuclei index (Fig.3A) is compared with the growth fraction of the liver tissue (Fig.3B) in the corresponding conditions. The growth fraction is defined as the number of labelled nuclei per 1000 nuclei after 7 injections of tritiated thymidine injected at 6 hours intervals.

Table 1. Hepatocarcinogenesis model (for details see ref.12				
Duration of DEN (10 mg/kg/ day) weeks	Subsequent treatment	Median time of death (in months)	Hepatomas at autopsy %	Promotion effect
2 (subcar- cinogen)	water	15	0	-
	partial hepatectomy	14	0	0
	Phenobarbi- tal continuous	15	80	+
	Phenobarbi- tal 8 weeks	15	0	0
6 (carcino- gen)	water	9	100	-
	partial hepatectomy	7	100	+
	Phenobarbi- tal continuous	5.5	100	+
	Phenobarbi- tal 4 weeks	5.5	100	+

A comparison between table 1 and Fig. 3 allows us to correlate, in each experimental condition : 1. the presence and persistence of preclasto- genic lesions susceptible to give rise to the formation of a micronucleus; 2. the growth fraction in treated but unoperated precancerous livers; 3. the carcinogenesis evolution.

In the control animals (Fig.3B), the growth fraction is already low in 2 months old rats and decreases with age. The mitoses induced by par- tial hepatectomy (Fig.3A) reveal no micronuclei except a few in 12 months old animals. This corresponds to the spontaneous DNA lesions accumulation occuring normally with the age. No hepatic tumor has been observed in this control group even when rats operated after 12 months were sacrificed at the age of 2 years (unpublished results).

DEN administered for only 2 weeks (subcarcinogenic treatment) initia- tes preneoplastic foci that are slowly growing but remain without any malignant transformation up to the time of death (table 1). In that case (Fig.3B) the growth fraction of liver cells is maintained at a low level after the DEN treatment. Partial hepatectomy (Fig.3A) performed 2 months after the beginning of the treatment does not reveal numerous micronuclei and does not promote carcinogenesis (table 1). The number of micronuclei expressed by the regenerating process is getting higher when partial he- patectomy is performed 4 months after the beginning of the treatment but remains at about the same level when the operation is delayed further (Fig.3A).

Phenobarbital given chronically after the same subcarcinogen DEN treatment promotes tumorigenesis so that 80% of rats die with hepatic can- cer after about 15 months (table 1). But, in this case (Fig.3B), the growth fraction of precancerous livers is higher than after DEN alone and

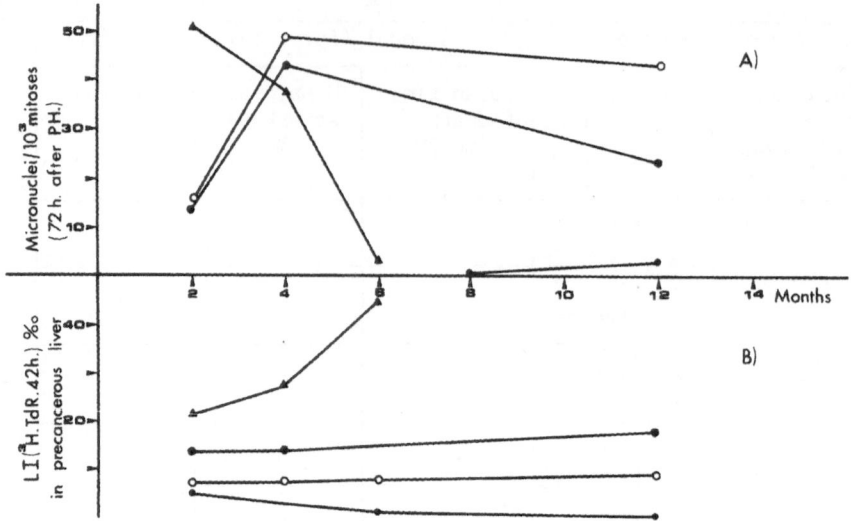

Fig.3. Micronuclei index (see the text) produced by partial hepatec-
       tomy (A) and the growth fraction (see the text) in unoperated
       corresponding livers against the months following the DEN
       treatments.
       Experimental groups :(●) untreated controls; (o) DEN for
       2 weeks; (◉) DEN for 2 weeks followed by a continuous pheno-
       barbital treatment; (▲) DEN for 6 weeks. Compare with
       table 1.

micronuclei produced by partial hepatectomy (Fig.3A) are significantly decreased when the operation is performed later than at the 4th month. On the
contrary, phenobarbital administration limited at about the 2d month
after the beginning of the DEN treatment (phenobarbital for 8 weeks,
table 1) does not promote the carcinogenic process . During this period
(Fig.3A) the micronuclei even revealed by partial hepatectomy remain low.
     After 6 weeks of DEN administration, 100% of animals die with
hepatomas about 9 months after the beginning of treatment (table 1). In
this case (Fig.3B), the growth fraction of precancerous liver is already
higher than in all the other conditions soon after the end of treatment
and increases up to the 6th month. Inversely (Fig.3A) a very important
number of micronuclei is observed when partial hepatectomy is performed
soon after the carcinogen administration but decreases rapidly to a very
low level when the operation is delayed up the 6th month. In this condition (table 1) partial hepatectomy performed soon after the end of the
DEN treatment accelerate the carcinogenesis but this operation reveals an
important number of micronuclei (Fig.3A). In the same conditions, phenobarbital given for only 4 weeks after the carcinogen administration or
continuously promotes carcinogenesis by about 3,5 months (table 1). Both
treatments double the growth fraction observed after DEN alone[12] and the
production of micronuclei is very high in presence of mitotic activity
induced by partial hepatectomy soon after the DEN treatment (Fig.3A).
     These results clearly show that nuclear lesions, susceptible to give
rise to micronuclei in growing cells, can be accumulated and can persist

for a long time after the DEN administration in non-growing cells.

Moreover in the different experimental conditions, there is a good relationship between the mitotic expression of micronuclei and the promotion of carcinogenesis. The number of cells containing micronuclei decreases in a few days. The mechanism is either that they suffered damages incompatible with cell life or that the micronuclei are eliminated by internal digestion or by a subsequent mitosis. This suggests that, in surviving cells, micronuclei are the sign of important chromosome deletions and are also a good "indicator" of the amount of other chromosome rearrengements. Such mechanisms are now considered as involved in oncogene activation inducing malignant transformation[17-19]

Table 2. Labeling index (LI : 7 tritiated-thymidine injections at 6 hours intervals) in preneoplastic areas and in the phenotypically normal adjacent parenchyma

Experimental conditions	LI in normal parenchyma	LI in preneoplastic areas
DEN for 2 weeks followed by water for 12 months	12	15
DEN for 2 weeks followed by Phenobarbital for 12 months	17	44
DEN for 6 weeks followed by water for 1,5 months	22	41
DEN for 6 weeks followed by Phenobarbital for 1,5 months	41	78

In fact, our observations show that the experimental conditions where the number of cancers is highest, are not those where there are a large number of lesions giving rise to numerous micronuclei but those where the decrease in their number is the most important.

This strengthens our previous observations that, the malignant transformation implies a disturbance of the mitotic control after the DEN initiation[7-12]. In our model, an efficient promoting effect can be obtained either by protracting the DEN feeding for 6 weeks or by switching to other promoting interventions (partial hepatectomy, phenobarbital administration). They all have the common property to induce an important growth by disturbing the mitotic control, so that, micronuclei can be produced in large number and thereafter eliminated.

This could explain the observed correlation between the mitotic control disturbance, the micronuclei production and the promotion of malignancy. However, these long term nuclear damages are observed in the whole liver parenchyma while the malignant transformation is supposed to occur in preneoplastic areas[23]. It must be pointed out that, the cells of these precancerous lesions present, in any case, a proliferative advantage[24] over the phenotypically normal adjacent parenchyma (table 2).

In the light of the present results, it could be speculated that this selective growth, which increases the amount of chromosomal damages, makes them a likely first microenvironment favouring the oncogene expression and thus malignancy.

The tumor promoting effect could thus consist in a disturbance of the cell growth control, which enhances the mitotic activity during the precancerous stage. This is more important in precancerous cells and could then favours the emergence of chromosome aberrations involved in the malignant transformation[17-19].

References

1. M.F. Rajewsky, L.H.Angenlicht, H.Biessman, R.Goth, D.F.Hulser , O.D. Laerum and L.Y.Lomakina, Nervous-system-specific carcinogenesis by ethylnitrosourea in the rat : molecular and cellular aspect, in : "Origin of human cancer", H.H.Hiatt, J.D.Watson, J.A.Winsten, eds., Cold Spring Harbor, New York (1977).
2. P.D.Lawley, DNA as target of alkylating carcinogens, Brit.Med.Bul. 36:19 (1980).
3. J.V.Frei, D.A.Swenson, W. Warren and D.Lawley, Alkylation of deoxyribonucleic acid in vivo in various organs of C57BL mice by carcinogens : N-methyl-N-nitrosourea, N-ethyl-N-nitrosourea and ethyl methanesulfonate, Biochem.J. 174:1031 (1978).
4. H.Barbason, A.Fridman-Manduzio and E.H.Betz, Long term effect of a single dose of dimethylnitrosamine on the rat liver, Z.Krebsforsch. 84:135 (1975).
5. A.Renard, M.Lemaître and W.Verly, Repair O^6-alkylguanine lesions in DNA by chromatin enzymes, Biochimie 64:803 (1982).
6. L. Den Engelse, G.J.Menkveld, R.J. De Brij and D. Tates, Formation and stability of alkylated pyrimidines and purines (including imidazole ring-opened 7-alkylguanine)and alkylphosphotriesters in liver DNA of adult rats treated with ethylnitrosourea or dimethylnitrosamine, Carcinogenesis 7:393 (1986).
7. J.Van Cantfort and H.Barbason, Influence of a chronic administration of diethylnitrosamine on the relation between specific tissular and division functions in the rat liver, Europ.J.Cancer 11:531 (1975).
8. H.Barbason, Correlation between the circadian rhythms of division and tissue functions in the liver of rats in normal and precancerous state, Acta Histochem. XVI:99 (1976).
9. H.Barbason, A.Fridman-Manduzio, P.Lelièvre and E.H.Betz , Variations of liver cell control during diethylnitrosamine carcinogenesis, Europ.J.Cancer13:13 (1977).
10.H.Barbason, V.Smoliar and J.Van Cantfort, Correlation of liver growth and function during liver regeneration and hepatocarcinogenesis, Arch.Toxicol. suppl.2:157 (1979).
11. H.Barbason and E.H.Betz, Proliferation of preneoplastic lesions after discontinuation of chronic DEN feeding in the development of hepatomas in rat, Br.J.Cancer 44:561 (1981).
12. H.Barbason, C.Rassenfosse and E.H.Betz, Promotion mechanism of phenobarbital and partial hepatectomy in DENA hepatocarcinogenesis, cell kinetics effect, Br.J.Cancer 47:517 (1983).
13. A.D.Tates and L.Den Engelse, Time dependent induction of chromosome damage in rat hepatocytes in relation to alkylation damage of DNA. "Progress in Mutation Research", Natarajan, ed., Elsevier Biomedical Press (1982).
14. D.Tates, I.Neuteboon, A.H.M.Rotteveel, N. de Vogel, G.J.Menkveld and L.Den Engelse, Persistence of preclastogenic damage in hepatocytes of rat exposed to ethylnitrosourea, diethylnitrosamine, dimethylnitrosamine and methyl methanesulfonate,correlation with DNA O-alkylation, Carcinogenesis 7:1053 (1986).
15. H.Barbason,Réparation des altérations nucléaires induites dans le foie de rat par une irradiation X, Int.J.Rad.Biol. 16:233 (1969).

16. H.Barbason, Long term effect of X-rays or dimethylnitrosamine upon rat liver, Int.J.Rad.Biol. 38:114 (1981).
17. M.Barbacid, Oncogens and human cancer : cause or consequence ? Carcinogenesis 7:1037 (1986).
18. H.Harris, Malignant tumors generated by recessive mutations, Nature 323:582 (1986).
19. S.H.Friend, R.Bernards, S.Rogelj, R.A.Weinberg, J.M.Rapaport, D.M. Albert and Th.Dryja, A human DNA segment with properties of the genes that predisposes to retinoblastoma and osteosarcoma, Nature 323:643 (1986).
20. P.S.Miller, S.Chandrasegaran, D.L.Dow, S.M.Pulfort and L.S.Kan, Synthesis and template properties of an ethyl phosphotriester modified decadeoxyribonucleotides, Biochemistry 21:5468 (1982).
21. P.S.Miller, J.C.Barrett and P.O.P. Ts'o, Synthesis of oligodeoxyribonucleotides ethyl phosphotriesters and their specific complex formation with transfer ribonucleic acid, Biochemistry 13:4887 (1974).
22. Y.Takeda, D.H.Ohlendorf, W.F.Anderson and B.W.Matthews, DNA-binding proteins, Sciences 221:1020 (1983).
23. H.M.Rabes, Th.Bucher, A.Hartman, I.Linke and M.Dunnwald, Clonal growth of carcinogen-induced enzyme-deficient preneoplastic cell population in mouse liver, Cancer Res. 42:3220 (1982).
24. H.M.Rabes and R.Szymkowiak, Cell kinetics of hepatocytes during the preneoplastic period of diethylnitrosamine-induced lievr carcinogenesis, Cancer Res. 39:1298 (1979).

NUCLEAR ALTERATIONS DURING HEPATOCARCINOGENESIS:

PROMOTION BY 2-ACETYLAMINOFLUORENE

Per O. Seglen, Gunnar Sæter and Per E. Schwarze

Institute for Cancer Research
The Norwegian Radium Hospital
Montebello, 0310 Oslo 3, Norway

Normal liver growth takes place partly by ordinary cell division, partly by polyploidization. The latter mechanism becomes increasingly dominant as the animal matures and ages. In adult rats of the Wistar Kyoto strain, the majority of the hepatocytes (60%) are tetraploid, 20-25% are octoploid, and about 15% are diploid. The latter, being of small size, make up less than 10% of the liver mass. Fig. 1A shows the increase in absolute hepatocyte numbers, and Fig. 1B the contribution of the various cell ploidy classes to liver weight following a 2/3 partial hepatectomy in the young (70-100 g) animal. There is a rapid increase in all mononucleated cell types during the regeneration phase (the first week); subsequent liver growth is dominated by polyploidization and tetraploid cell division, and there is actually a decrease in the number of diploid cells.

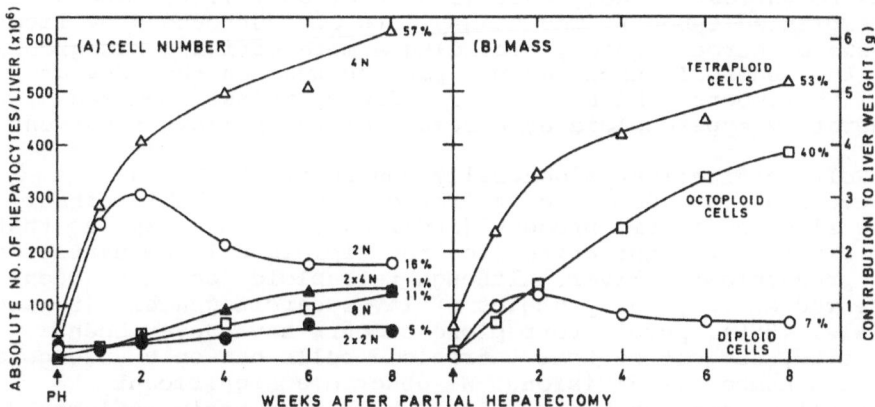

Fig. 1. Development of hepatocellular ploidy after partial hepatectomy in young rats. (A), Absolute number of hepatocytes within each ploidy class; (B) contribution of each major ploidy category to liver mass. Values were calculated by computer on the basis of flow-cytometry (isolated cells and nuclei), binuclearity counts and liver weight determinations.

Table 1. Ploidy of tumours induced by PH+DEN+AAF (4-8 months)

	Mo.	% Diploid nuclei	% Diploid cells[a]
Normal liver	4	21.6 ± 2.0 (5)	7.6 ± 1.9 (6)
Nodules < 2.5 mm	4	65.8 ± 2.4 (16)[b]	64.3 ± 3.0 (2)
Nodules ≥ 2.5 mm	4	81.4 ± 2.4 (13)[b]	80.5 ± (1)
Carcinomas	5-8	83.5 ± 1.5 (13)	79.9 ± 4.1 (3)

[a]Flow cytometric measurements, uncorrected for aggregates.
[b]$P < 0.001$ for difference between large and small nodules.

Abnormal proliferation kinetics in hepatic tumours: replacement of polyploidization by diploid cell division

Hepatic carcinomas and nodules, induced within 3-8 months by treatment of partially hepatectomized rats with diethylnitrosamine (DEN) as initiator and 2-acetylaminofluorene (AAF) as promoter (Schwarze et al., 1984), show a characteristic abnormality in their growth pattern: in contrast to normal adult liver tissue, the tumours appear to grow predominantly by diploid cell division. An uncorrected flow-cytometric analysis (which because of aggregate formation somewhat underestimates the number of diploid cells) indicates that there are less than 10% diploid hepatocytes in the normal adult liver as compared to 65-85% in tumours (Table 1). The percentage values for diploid nuclei are somewhat higher, reflecting the presence of binucleated cells (2x2N) as well as of aggregates in normal hepatocyte suspensions. The two sets of values are, however fairly similar in the case of the tumours, indicating that neither 2x2N cells nor aggregates are quantitatively important in the tumour cell suspensions.

A diploid growth pattern is also seen in tumours arising after transplantation of hepatocytes from carcinogen-treated rats to untreated recipients (Seglen et al., 1986), and in transplanted tumours. The transplants are surrounded by liver tissue of normal ploidy, providing a more striking background for the abnormal tumour growth pattern than in the case of primary tumours, which are surrounded by tissue rendered moderately hyperdiploid as a result of the primary treatment.

Polyploidization is generally considered to be an irreversible process, i.e. tetraploid cells probably cannot give rise to diploid progeny (Nadal, 1970). This implies that diploid tumours must arise from the diploid cell population in the preneoplastic liver. Although tetraploid foci have been observed at very early stages of liver carcinogenesis (Sarafoff et al., 1986), purely tetraploid tumours have never been reported, suggesting that tetraploid cells can only undergo a limited number of divisions. We observe a significant correlation between tumour size (which presumably reflects growth rate) and percentage of diploid cells in early nodules (Table 1), which indicates that polyploidization may be associated with a progressively diminishing growth potential. We therefore suggest that the reduced polyploidization tendency generally seen in hepatic tumours corresponds to an increased growth fraction, giving the tumours a proliferative advantage correlating with their percentage of diploid cells.

Both early outgrowth of phenotypically altered hepatocytes and development of tumours is promoted by AAF

In our carcinogenic regimen DEN is given as a non-necrogenic dose (50 mg/kg body wt.) to young Wistar Kyoto rats (70-100 g) 24 h after a 2/3 partial hepatectomy. After a one-week interval the animals are given a diet containing 0.02 % AAF for four weeks. Although AAF is a known hepatocarcinogen and produces small liver nodules after eight months in the absence of DEN initiation, we have never seen hepatocarcinomas within this period with AAF alone, and will - in the present context - regard it primarily as a promoter of DEN carcinogenesis. In contrast, DEN alone - after partial hepatectomy - induces cancer in two-thirds of the animals at eight months.

AAF strongly promotes the early outgrowth of phenotypically altered hepatocytes, as exemplified by cells staining positively for gamma-glutamyltranspeptidase, GGT. In preparations of purified hepatocytes, isolated by collagenase perfusion, there are no GGT-positive cells six weeks after DEN alone, whereas 30% of the cells are positive after DEN + AAF (Fig. 2). Although some of the GGT-positive cells (inducible expressors?) subsequently lose their stainability quite rapidly, approximately one-half (constitutive expressors?) maintain GGT expression even at 16 weeks. With AAF alone, only 3% of the cells are GGT-positive at six weeks, and approximately 1% thereafter.

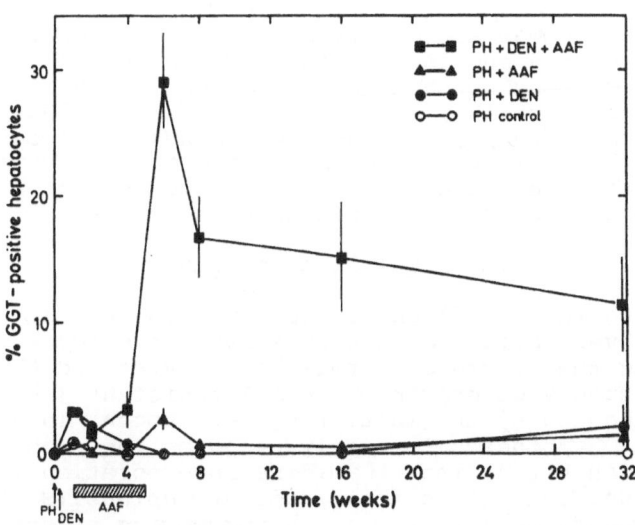

Fig. 2. Induction of GGT expression in hepatocytes by DEN+AAF. Enzymatic activity was measured cytochemically in hepatocytes isolated by collagenase perfusion at various times after partial hepatectomy.

Table 2. Effect of AAF on development of liver tumours after initiation of carcinogenesis by PH+DEN

Tumour type and time after PH+DEN	Tumours per animal			
	- AAF		+ AAF	
Small nodules (<1 mm)				
8 weeks	15 ± 8 (6)		6 ± 4 (11)	[d]
4 months[a]	124 ± 35 (5)	[b]	26 ± 13 (11)	
8 months[a]	120 ± 30 (5)	[b]	1.7 ± 1.7 (6)	[c]
Large nodules (≥1 mm)				
8 weeks	0.2 ± 0.2 (6)		8 ± 4 (11)	
4 months[a]	1.4 ± 0.5 (5)		14 ± 3 (11)	[e]
8 months[a]	69 ± 45 (5)		50 ± 14 (6)	
Hepatocarcinomas				
8 weeks	0 ± (6)		0 ± (11)	
4 months	0 ± (5)		0.4 ± 0.2 (11)	
8 months[a]	0.8 ± 0.3 (6)		2.4 ± 0.4 (8)	[e]

[a]Some of the animals became moribund and were sacrificed before eight months.
[b]When the number of small nodules exceeded one hundred per liver, only approximate values were recorded.
[c]$P<0.005$; [d]$P<0.01$; [e]$P<0.02$ for significance of AAF-effect according to the t-test.

AAF also promotes the outgrowth of liver nodules (Table 2). Although DEN alone induces numerous very small nodules, at eight weeks nodules larger than 1 mm in diameter are only seen after combined treatment (DEN + AAF). Even at four months the number of nodules larger than 1 mm is ten times higher after AAF promotion.

Hepatocarcinomas are observed in one-third of the animals after hepatectomy and four months with the combined treatment (DEN+AAF), whereas no carcinomas are seen at this time with DEN alone. At eight months, the majority of animals have cancer in both treatment groups, but the average number of carcinomas per animal is three times as high after the combined treatment. AAF promotion of liver carcinogenesis is thus evident at all observable stages of the carcinogenesis process.

AAF does not inhibit normal liver growth

According to an influential current hypothesis, AAF promotes liver carcinogenesis by selective cytotoxicity, suppressing the growth of normal hepatocytes and thus favouring the compensatory outgrowth of an AAF-resistant (mutant?) cell minority induced by the initiating carcinogen. This "resistant hepatocyte" hypothesis is mainly based on the reported ability of AAF to inhibit nuclear thymidine incorporation in normal liver tissue, but not in focal/nodular lesions (Solt et al., 1977). However, despite the strong promoting effects of AAF in our system, we have not observed any inhibition of liver growth by this drug. Liver weight, DNA and protein content increase at the same rate in the presence or absence of AAF, and regardless of whether carcinogenesis has been initiated by DEN or not

(Fig. 3). Body weight gain is somewhat retarded by AAF feeding, but the drug is apparently not hepatotoxic in Kyoto rats at the dose level used.

It is thus clear that the promoting effects of AAF cannot be accounted for by selective cytotoxicity in our system. Even in the model system from which the "resistant hepatocyte" hypothesis was derived, i.e. Fischer rats given AAF before and after a partial hepatectomy, we observed, without applying an initiating carcinogen, a doubling of the liver mass during the week of AAF feeding following hepatectomy.

AAF inhibits polyploidization and expands the diploid hepatocyte population

We have previously reported that the combined carcinogen treatment (DEN+AAF) induced a large increase in the fraction of diploid hepatocytes at a very early stage of hepatocarcinoge-nesis, i.e. in the preneoplastic liver at eight weeks (Schwarze et al., 1984). It now turns out that most of this effect is due to AAF, and that AAF alone (with or without a preceding partial hepatectomy) can induce a severalfold increase in the proportion of diploid cells in the liver. Fig. 4 shows the time course of change in the percentage of diploid cells (Fig. 4A) and nuclei (Fig. 4B), and the effects of carcinogens alone or in combination. The diploid cell fraction increases rapidly when AAF treatment is initiated, and declines slowly after withdrawal of AAF. With the combined treatment (DEN+AAF) the diploid cell fraction remains elevated throughout the study period.

Table 3 shows the changes in absolute cell numbers within the various ploidy classes during the period of AAF treatment (four-week treatment, measurements at 0 and 5 weeks). It can be seen that AAF strongly suppresses the accumulation of binucleated cells and octoploid mononucleated cells, whereas

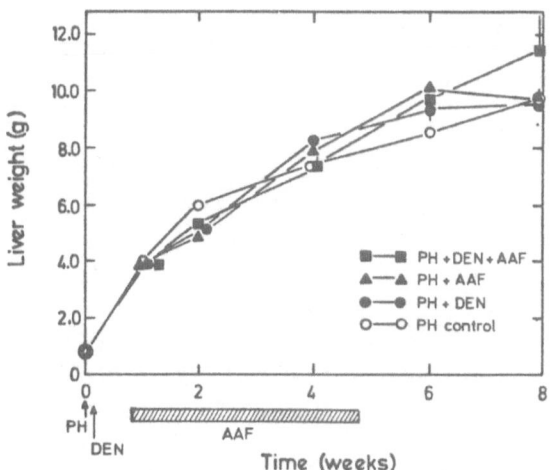

Fig. 3. Lack of effect of carcinogens on liver growth. Livers were excised and weighed at various times after partial (2/3) hepatectomy.

Table 3. Effect of carcinogens on changes in absolute hepatocyte numbers within various ploidy classes during five weeks of liver growth.

	Ploidy class (million cells)				
	2N	2x2N	4N	2x4N	8N
PH control	-73	46	220	102	70
DEN	16	87	203	120	81
AAF	360	6	482	10	34
DEN+AAF	649	27	326	13	10

Values represent net changes in cell numbers 1-6 weeks after partial hepatectomy. AAF treatment 1-5 weeks. Cell numbers are calculated by computer on the basis of flow cytometry (cells and nuclei), binuclearity counts and liver weight determinations.

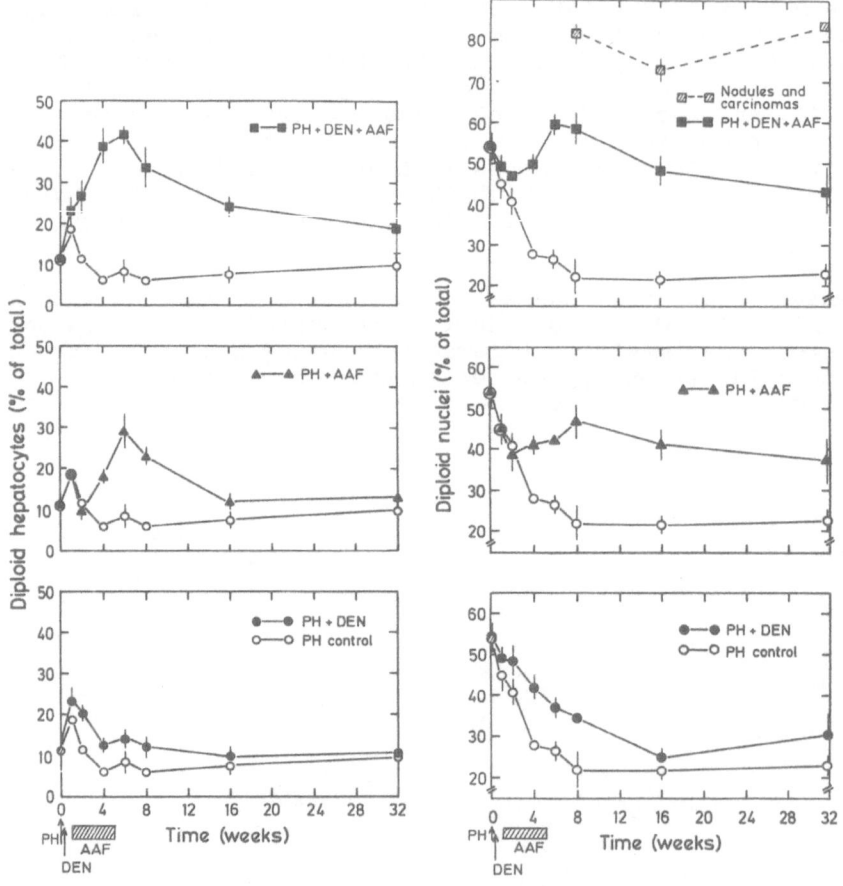

Fig. 4. Effect of carcinogens on the fraction of diploid hepatocytes (A) and diploid hepatocellular nuclei (B) after partial hepatectomy and during subsequent liver growth. Flow-cytometric analysis of collagenase-isolated hepatocytes and their nuclei, not corrected for aggregate formation.

accumulation of mononucleated diploid and tetraploid cells is stimulated. It thus seems as if AAF inhibits polyploidization, i.e. the formation of binucleated cells and the consequent flow of cells from the diploid to the tetraploid population, and from the tetraploid to the octoploid population. Cell division within the diploid and tetraploid populations appears, however, to be unaffected, resulting in a relative expansion of these populations due to blockade of the exit flow (binucleation).

A study of the time course of changes in binucleation following partial hepatectomy confirms the role of AAF as an inhibitor of polyploidization. AAF prevents, in large measure, both the rapid decrease in binucleated cells following hepatectomy, and the subsequent recovery (Fig. 5). This means that AAF interferes both with the formation of binucleated cells and with their subsequent conversion to mononucleated cells of a higher ploidy class. In other words, AAF does not just interfere with some biochemical step related to binucleation, but appears to repress the whole polyploidization programme in a hormone-like fashion.

By centrifugal elutriation it is possible to prepare fractions enriched in diploid and tetraploid hepatocytes, respectively (Schwarze et al., 1986a). Biochemical analysis of such fractions indicates that diploid and tetraploid cells are functionally similar, even with respect to some properties which are specifically altered by carcinogen treatment. However, there is one notable difference: the fraction of carcinogen-induced GGT-expressing cells is significantly higher in the diploid hepatocyte population (Schwarze et al., (1986b).

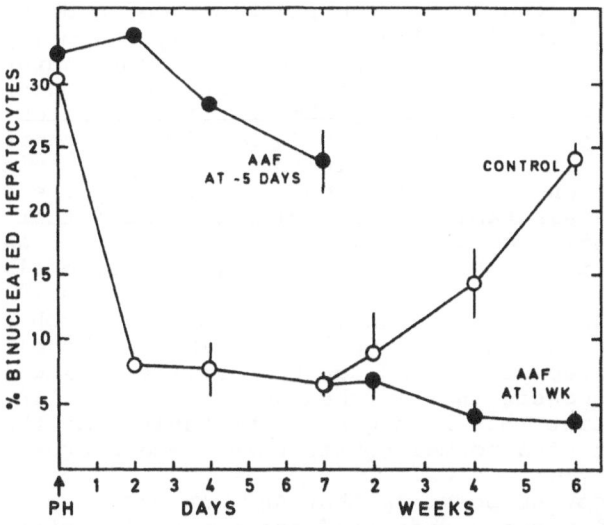

Fig. 5. AAF inhibits both the disappearance of binucleated cells after partial hepatectomy and their subsequent re-appearance.

Possible mechanisms for the promoting effects of AAF

Diploid expansion. Being the only ploidy class containing cells with an unlimited growth potential (i.e., stem cells), the diploid hepatocytes can be regarded as a precursor population for subsequent tumour development. A several-fold expansion of this population, as induced by AAF, would therefore be expected to increase the carcinogenic risk in a general way. Furthermore, most of the mutant phenotypes induced by the initiating carcinogen, DEN, are likely to originate within the diploid population (the tetraploid genome, carrying four alleles of each kind, would be extremely well protected against the expression of recessive mutations, including oncogenic lesions which are generally recessive, cf. e.g. Klein & Klein, 1986). In the presence of AAF, diploid mutants get a chance to form diploid clones of some size, rather than to undergo irreversible differentiation (polyploidization). If overall liver growth is slowing down by the time of AAF withdrawal, the clones may persist as diploid risk populations for considerable lengths of time. Were the mutants allowed to polyploidize, they would lose their potential for unlimited growth as well as their change to undergo additional expressible oncogenic mutations. AAF may thus act both to preserve the proliferative potential of initiated cells, and to increase the risk for further carcinogenic progression among mutant and normal cells alike.

Constitutive hyperproliferation and hypopolyploidization. During the period of rapid liver growth, hyperproliferative lesions will of course expand particularly rapidly. Constitutive hyperproliferation would furthermore be expected to be a prerequisite for subsequent clonal expansion in the absence of exogenous growth stimuli. However, unless the hyperproliferative clone is of stem cell origin, or has secondarily acquired a reduced polyploidization probability (i.e., below 0.5), it will gradually polyploidize, lose its oncogenic potential, and eventually stop growing as the proliferative potential of the polyploid cells becomes exhausted. Acquisition of a constitutively low polyploidization probability would therefore be one of the more advantageous secondary alterations an initiated clone could undergo (it could also arise as a primary abnormality, in which case subsequent diploid expansion would be of no further consequence). It is conceivable that AAF, by activating polyploidization-suppressive genes, could make the same genes particularly vulnerable (accessible) to damage that may render them permanently active. It is also possible that AAF may induce constitutive hypopolyploidization by eliciting the expression of polyploidization-suppressive genes in mutant cells which have lost the ability to shut off such genes. The fact that AAF-induction of GGT expression is largely restricted to DEN-initiated cells, and can be persistent as well as transient, suggests that induced gene activation in repression-defective mutants may be a general mechanism for the establishment of abnormal constitutive gene expression.

It is of course possible that AAF may use other promotional mechanisms than those discussed above. AAF is, after all, a carcinogen, and is likely to inflict mutational damage upon the cells during the proliferation phase. The induction of new oncogenic lesions in addition to those already induced by DEN would be difficult to distinguish from a pure promotional effect indirectly favouring the establishment of such lesions. Furthermore, in its role as hormone-like gene activator, AAF could affect genes more directly involved in proliferation than those associated with polyploidization or GGT expression, perhaps functioning as a growth factor for a minority of mutant cells. AAF-dependent hyperproliferative phenotypes would proliferate selectively in the presence of AAF, establishing expanded clones which would be at increased risk of taking an additional step from AAF-dependence to AAF-independence, in analogy with the stepwise progression of tumours towards increasing independence of hormones and growth factors (Klein & Klein, 1986). The relative importance of (1) generalized diploid expansion, (2) constitutive hypopolyploidization, (3) AAF-dependent hyperproliferation and (4) constitutive hyperproliferation, in the carcinogenesis-promoting effect of AAF, can only be elucidated by future studies.

Acknowledgement

This work has been generously supported by The Norwegian Cancer Society.

References

Klein, G., and Klein, E., 1986, Conditioned tumorigenicity of activated oncogenes, Cancer Res. 46: 3211.

Nadal, C., 1970, Polyploïdie hépatique du rat. Mode de formation des cellules binucléées, J. Microscopie 9: 611.

Sarafoff, M., Rabes, H.M., and Dörmer, P., 1986, Correlations between ploidy and initiation probability determined by DNA cytophotometry in individual altered hepatic foci, Carcinogenesis 7: 1191.

Schwarze, P.E., Pettersen, E.O., Shoaib, M.C., and Seglen, P.O., 1984, Emergence of a population of small, diploid hepatocytes during hepatocarcinogenesis, Carcinogenesis 5:1267.

Schwarze, P.E., Pettersen, E.O., and Seglen, P.O., 1986a, Characterization of hepatocytes from carcinogen-treated rats by two-parametric flow cytometry, Carcinogenesis 7:171.

Schwarze, P.E., Pettersen, E.O., Tolleshaug, H., and Seglen, P.O., 1986b, Isolation of carcinogen-induced diploid rat hepatocytes by centrifugal elutriation, Cancer Res. 46:4732.

Seglen, P.O., Schwarze, P.E., and Sæter, G., 1986, Changes in cellular ploidy and autophagic responsiveness during rat liver carcinogenesis, Toxicol. Pathol. 14:342.

Solt, D.B., Medline, A., and Farber, E., 1977, Rapid emergence of carcinogen-induced hyperplastic lesions in a new model for the sequential analysis of liver carcinogenesis, Am. J. Pathol. 88:595.

M.Kirsch-Volders[1],S.Haesen[1],A.Deleener[1],Ph.Castelain[1],H. Alexandre[2,3] and V.Preat[4]

[1].Lab.Antropogenetika,Vrije Universiteit Brussel,Brussels,Belgium
[2].Lab. de Cytologie et Embryologie moléculaires,Université Libre de Bruxelles,Brussels,Belguim.
[3].Research Associate of the National Fund for Scientific Research, Belgium
[4].Lab. de Biochimie Toxicologique et Cancérologique, Université Catholique de Louvain, Brussels, Belgium

INTRODUCTION

The study of the cancer phenotype, should from the theoretical point of view, be considered as the study of any other phenotype. It is |the result of the interaction between genotype and environment; of course this does not exclude that environmental factors can modify the inherited genotype. The cancer phenotype is dependent on the interaction of one (monogenic inheritance) or more (polygenic inheritance)"cancergenes", which may be dominant or recessive, with the surrounding conditions which may or may not favor the progression of the pre-malignant cells. As far as the polygenic model is concerned, the expression of the cancerphenotype may be understood as the probability to combine in a given cell, the expression of a given set of genes; due to the number of cancergenes, different combinations of genesets can be responsible for the (pre)-malignant status.

The dominant cancer genes, usually known as oncogenes, are genes which are expressed in normal cells (c-myc, c-ras family, etc...) but expressed in a modified way or overexpressed in tumor cells (for review[1,2]). The recessive "cancer genes" are genes which are not expressed in normal cells but are expressed in tumor cells; their existence was demonstrated by cellfusion experiments [3,4,5] and confirmed by the study of familial cancers [6] as retinoblastoma and Wilm's tumor.

This theoretical approach of cancer genetics nicely agrees with the description of carcinogenesis as a multistep, multifactorial process involving genetic as well as epigenetic factors. It is clear indeed, that although this paper is essentially concerned with the importance of genetic alterations, epigenetic factors are of crucial importance in carcinogenesis (for review[7]).

The question addressed to the geneticist concerned with the study of carcinogenesis is which genetic alterations or combination of genetic alterations may lead to the modified or enhanced expression of dominant oncogenes and to the expression of recessive cancer genes. Gene mutations are considered as responsible for the initial event by which some oncogenes express a modified protein and by which recessive cancer genes are induced; chromosomal rearrange-

ments as translocation, amplification, chromosome loss or modifications of
ploidy level are involved in further step(s) which lead to overexpression
of dominant oncogenes and expression of recessive cancer genes.

Our aim is to perform a sequential analysis of chromosomal rearrangements
and gene expression in an in vivo model for liver carcinogenesis, which requires
a synchronisation of the events leading to carcinogenesis. Recently, several
procedures allowing a better synchronisation have been described for hepatocarcinogenesis in the rat. SOLT and FARBER[8] developed a procedure that consists of the administration of an initiating dose of diethylnitrosamine (DENA)
followed by a selection with a short exposure to 2-acetylaminofluorene (2-AAF)
in combination with a proliferative stimulus, such as CCl_4 administration (I+S
protocol). Finally, this procedure can be completed with a promotion phase by
phenobarbital (PB) treatment [9] which causes an acceleration of the carcinogenic
process (I+S+P protocol).

In this study different genetic parameters were analysed during hepatocarcinogenesis induced by the I+S and I+S+P protocols.
- Frequencies of mono- and binucleated hepatocytes on hematoxylin-eosin stained
  liver slices
- DNA content of nuclei after Feulgen staining of liver slices
- Counting and karyotyping of chromosomes in metaphases obtained after liver
  perfusion
- Expression of the C-Ha-ras oncogene measured by Northern blotting of purified
  mRNA from normal, nodular or non-nodular, cancerous or non-cancerous liver
  parenchyma.

MATERIAL AND METHODS

a) Treatment of the animals

The experimental protocol is that described by LANS et al.[9]. Adult Male
Wistar rats (age 2,5-3 months) outbred WI (IOPS AF) HAN, IFFACREDO, France
were injected i.p. with a single necrogenic dose of DENA (200 mg/kg dissolved
in 0.9% NaCl). Two weeks later, a selection similar to that described by SOLT
and FARBER[10] was applied by giving the animals a diet containing 0.03% 2-acetyl-
aminofluorene (2-AAF) for two weeks. In the middle of this period, a necrogenic
dose of CCl_4 (2ml/kg, v/v in corn oil) was given by gavage in order to stimulate
the selective division of the initiated cells. One week after 2-AAF selection,
the animals received a basal diet (group I+S) or a 0.05% phenobarbital supplemented diet (group I+S+P) up to the end of the experiment. For each type of
treatment, 3 to 5 animals were analyzed.

Depending on the type of experiments, treatment and sampling were performed in different ways
1) measurement of DNA-content in nuclei and determination of frequencies of
   mono- and polynucleated hepatocytes.
   The rats received either an I+S or an I+S+P treatment; the PB treatment
   varied from 2 days to 5 months. Liver was removed and analyzed histologically.
2) counting and karyotyping of metaphase chromosomes.
   Animals were submitted to I+S or I+S+P+ protocols; the PB treatment varied
   from 2 to 3 days. Control animals at the age of 2.5 months received either
   the same basal diet without carcinogens (N.D.) or a 0.05% phenobarbital
   supplemented diet (PB) for 2 days.
   Metaphases were studied on isolated hepatocytes obtained after perfusion;
   the perfusion was preceded or not by a two-thirds partial hepatectomy (P.H.)
       32 hours before killing.

3) determination of changed c-Ha-ras expression

Adult control anaimal for this experiment received no treatment. Some of them were submitted to a two-thirds partial hepatectomy (P.H.) and killed 6h or 30h later. Others didn't undergo the P.H. Treated animals received the I+S+P (0.05% PB) protocol for 4 weeks, 5 months and 7 months.

b) histology

The liver was sliced and fixed in Carnoy solution (acetic acid: chloroform: ethanol; 1:3:6). The embedded liver slices were cut as serial sections and stained with hematoxylin - eosin or with Feulgen.

The livers of animals killed after I+S+7 days N.D. or 15 days N.D. showed distinguishable foci. The respons of the different animals was however very heterogeneous and some of the animals showed no lesions at all. 3 weeks N.D-livers displayed an altered liver morphology, with or without nodules. After 5 months of N.D. however, regression of the nodules had occured and only appearantly normal tissue could be observed.

For the animals which received PB instead of N.D., the same heterogeneity in respons is found shortly after I+S: no lesions were found in the 6 days PB treated rats, while the 8 day PB treated animals all showed foci. After 3 weeks PB treatment a very high number of so called pseudonodules was observed, so that in the surrounding or non-nodular portion of the liver parenchyma no clearcut sample could be taken. After 3 months PB treatment however, a regression of the pseudonodules had occured and all 3 animals showed small nodules in "normal" surrounding parenchyma. Animals that were fed PB for 5 months after I+S had developed either carcinoma or late nodules.

c) cytodensitometric measurements of the nuclear DNA content

The DNA content of the Feulgen-stained cell nuclei was measured using a Vickers densitometer M85 at 570 nm on interphase nuclei using the background substractive method. Per animal one or two random samples were taken in the -appearantly - normal liver parenchyma, while in animals presenting focal or nodular lesions, one to four lesions were analysed by measuring one sample (50 to 100 nuclei) in the lesion in addition to one sample (50 to 100 nuclei) of the parenchyma that closely surrounded the lesion.

The DNA histograms of nuclei contained within a liver section do not reflect the true nuclear ploidy distribution, because by the sectioning procedure nuclei may be sliced and therefore in some cases only a part of the nucleus will be measured, moreover, the diploid (2N) nuclei may be either in G1 (2C value) or in G2 (4C value): however 2N, 4C nuclei and 4N, 4C nuclei can not be distinguished. In order to calibrate the different ploidy levels, liver printing was performed and the liver print preparations so obtained were fixed in Carnoy solution, stained by the Feulgen reaction and measured for DNA content [11]; furthermore, isolated rat spermatozoa (possesssing haploid (IC) nuclei) were stained in a similar way. The defined population of diploid nuclei will althus be described here by the symbol (2C<->4C).

d) isolation of hepatocytes by perfusion

To isolate parenchymal cells at different times, rats were submitted to a chemical enzymatical liver perfusion derived from BERRY and modified by KRACH et al.[12]. After the enzymatic liver perfusion, the cell suspension obtained was incubated with colcemid (0.1 mg/ml) for 1.5 h at 37°C. Air-dried slides were obtained by routine processing through hypotonic solution (15 min; 0.075 M KCL) fixation (3:1methanol: acetic acid) and spreading of the cells on precleaned slides.

233

e) staining of metaphases

For chromosome counting, the hepatocytes obtained after perfusion were stained with Giemsa (5% aqueous Giemsa for 5 min.)

For karyotyping, two week old preparations were trypsin digested (0.01% solution of trypsin 1:250 in Hanks solution without Ca^{++}, Mg^{++} and phenol red) for about 90 sec at room temperature. After rinsing in distilled water and Hanks solution, the preparations were stained with Giemsa (2% aqueous Giemsa for 10 min.). The difficulty of obtaining enough well spread and well banded metaphases of rat hepatocytes led to quite low efficiency.

f) analysis of the chromosome data

Hepatocytes, even after partial hepatectomy, show a relatively low percentage of metaphases (in this work 2‰); moreover, an important fraction of them are tetraploid or octaploid. For these reasons, metaphases where the individual chromosomes can clearly be counted, are not easy to obtain.

To avoid the selection of the well-spread metaphases, 20 consecutive metaphases were photographed per animal. According to the quality of the chromosome spreading on each metaphase, the metaphases were classified:
  a) if not exact chromosome counting was possible, approximatively into
     haploid (N), diploid (2N), tetraploid (4N) or octaploid (8N) classes.
  b) if exact chromosome counting was possible, precisely according to the
     exact number of chromosmes counted.
In this case, the ploidy level of these metaphases was additionally defined according to the following schema :

10-31 chromosomes	N
32-52 chromosomes	2N
53-73 chromosomes	3N
74-94 chromosomes	4N
95-115 chromosomes	5N

In this paper, only the data obtained on the frequencies of diploid or circa-diploid metaphases (2N) were selected to be compared with the frequencies of 2C<->4C nuclei.

g) northern blotting of purified mRNA

Isolation of total RNA from rat/liver was performed according to the method of Glisin et al.[13] and Chirgwin et al.[14]. Selection of mRNA was carried out essentially as described by Aviv and Leder[15] on an oligo (dt) cellulose column. mRNA's were separated by electrophoresis in a denaturing 1.0% agarose gel and blotted on an Amersham nylon membrane. The probe (v-bas, 0.62 kb Bam HI-Hind III fragment, Dr. J. Merregaert, Dep. Bioch., U.I. Antwerp) was labelled with ^{32}P by nicktranslation to a specific activity of $4.8.10^7$ cpm/ug DNA. Hybridisation was carried out overnight, the filters were washed and exposed to Amersham hyperfilm.

RESULTS

1) Frequencies of diploidy in interphase nuclei and in metaphases

The genetic complement of a cell can be defined by quantification of the DNA content (2C, 4C etc...) and/or by counting the number of chromosomes (2N= diploid cell, 4N = tetraploid cell ....etc). This implies that a diploid (2N) cell may correspond either to a 2C DNA content (G1 phase) or to a 4C content (G2 phase).

234

On liver slices, one must however realize that the estimated DNA content is always approximative since in some cases, only a part of the nucleus will be measured; counting of chromosomes obtained after liver perfusion,on the other hand, allows no identification of the karyotyped cell.Genetic analysis of the liver is moreover complicated by the existence of tetraploid and octaploid hepatocytes in adult rats. A correct estimation of the exact ploidy is thus only possible by combining measurements of DNA content,here on liver slices, with counting of chromosomes from metaphases obtained after liver perfusion. Results obtained from both types of quantification are summarized on figure 1 for the I+S protocol and on figure 2 for the I+S+P protocol. The horizontal axis shows the stage of the treatment and the vertical axis gives the percentage of circa-diploid (2N) metaphases with or without hepatectomy (below) and the percentage of (2C<->4C) nuclei in normal tissue or in focal nodular and surrounding tissue (above).

As far as the I+S protocol is concerned, it is clear that it induces already 7 days after the end of the selection phase an increase of diploid metaphases (71%) as compared to the controls (47%); this increase is higher with hepatectomy than without. The frequencies of (2C<->4C) nuclei are very low, even lower than in non-treated animals, until 3 weeks after the end of the selection procedure; the diploid nuclei represent at this stage about 25% of the nuclei and are essentially observed in nodules when they are present.

Treatment with phenobarbital alone on the contrary reduces the frequency of diploid metaphases (33%); also in the I+S+P protocol, a 3-days treatment with PB shows a lower frequency of diploid metaphase (42%) than in the absence of PB (62%). The percentage of (2C<->4C) nuclei in the I+S+P treated rats are similar to the frequencies observed in the I+S protocol. However, the increase of (2C->4C) nuclei and the decrease of these nuclei at later stages starts earlier in the I+S+P protocol than in the I+S protocol.

2) Frequencies of mononucleated and binucleated hepatocytes on liver slices

Table 1 summarizes the data obtained on the frequencies of binucleated cells in treated and untreated animals. Untreated young rats show a high frequency of binucleated cells (about 30% in 4 weeks aged animals); this frequency decreases to reach a value of 7% in 10 weeks aged animals. In treated rats, most of the studied cell populations(normal tissue, lesions and surrounding parenchyma) show a relatively low percentage of binucleated cells (from 3.5 to 9.5%). However, 3 weeks after completion of the I+S protocol, a higher frequency (15.5%) of binucleated cells is found in the nodules. The same increase is found if a phenobarbital treatment was added to the I+S protocol for 3 weeks; after a 5 months period in the I+S or I+S+P protocols such high frequencies of binucleated cells are no more observed.

3) Frequencies of chromosome aberrations

Metaphases were rare in hepatocytes from animals which did not receive a mitotic stimulus as partial hepatectomy or CCl_4 treatment. To make the different samples comparable, all treated and untreated animals were submitted to a partial hepatectomy before performing the perfusion. Despite the relatively large number (5) of rats analysed per treatment, the yield of well banded metaphases was low; therefore the obtained karyotypes will only be considered as indicative.

The data collected from these experiments are shown on table 2. They show a clear tendency of disappearance of tetraploid metaphases just after the initiation/selection treatment (with or without phenobarbital). The frequencies of hypodiploid metaphases are much more important than.the frequencies of hyperdiploid cells in all treated samples. However, within the circa-diploid metaphases, no preferential loss or gain of a specific chromosome was observed.

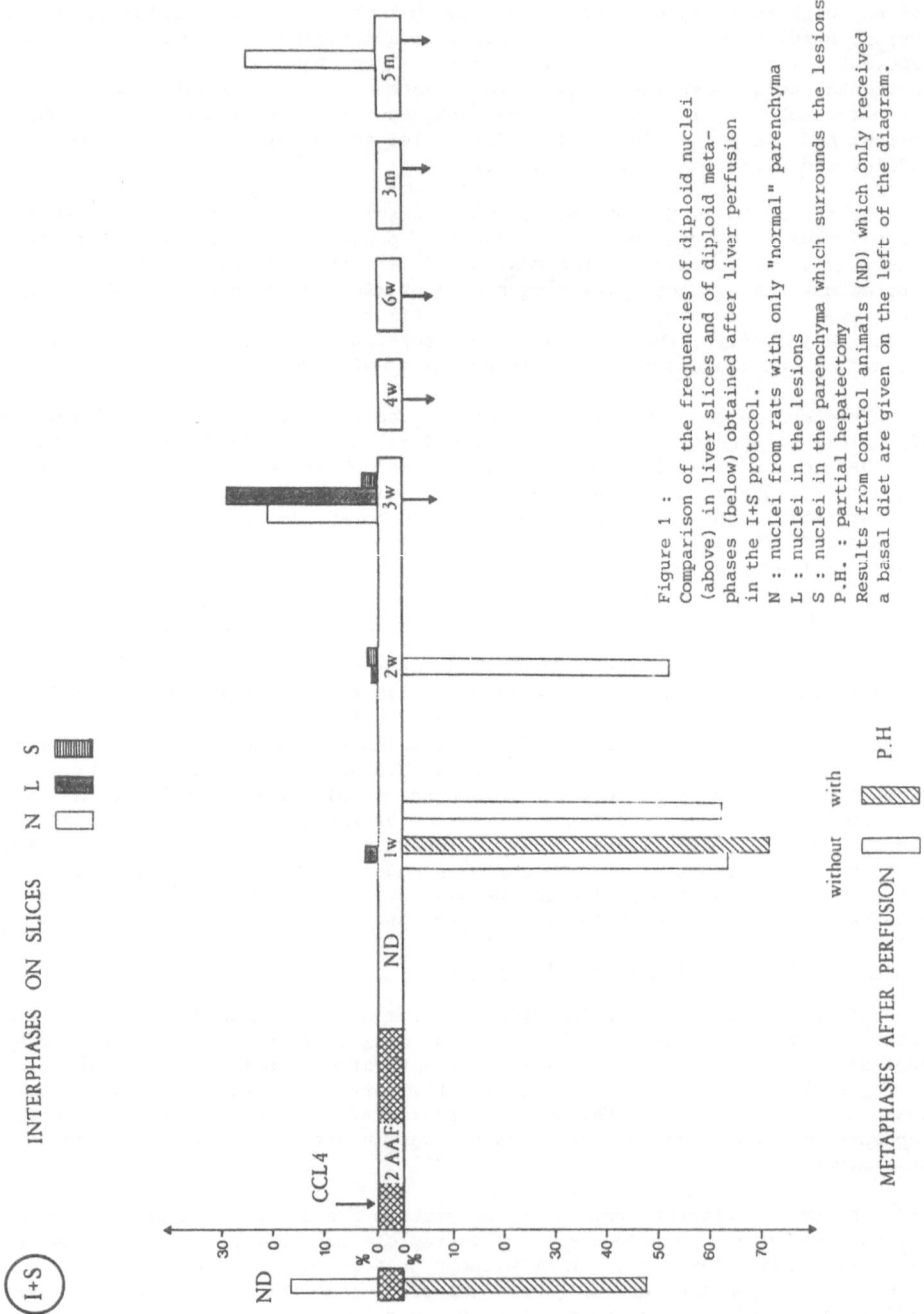

Figure 1 :
Comparison of the frequencies of diploid nuclei
(above) in liver slices and of diploid meta-
phases (below) obtained after liver perfusion
in the I+S protocol.
N : nuclei from rats with only "normal" parenchyma
L : nuclei in the lesions
S : nuclei in the parenchyma which surrounds the lesions
P.H. : partial hepatectomy
Results from control animals (ND) which only received
a basal diet are given on the left of the diagram.

INTERPHASES ON SLICES

N   L   S

METAPHASES AFTER PERFUSION

without   with   P.H

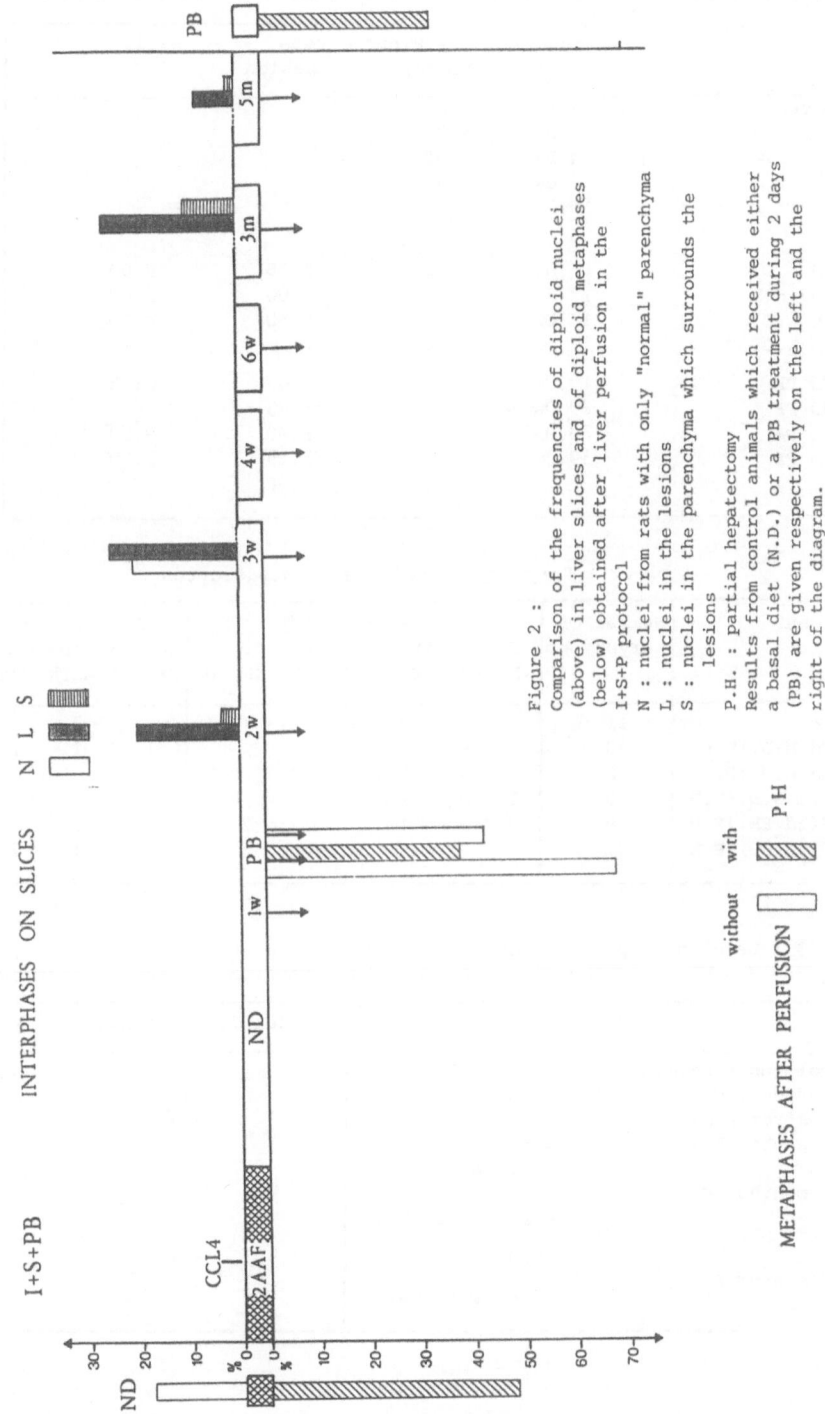

Figure 2 :
Comparison of the frequencies of diploid nuclei
(above) in liver slices and of diploid metaphases
(below) obtained after liver perfusion in the
I+S+P protocol

N : nuclei from rats with only "normal" parenchyma
L : nuclei in the lesions
S : nuclei in the parenchyma which surrounds the
    lesions

P.H. : partial hepatectomy
Results from control animals which received either
a basal diet (N.D.) or a PB treatment during 2 days
(PB) are given respectively on the left and the
right of the diagram.

Table 1 : Percentage of binucleated cells: treated and untreated rats

	Age	% Binucleated Normal	Lesion	cells Surr.
Untreated	3.5w	15.05		
	4.0w	29.20		
	4.5w	25.00		
	7.0w	11.45		
	10.0w	7.20		
Treated				
I+S+7d N.D.	16.0w	6.50	5.25	8.00
I+S+15d N.D.	17.0w	6.75	6.00	5.00
I+S+3w N.D.	19.0w	5.00	15.50	4.00
I+S+5m N.D.	39.0w	11.87	-	-
I+S+8d PB	17.0w	-	8.33	6.25
I+S+3w PB	19.0w	3.50	15.93	-
I+S+3m PB	30.0w	-	9.00	9.50
I+S+5m PB	39.0w	-	5.25	3.70
		carc. :	6.50	

Table 2 : Karyotypic analysis of hepatocytes

Treatment	Number of karyotypes	C. N	circa <2N	2N	>2N	c. 3N	c. 4N	c. 8N	Transl.	Mark.	Frag.
P.H.	11			2	1		7	1		3	
I+S+7d N.D.+P.H.	20		6	13	1				1	1	1
I+S+9d N.D.+P.H.	10	1	4	1		4					2
I+S+15d N.D.+P.H.	8	1	5	2							
I+S+P(2d PB)+P.H.	9	3	3	1			2				
I+S+P(8d PB)+P.H.	21	3	9	4	2		3		1	1	2

Table 3 : Level of expression of the c-Ha-ras oncogene, as measured by Northern blot hybridisation of the mRNA with ^{32}p labelled probes

	Expression of c-Ha-ras
Control (no treatment)	+
+ 6h after P.H.	+
+ 30h after P.H.	+ +
I+S+4 weeks PB (no lesions isolated)	+ +
I+S+5 months PB — Nodules	+ + +
I+S+5 months PB — surr. parenchyma	+ + +
I+S+7 months PB — Nodules	+ +
I+S+7 months PB — surr. parenchyma	+ +

As far as chromosome aberrations are concerned, a metacentric marker chromosome is found in treated and untreated rats as well. Besides this, acentric fragments and translocations were found but with frequencies which are difficult to interprete.

4) Expression of c-Ha-ras oncogenes.

In table 3 the results for the Northern blotting experiments with c-Ha-ras are summarized. No increase in the amount of ras-transcripts is observed shortly after partial hepatectomy (6h) as compared with control animals. 30h after PH, a relative increase in the number of transcripts is found, as shown by the increasing intensity of the band on the autoradiography.

In the liver of animals submitted to the I+S+P protocol, the level of c-Ha-ras expression is elevated in the 4 weeks PB-treated animals as well as in the 7 months PB treated animals. A markedly sharp increase is seen after 5 months PB treatment. Interestingly, however no difference in expression level is observed in the late nodules or carcinomas and their surrounding parenchyma (5 months PB and 7 months PB).

DISCUSSION

1) Evidence for the increase of the frequency of diploid cells during hepato- carcinogenesis.

The observation that the frequency of 2C nuclei (and not 2N metaphases) increase after in vivo treatment of liver cells by carcinogens is not new. It was found after treatment with different carcinogens (aflatoxine B_1, thioaceta-metide, 2AAF, DENA, 3'M) and with different technical approaches as zonal centri-fugation (17, 18, 19, 20, 21), elutriation (21), flow cytometry (18, 22, 23), micro-spectrophotometry (24) and karyotyping (25). These observations clearly agree with the increase of (2c <->4c) nuclei observed by us after Feulgen-micro-densitometric analysis of liver slices obtained from rats treatment with the I+S protocol and the I+S+P protocol.

Our results on metaphases provide additional information.
1. Since the lesions essentially show mononucleated cells, one may assume that the observed diploid metaphases are not the result of the simultaneous division of the two nuclei of a binucleated cell but indeed the mitosis of a mononucleated diploid cell.

2. They indicate whether the 4C values observed on interphase nuclei cor-respond to G_2 phases of diploid (2N) nuclei or G_1 phases of a tetraploid (4N) nuclei. As far as the tetraploid metaphases are concerned one should however not forget that in the liver, a tetraploid (4N) metaphase may also result from a synchronized mitosis of a binucleated (2x2N) hepatocyte.

3. As a matter of fact, data collected on metaphases are specific for di-viding cells. Since the metaphase show a clear increase of diploidisation (2N) after I+S treatment, one may assume that these dividing cells are the precursors of the diploid lesions observed by densitometrical analysis of interphase nuclei.

Recently, Styles ey al. [26] demonstrated that genotoxic carcinogens induce a reduction in the frequency of binucleated cells, in male Alpk/Al rats. In our study with male Wistar rats, no decrease of the frequency of binucleated cells was observed after the treatment with the I+S or the I≠S+P protocol; our data show that binuclearity decreases with age and that some increase of binuclea-rity is observed in the nodules 3 weeks after the completion of the selection procedure. From the comparison of their data on nuclearity and on diploidisation, Styles et al. [26] suggested that non-genotoxic carcinogens stimulate the production of 4C or 4N mononucleated cells but that genotoxic carcinogens induce an increase of mononucleated 2C cells. However since no results on metaphases were available, it was difficult for them to conclude on the exact nature of the so-called diploid cells.

As far as our results are concerned, we are able to compare data on nuclearity, on DNA content of interphase nuclei and on ploidy level of dividing cells. This comparison confirms that binucleated cells form an essential step towards polyploidisation but also that an important distinction has to be made between chromosome number (2N,4N) and DNA content (2C,4C). According to this, new diagrams can be proposed to describe polyploidization during liver maturation and the shift from 4N to 2N induced by genotoxic carcinogens. Due to the well known existence of binucleated hepatocytes, it is logic to assume (Fig. 3) that during liver maturation the absence of cytokinesis leads to a binucleated (2x (2N,2C)) cell which after S phase and mitosis on one spindle may be converted to two tetraploid (4N, 4C) cells. Under the influence of a genotoxic carcinogen, the shift from 4C to 2C (fig. 3B) may occur either by mitoses of G2 arrested (2N,4C) cells or by cytokinesis of a binucleated (2x (2N,4C)) cell into two diploid mononucleated cells (2N,4C), followed by a normal mitosis (2 cells with each 2N, 2C values); this of course, as far as we still have to assume that reduction of chromosome number (meiosis) is impossible in somatic cells.

If one takes into account the previous comments it is possible to interprete our results in the following way. The increase of 2N and the relative decrease of 4N metaphases underline the fact that the Initiation/Selection protocol for hepatocarcinogenesis does not convert directly tetraploid (4N) cells into diploid (2N) cells but inhibits further progression from diploidy to tetraploidy and/or stimulates cytokinesis of binucleated diploid (2x2N,4C) hepatocytes. These diploid dividing cells would further give rise to the lesions responsible for cancer progression.

Although attractive, this hypothesis leaves us with many unanswered questions. As an example,3 months after the termination of the I+S procedure animals treated with I+S or I+S+P protocols show in the nodules an increase of diploidisation and a relatively higher frequency of binucleated cells.

2) No evidence for the presence of visible chromosome rearrangements or specific monosomies, during the early stages of hepatocarcinogenesis

As far as the chromosome aberrations are concerned,some metaphases show chromosomal rearrangements and moreover some treatments (I+S+7days N.D.+P.H., I+S+P (8days PB) + P.H) induce higher frequencies of chromosome aberrations. However the samples are too small to consider these observations as significant. Besides these data on the increase of chromosome mutations during the first steps of hepatocarcinogenesis,it is worthwhile to underline the presence of a marker chromosome in control and treated animals of the studied Wistar strain.

Since monosomy clearly favors the expression of a recessive allel, we carefully identified the monosomies, nullosomies and trisomies in the circadiploid metaphases. However no specific chromosome loss (or gain) was observed.

3) Increase in the expression of c-Ha-ras oncogene during hepatocarcinogenesis

Northern blot hybridisation shows that there is an increase in the level of Ha-ras transcripts, relative to the level in normal hepatocytes,30h after a 2/3 hepatactomy of the liver. This increase has not yet started 6h after P.H.,which may indicate that a change in Ha-ras-transcription coincides with the onset of DNA-synthesis (peak around 24 hours after P.H.)[27]. The same increase is observed in the livers of animals treated for 4 weeks with PB after I+S, as well as in the late nodules and their surrounding parenchyma (5 months PB) and in the carcinoma and surrounding parenchyma (7 months PB). These observations are in accordance with the reports of Corcos et al.[28] and Makino et al.[29].

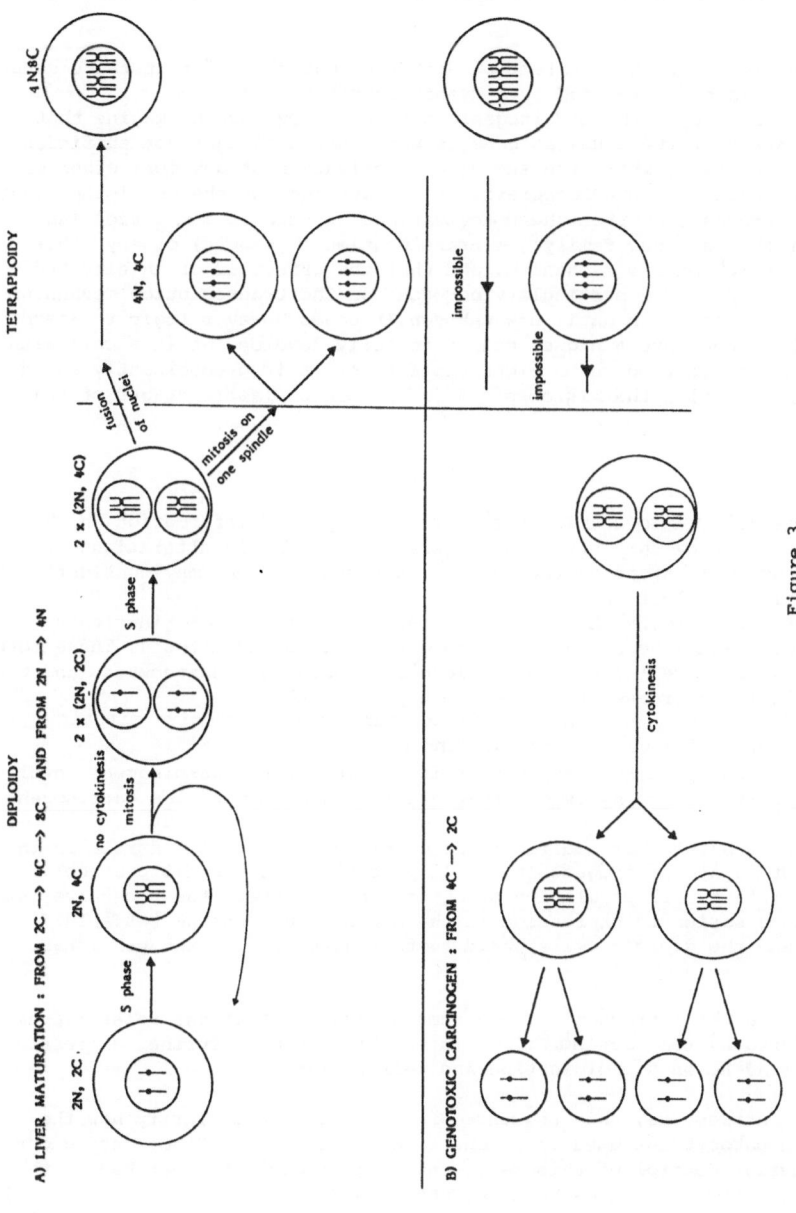

Figure 3.

Hypothetic diagrams illustrating the changes in DNA amount (C values) and chromosome numbers (N values) during liver maturation (A) and after treatment with a genotoxic carcinogen (B).

As suggested by others[29,30] the increase of c-Ha-ras transcripts points to the proliferation of hepatocytes,which takes place as well in regenerative processes (after P.H.) as in carcinogenesis of the liver. This overexpression of c-Ha-ras seems however not to be the determining factor to cause the outgrowth of preneoplastic foci and nodules, since there is also an overexpression observed in the perinodular and tumour surrounding parenchyma. This could suggest that the c-Ha-ras oncogene acts in a dominant way,since the lesion - surrounding parenchyma seems to have a predominantly polyploid DNA-constitution.

The probable synergistic effect of different oncogenes,for instance c-Ha-ras and c-myc, has been proposed as a major contribution to the onset and maintenance of the carcinogenic process[31]. One could imagine that the overexpression of the c-Ha-ras gene is necessary althought not sufficient for cell-proliferation, where the subsequent activation of one more other oncogenes can be regarded as a cooperative factor,reflecting the multistep nature of the cancer process. Whether these activations are due to a mutation (as described for the ras-gene family), a translocation (myc-gene) or any other genetic or even epigenetic mechanism, and what the effect is of an elevated level of transcripts of a particulary oncogene on the transcription mechanism of another (onco-)gene, is until now unknown.It seems however logic to assume that these phenomena have a higher chance to fully development in a cell with a diploid DNA-constitution,which might explain why it is predominantly an outgrowth of diploid cells that is observed in the preneoplastic stages of rat hepatocarcinogenesis.

4) Conclusion

If one is allowed to combine the different types of information which were made available by this study and others on the genetic alterations occuring during the early steps of rat hepatocarcinogenesis, one may consider that after initiation + selection

1. G2 arrested (4C,2N) hepatocytes undergo mitosis and/or binucleated diploid (2x2N) hepatocytes undergo cytokinesis and mitosis. These result into a relative increase of diploid mononucleated hepatocytes (and thus a relative decrease of tetraploid hepatocytes)
2. the diploid hepatocytes proliferate further by succesive mitotic divisions and give rise to foci and nodules
3. no visible chromosome aberration is induced by the carcinogens involved
4. no specific monosomy is observed after treatment with the carcinogens.

This data suggest that modifications of ploidy levels play a role in the early steps of hepatocarcinogenesis. It is probable that the I+S protocol selects a resistant cell population of mutated hepatocytes; the recessive mutation would come easier to expression in the diploid than in the tetraploid hepatocytes and the diploid cells would further give rise to the persistant nodules.

Refering to the introduction, one should consider that the recessive cancer gene was induced by some gene-mutation in the livergenome; further expression should be dependent on diploidisation and cellcycling.

Although attractive, this sequence of events does not clarify how the binucleated hepatocyte assumed to evaluate te tetraploidy (4N), at once undergoes cytokinesis. Control of this key event must probably be searched at the level of epigenetic factors as hormones etc... Additionally or complementarily to the described events one cannot neglect a possible role of the dominant oncogenes in hepatocarcinogenesis. It is not excluded that the cooperation of 2 or more activated oncogenes at some sites of the liver parenchyma provides precisely the surrounding in which diploidisation can occur.

ACKNOWLEDGEMENTS

    We thank Mrs. G.Plas, Mrs. K. Hamelrijck and Mr. R. Wellens for skillful
technical help. We also thank Dr. L. Michiels from the U.I.Antwerp for helpful
scientific advise. S. Haesen is a doctoral fellow of I.W.O.N.L. Belgium.

REFERENCES

1. H. Varmus, The Molecular genetics of cellular oncogenes, Ann. Rev. Genet.
   18:553 (1984)
2. J. Bischop, Trends in Oncogenesis, Trends in Genetics, 245 (1985)
3. H. Harris,cellfusion and the analysis of malignancy, Proc. R. Soc. Lond.
   B. Biol. Sci., 179: 1 (1971)
4. E.P. Evans, M.D. Burtenshaw, B.B. Brown, R. Hennion and H. Harris, The
   analysis of malignancy by cell fusion. IX Re-examination and clarification of the cytogenetic problem, J. Cell. Sci. 56:113 (1982).
5. E.S. Srivatsan, F.B. William and E.J. Stanbridge, Implication of chromosome 11 in the suppression of neoplastic expression in human cell
   hybrids, Cancer Res. 46:6174 (1986)
6. A.G. Knudson, Genetics of human cancer, Ann. Rev. Genet. 20:231 (1986)
7. G. Klein and E. Klein, Evolution of tumours and the impact of molecular
   oncology, Nature 315: 190 (1985).
8. D.B. Solt and E. Farber, New principle for the analysis of chemical
   carcinogenesis, Nature 363:701 (1976).
9. M. Lans, J. de Gerlache, H.S. Taper, V. Preat and M.B. Roberfroid, Phenobarbital as a promotor in the initiation/selection process of experimental rat hepatocarcinognesis, Carcinogenesis 4,2:141 (1983)
10.D.B. Solt, A. Medline and E. Farber, Rapid emergence of carcinogen-induced
   hyperplastic lesions in a new model for sequential analysis of liver
   carcinogenesis, Am. J. Pathol. 88:595 (1977).
11.A. Deleener, Ph. Castelain, V. Preat, J. de Gerlache, H. Alexandre and M.
   Kirsch-Volders, Changes in nucleolar transcriptional activity and
   nuclear DNA content during the first steps of rat hepatocarcinogenesis.
   Carcinogenesis, 8,2:195 (1987).
12.G. Krack, O. Gravier, M. Roberfroid and M. Mercier, Subcellular fractionation of isolated rat hepatocytes : A comparison with liver homogenate,
   Biochim Biophys Acta 632:619 (1980).
13.V. Glisin, R. Crkvenjakov and C. Byus, Ribonucleic acid isolated by cesium
   chloride centrifugation, Biochemistry 13:2633 (1974).
14.J. Chirgwin, A. Przybyla, R. MacDonald and W. Rutter, Isolation of biologically active ribonucleic acid from sources enriched in ribonuclease,
   Biochemistry 18:5294 (1979).
15.H. Aviv, P. Leder, Purification of biologically active globin messenger
   RNA by chromatography on oligothymidylic acid-cellulose, Proc. Natl.
   Acad. Sci. 69:1408 (1972).
16.M. Goyette, C. Petropoulos , P. Shank and N. Fausto, Regulated transcription of c-Ki-ras and c-myc during compensatory growth of rat liver, Mol.
   and cell. Biol. 4: 1493 (1984).
17.H. Godoy, D. Judah, H. Arora, G. Neal, G. Jones, The effects of prolonged
   feeding with aflatoxin B_1 on adult rat liver, Cancer Res. 36:2399(1976).
18.F. Gonzaler-Mujica, A. Mathias, Studies of nuclei separated by zonal centrifugation from liver of rats treated with thiocetamide, Biochem. J.132:
   163 (1973).
19.G. Neal, H. Godoy, D. Judah, W. Butler, Some effects of acute and chronic
   dosing with aflatoxin on rat liver nuclei, Cancer Res. 36:1771 (1976)
20.G. Neal, W. Butler, A comparison of the changes induced in rat liver by
   feeding low levels of aflatoxine or an azo dye, Br. J. Cancer 37:455
   (1978).
21.P.E. Schwarze,E.O. Petterson, H. Tolleschaug, P.O. Seglen, Isolation of
   carcinogen induced diploid rat hepatocytes by centrifugal elutriation,
   Cancer Res. 46:4732 (1986).

22. V.Digernes, O. Iversen, Flow cytometry of nuclear DNA content in liver tumors in rats exposed to acetylaminofluorene, Virchows Ach (Cell Path) 4:139 (1984)

23. J. Styles, B. Elliot, P. Lefevre, M. Robinsom, N. Tritchard, D. Hart, J. Ashby, Irreversible depression in the ratio of tetraploid-diploid liver nuclei in rats treated with 3'-methyl-4-dimethyl-aminoazobenzene (3'M) Carcinogenesis 6:21 (1985).

24. H. Mori, T. Tanaka, S. Sugie, M. Takhahashi, G. Williams, DNA content of liver cell nuclei of N-2-fluorrenylacetamide -induced altered foci and neoplasms in rats and human hyperplastic foci, J. of Natl. Cancer. Inst. 69: 1277 (1982).

25. F.F. Becker, R.A. Fox, K.M. Klein, S.R. Wolman, Chromosome patterns in rat hepatocytes during N-2 fluorenylacetamide carcinogenesis. J. of Natl. Cancer Inst. 46:1261 (1971).

26. J.A. Styles, M. Kelly, C.R. Elcombe, A cytological comparison between regeneration, hyperplasia and early neoplasia in the rat liver. Carcinogenesis 8,3:391 (1987).

27. M. Goyette, C. Petropoulos, P. Shank, N. Fausto, Expression of a cellular oncogene during liver regeneration, Science 219;510 (1983)

28. D. Corcos, N. Defer, M. Raymondjean, B. Paris, M. Corral, L. Tichonicky, J. Kruch, D. Glaise, A. Saulnier and C. Guguen-Guillaouza, Correlated increase of the expression of the c-ras genes in chemically induced hepatocarcinomas, Biochem. and Biophys. Res. Comm. 122; 259 (1984).

29. R. Matrino, K. Hayashi, S. Sato and T. Sugimura, Expression of c-Ha-ras and c-myc genes in rat liver tumors, Biochem. and Biophys. Res. Comm., 119:1096 (1984).

30. P. Jaswen, M. Goyette, P. Shank and N. Fausto, Expression of c-Ki-ras, c-Ha-ras and c-myc in specific cell types during hepatocarcinogenesis, Mol. and Cell. Biol., 5:780 (1985).

31. H. Land, L. Parada, R. Weinberg, Cellular oncogenes and multistep carcinogenesis, Science 222:771 (1983).

ROLE OF ONCOGENES IN HEPATOCARCINOGENESIS

C. GUGUEN-GUILLOUZO, G. BAFFET, P.L. ETIENNE and D. GLAISE
N. DEFER[*], M. CORRAL[*], D. CORCOS[*] and J. KRUH[*]

INSERM - U 49 - Hôpital Pontchaillou - 35033 RENNES Cédex
[*]Institut de Pathologie Moléculaire - 24, rue du Faubourg
St Jacques - 75014 PARIS - FRANCE

INTRODUCTION

Oncogenes are a set of genes which have been implicated in carcinogenesis. They are activated forms of proto-oncogenes which are part of the genetic complement of all normal cells. These genes are highly conserved during evolution suggesting that they play a critical role in some fundamental phenomena in life.

Evidence has accumulated supporting the view that several oncogenes can be involved in carcinogenesis, each of them being characteristic of one of the steps during the multi-stage carcinogenesis process. However, a single properly activated oncogene can also trigger the whole process of malignant conversion of a normal cell. Consequently, both the oncogene-one gene and the multigene-one cancer hypotheses may be currently proposed.

Hepatocarcinogenesis proceeds along several steps, following the general pathway of initiation, promotion and progression. First, expression of oncogenes during the course of hepatocarcinogenesis will be reported. Then, we shall attempt to analyse the biological significance of these observations in the light of :
- the generality of oncogene activation in hepatocarcinogenesis ;
- similarities between the patterns of oncogene expression which characterize hepatocarcinogenesis and those which may occur in normal tissue ;
- homologies between these oncogenes and other known cellular genes.

I - EXPRESSION OF ONCOGENES IN DENA-INDUCED HEPATOCARCINOGENESIS

We have chosen to examine the expression of twelve different oncogenes in the liver of rats subjected to a short diethyl-nitrosamine (DENA) treatment after a two-third partial hepatectomy[1,2,3]. Indeed, this simple basal model is suitable for studying the successive steps of hepatocarcinogenesis since the carcinogen is given for only 3 consecutive days and the cancer developpes slowly during several weeks, without additional treatment, by transformation of hepatocytes and without proliferation of "oval cells"[4]. C-mos, c-abl, c-myc, c-sis and c-src oncogenes were found weakly expressed in hepatocytes from both normal and

DENA-treated rats. In contrast, c-fos, c-myc, N-myc and the ras gene
family were activated with a partly different time-course. Transcripts of
c-fos and N-myc were first increased.

A 2-fold increase in c-fos expression was observed in the
hepatocytes as early as 8 days after treatment[1]. This expression
increased with time and reached a level corresponding to 5- to 6- fold
the basal level after 2-4 months. This increase was maximal after 70
weeks. At this late stage, hepatocytes from the non-tumoral zone could be
separated from tumor nodules by the collagenase perfusion technique and
cell filtration on a nylon mesh ; undissocated nodules being retained on
the filter. Using this technique, overexpression of c-fos was
demonstrated not only in malignant nodules but also in the apparently
untransformed non-nodular hepatocytes.

It is then clear that the increase of oncogene expression occurs as
well in the non tumoral part of liver as in malignant nodules.

N-myc gene expression also increased early during DENA-induced
carcinogenesis, and reached its maximal level on the first month[2]. It is
interesting to notice that it is one of the first observations of an
increased expression of N-myc in tumors from non-neural origin.

Overexpression of c-myc occured later, 5 to 7 months after DENA
treatment. The same observation was made for the 3 ras genes which were
overexpressed from 6 months after treatment to late stages of
carcinogenesis, as well in the non tumoral zones as in cancerous
nodules[3]. It is important to note that there is a coordinated expression
of these 3 genes, suggesting that their abnormal expression may result
from some epigenetic mechanisms. A parallel overexpression of the 3 ras
genes is unusual in other tissues.

II - GENERALITY OF ONCOGENE ACTIVATION IN HEPATOCARCINOGENESIS

One approach for determining the biological significance of oncogene
activation in hepatocarcinogenesis is to provide informations on the
generality of these alterations.

A) - We have first analysed the observations made by several groups
using various animal models of liver carcinogenesis, including a choline-
deficient diet containing ethionine[5], a protein-free diet[6], or administration of 3'methyl-4-dimethylaminoazobenzene (3'-Me-DAB)[7] and aflatoxin
B_1[8]. It may be concluded that c-abl, c-mos and c-src remained unchanged
during hepatocarcinogenesis in rats and mice. In contrast, c-myc, c-Ki-
and c-Ha-ras oncogenes appeared to be increased in all cases. Up to now
the number of studies devoted to c-fos oncogene is more limited. However,
an increased expression of this gene was often demonstrated[9]. An increase
of N-myc oncogene activity has recently been reported in DENA-treated rat
liver[2] and activation of c-raf oncogene has also been found in one
case[10].

It may be noted that the abundance of c-myc, cKi- and c-Ha-ras
transcripts increased as early as 2 weeks after starting the choline-
deficient diet. This overexpression is observed earlier than with DENA
treatment. This could be explained in this case by the proliferation of
"oval cells". Indeed, in contrast to DENA administration, both this
choline-deficient diet and 3'-Me-DAB treatment induced proliferation of
stem cells or "oval cells"[11]. Evidence has been provided suggesting that
expression of c-Ki-ras and c-myc oncogenes was high in these "oval
cells"[5].

B) - These observations have been extended to human hepatocarcinomas. Biopsies from 25 patients have been studied. We found, in contrast
to the results obtained with rats, a preferential activation of N-ras, an
activation of other ras genes in half of the cases and an elevated amount
of c-fos transcripts only in two cases. N-ras and c-Ki-ras were expressed
as well in non tumoral parts of the liver as in the tumors (Fig. 1).

Transcripts of c-erb-A, c-erb-B and c-sis remained very low in
fragments from both normal livers and carcinomas. However, a recent study
has reported that abnormal c-erb-B oncogene expression might occur in
human cirrhotic livers and in hepatomas[12].

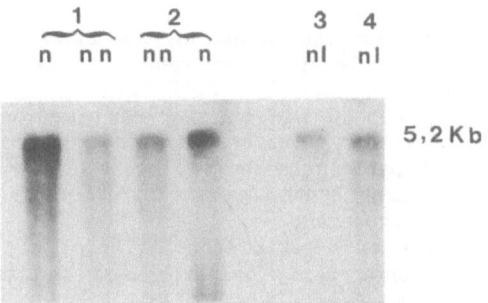

Figure 1 : Relative levels of N-ras transcripts (10 µg) in human
hepatocarcinomas from two patients (lanes 1 and 2) and in
normal liver (lanes 3 and 4). RNAs were extracted from tumor
nodules (n) and non-nodular parts of liver (nn) and analyzed
by Northern-blot.

C) - We have also extended our study to two in vitro models. The
first one was concerned with the spontaneous transformation of liver
cells in vitro. Liver epithelial cells, presumably derived from primitive
biliary cells, can be cultured in a proliferative state. However, after
several months they gradually undergo spontaneous transformation as
evidenced by their ability to grow in soft agar and by induction of
tumors after injection to syngenic rats[13]. By comparing these cells at
different passages, we found a progressive increase of the c-Ki-ras
expression, a constant expression of c-Ha-ras and no expression of N-ras,
c-fos and c-myc. Interestingly, gradual changes of expression of several
cytoskeleton proteins and of their phosphorylation activities were
observed concomitantly[14]. Similar observations have been reported in
vivo. Thus, an active cellular oncogene was demonstrated in
hepatocellular neoplasms arising spontaneously in 24 month-old B6C3F1
mice[15].

It is then evident that overexpression of at least one oncogene
accompanies the gradual spontaneous transformation process of liver cells
as well in vitro as in vivo.

The second model was made of human differentiated hepatocarcinomas which are usually not easy to establish in culture. When we succeeded to set up an hepatoma cell line, we observed that 3 to 4 months were needed to get cell proliferation and, surprisingly, that growth of small colonies occured at the same time in all dishes of the experiment. More interesting was the observation that expression of c-myc transcripts was highly increased in all the clones which were established, independently of their differentiated state (Fig. 2).

This observation strongly suggests that these cells need to escape from mechanisms which regulate their growth in vivo to be able to proliferate in vitro. Furthermore, it emphasizes the role of oncogenes as regulators in these processes.

Thus, four major characteristics are currently emerging from these different observations :
i) the constant oncogene activation during the liver cancer process in vivo and in vitro ; at least 2 oncogenes being overexpressed in hepatocarcinomas in vivo ;
ii) the variability in the nature of the overexpressed oncogenes. Indeed, increased expression of either c-fos or c-myc or c-Ha-ras, although being a frequent feature in hepatocarcinomas, is not necessarily required for the maintenance of the tumor state, making it difficult to define their role in the liver cancer process ;
iii) the apparent absence of hepatic specificity of the oncogenes which are activated, all of them being overexpressed in tumors from other tissues ;
iiii) the impossibility, at the present time, to associate an activated oncogene with a specific stage in hepatocarcinogenesis. Conflicting conclusions may arise from variations in oncogene activation from one species to another, from differences in the carcinogens used and also from the cellular heterogeneity due to the different effects of the various carcinogens on the induction of hyperplastic cell growth and hyperplastic foci. Indeed, variations in the number and size of neoplastic foci have been extensively described. Furthermore, variations in the oncogene alterations from one foci to another through the liver, at the same time,is very likely.

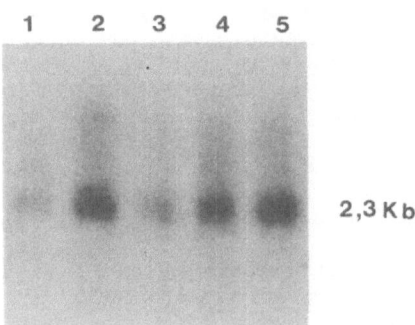

Figure 2 : Expression of c-myc transcripts in an established human
          hepatoma cell line. Four different clones (lanes 2 to 5) and
          the original tumor fragment (lane 1) were compared.

III - SIMILARITIES IN THE ONCOGENE EXPRESSION BETWEEN HEPATOCARCINOMAS AND NORMAL LIVER TISSUE.

Another way to determine the biological significance of oncogene activation in hepatocarcinomas is to search for a similar expression in their normal cell counterparts. An overexpression of various oncogenes can be observed in non cancerous tissues in several circonstances. Three different biological situations have been compared : pre- and post-natal development, regeneration after partial hepatectomy and liver cells in culture.

A) - Little is known about the presence of oncogene products in the liver during the fetal and early postnatal life. The available reports have examined the expression of the myc gene family, c-fos and c-Ha-ras in mice as well as in human fetuses[16,17,18], c-abl and c-mos in mice[16] c-erb-B, c-sis and c-Ki-ras in human fetuses[12], and ras oncoproteins in rats[19]. All reports have demonstrated :
(i) participation of cellular oncogenes (c-fos, c-myc, N-myc, c-abl, c-sis, c-ras) in normal developmental processes ;
(ii) differential activities of these oncogenes during pre- and post-natal development. Thus, c-fos was first highly expressed in extra embryonal tissues and to a lower rate in the other tissues. In later stages of foetal life, it remained expressed in various tissues including liver, but at a low level[16]. In contrast, c-Ha-ras was found to be expressed at considerable and constant level at all stages of prenatal development in various organs ;
(iii) an organ-specific expression of the different ras genes during the period of post-natal development[19].

B) - Events occuring during the early stages of liver regeneration are also of interest because they may tell us how cells in vivo respond when they move from a differentiated resting state (Go phase) to a proliferative state. The first important results were given by the Fausto's group[20,21] and by Makino et al.[22]. They showed a successive and transient overexpression of c-fos and c-myc followed by a high expression of c-Ha-ras oncogene concomitant to the peak of thymidine incorporation. In a similar study we have compared the c-fos, c-myc and N-myc transcripts, particularly at the first hours following partial hepatectomy[1,2]. We have evidenced an early expression of c-fos and c-myc with variations in their levels according to time. C-myc appeared very highly expressed 3 and 9 h after operation.

We may emphasize the high expression of N-myc in regenerating liver with a peak at 3 h[2]. Indeed high expression of N-myc has been observed in tumors from neural origin and in fetal tissues[18]. This is the first evidence for an involvement of N-myc in cell proliferation.

Transcripts of these all activated oncogenes returned to their basal levels by 96 h. The abundance of c-src and c-abl transcripts was unchanged during liver regeneration whereas mos gene transcripts were not detected.

C) - The third situation is represented by adult non-dividing hepatocytes isolated and maintained in culture. Indeed, in vitro systems are useful for determining events which may induce oncogene expression in normal liver cells. We have looked for possible changes in c-fos, c-myc and c-Ha-ras oncogene expression in normal non-dividing adult hepatocytes following their isolation and seeding and in relation with culture conditions. This study has shown that cell isolation by perfusion of either collagenase or EDTA specifically activated c-fos oncogene at a very high level within 20 min (Fig. 3). Similar results were obtained by detaching cultured cells in the presence of collagenase.

This strongly suggests that expression of c-fos has something to do with cell-cell interactions.

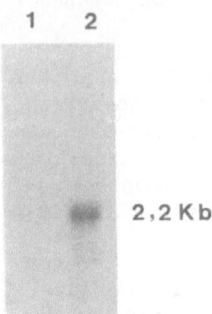

Figure 3 : Northern-blot analysis of the c-fos expression in normal rat
liver (lane 1) and in freshly isolated hepatocytes after
20 min. Collagenase perfusion (lane 2). 10 µg of each total
RNA were used.

Furthermore, an abnormal and constant overexpression of c-myc and
c-Ha-ras genes was found, independently of the culture conditions. These
results are intriguing and their interpretation is unclear at this time.
This is one of the first examples of a constant expression of c-myc in
normal non-dividing cells.

Together these observations :
i) emphasize the role of oncogenes as regulators of cell proliferation
   and differentiation in normal liver ;
ii) confirm that, among the oncogenes which are abnormally activated in
    hepatocarcinomas, several are activated in the normal liver tissue
    during pre- and postnatal development and during liver regeneration.
    This could be consistent with the general notion that liver
    regeneration may function as a promoter in liver carcinogenesis ;
iii) give some evidence for a relationship between cell shape and/or
     membrane properties and the expression of c-fos oncogene. They
     suggest that alterations of cell-cell interactions could induce
     changes in oncogene expression and thus emphasize the role of
     cell-cell contacts in the cancer process. On this basis, a number of
     studies have previously shown that many cancerous cells lack the
     capacity to communicate[23] and let to the hypothesis that
     intercellular communication might play a role in cell proliferation
     and in the process of carcinogenesis[24].

IV - HOMOLOGIES WITH OTHER KNOWN CELLULAR GENES.

Another approach to determine the role of cellular oncogenes in
abnormal cells is to search for homologies between them and other known
cellular genes. This approach is certain to become increasingly popular
as more gene and protein sequences become known.
Expression of c-fos, c-myc and ras gene families has been mostly
studied in hepatocarcinogenesis. However, we have to admit that very
little is known yet on the mechanism of action of these oncogenes. C-fos

and c-myc transcripts correspond to nuclear proteins. These proteins may modulate the activity of the cell's transcriptional machinery[25], whereas the ras genes code for a membrane bound protein (P21) which has a GTPase activity[26]. The role of the ras gene products could be central to cell growth factors through their receptor. Interestingly, there are various lines of evidence suggesting that nuclear oncogenes collaborate with cytoplasmic oncogenes in malignant transformation[25].

Several other oncogenes are better known thanks to their homology with well defined cellular genes. It is the case for c-sis oncogene which has homology with PDGF[27], c-erb-B which presents homology with the receptor of EGF[28] and, as recently shown, c-erb-A which presents homology with a sequence common to thyroid hormone receptor and glucocorticoid receptor[29].

In addition, important observations have been made that integrated hepatitis B virus (HBV) DNA sequences could be detected in patients with hepatocarcinomas. The exact significance of integrated HBV sequences is not completely clear. However, the recent discovery of HBV sequence integrated at the level of erb-A oncogene[30], the supposed DNA-binding domain of the human glucocorticoid and oestrogen receptor genes, might suggest a mechanism of action of this virus on human liver cancer process.

CONCLUSION

It may be assumed that oncogenes alone are probably not responsible for hepatocarcinogenesis. This hypothesis is supported by recent observations which report abnormal expression of endogenous retrovirus-related DNA sequences, in addition to oncogenes, in both carcinogen-induced and spontaneous liver tumor formation[9]. Likewise, different complementary DNA clones for genes overexpressed in chemically induced rat hepatomas have been recently isolated[31]. Characterization of these sequences would help to progress in the understanding of the liver cancer process.

However, there is no doubt that oncogenes play an important role since their activation represents a common feature in liver carcinomas and since their expression is induced in several situations indirectly related to carcinogenesis like cell proliferation and cell-cell communications.

REFERENCES

1. M. CORRAL, L. TICHONICKY, C. GUGUEN-GUILLOUZO, D. CORCOS, M. RAYMONDJEAN, B. PARIS, J. KRUH and N. DEFER, Expression of c-fos oncogene during hepatocarcinogenesis, liver regeneration and in synchronized HTC cells, Exp. Cell Res. 160:427 (1985).

2. M. CORRAL, B. PARIS, C. GUGUEN-GUILLOUZO, D. CORCOS, J. KRUH and N. DEFER, Increased expression of N-myc gene during normal and neoplastic rat liver growth, Exp. Cell Res. (1987) in press.

3. D. CORCOS, N. DEFER, M. RAYMONDJEAN, B. PARIS, M. CORRAL, L. TICHONICKY, J. KRUH, D. GLAISE, A. SAUNIER and C. GUGUEN-GUILLOUZO, Correlated increase of the expression of the c-ras genes in chemically induced hepatocarcinomas, Biochem. Biophys. Res. Commun., 122:259 (1984).

4. E. SCHERER and P. EMMELOT. Foci of altered liver cells induced by a single dose of diethylnitrosamine and partial hepatectomy : their contribution to hepatocarcinogenesis in rat. Eur. J. Cancer, 11:145 (1975).

5. P. YASWEN, M. GOYETTE, P.R. SHANK and N. FAUSTO, Expression of c-Ki-ras, c-Ha-ras and c-myc in specific cell types during hepatocarcinogenesis, Mol Cell. Biol., 5:780 (1985).

6. S. HORIKAWA, K; SAKATA, M. HETANAKA and K. TSUDADA, Expression of c-myc oncogene in rat liver by a dictary manipulation. Biochem. Biophys. Res. Commun., 140:574 (1986).

7. R. MAKINO, K. HAYASHI, S. SATO and T. SUGIMURA, Expression of the c-Ha-ras and c-myc genes in rat liver tumors. Biochem. Biophys. Res. Commun., 119:1096 (1984).

8. F. TASHIRO, S. MORIMURA, K. HAYASHI, R. MAKINO, M. KAWAMURA, N. HORIKOSHI, K. NEMOTO, K. OHTSUBO, T. SUGIMURA and Y. UENO, Expression of the c-Ha-ras and c-myc genes in aflatoxin B_1 induced hepatocellular carcinomas. Biochem. Biophys. Res. Commun., 138:858 (1986).

9. T.A. DRAGANI, G. MANENTI, G. DELLA PORTA, S. GATTONI-CELLI and I.B. WEINSTEIN, Expression of retroviral sequences and oncogenes in murine hepatocellular tumors, Cancer Res., 46:1915 (1986).

10. F. ISHIKAWA, F. TAKAKU, M. OCHIAI, K. HAYASHI, S. HIROHASHI, M. TERADA, S. TAKAYAMA, M. NAGAO and T. SUGIMURA, Activated c-raf gene in a rt hepatocellular carcinoma induced by 2-amino-3-methylinidazo-[4,5,8] quinoline. Biochem. Biophys. Res. Commun., 132:186 (1985).

11. P. YASWEN, N.T. HAYNER and N. FAUSTO. Isolation of oval cells by centrifugal elutriation and comparison with other cell types purified from normal and preneoplastic livers Cancer Res., 44:324 (1984).

12. X.K. ZHANG, D.P. HUANG, D.K. CHIU and J.F. CHIU, The expression of oncogenes in human developing liver and hepatomas, Biochem. Biophys. Res. Commun., 142:932 (1987).

13. E. MOREL-CHANY, C. GUGUEN-GUILLOUZO, C. TRINCAL and M.F. SZAJNERT, Spontaneous neoplastic transformation in vitro of epithelial cells strains of rat liver : cytology, growth and enzymatic activities, Eur. J. Cancer, 14:1341 (1978).

14. G. BAFFET, M. RISSEL and GUGUEN-GUILLOUZO C. Synthesis and phosphorylation of cytoskeleton components during spontaneous neoplastic transformaiton of epithelial cells. Submitted.

15. T. R. FOX and P.G. WATANABE, Detection of a cellular oncogene in spontaneous liver tumors of B6C3F1 mice, Science, 228:596 (1985).

16. R. MULLER, D.J. SLAMON, J.M. TREMBLAY, M.J. CLINE and I.M. VERMA, Differential expression of cellular oncogenes during pre- and postnatal development of the mouse, Nature, 299:640 (1982).

17. T. IWANAGA, T. FUJITA, T. TSUCHIHASHI, K. YAMAGUSHI, K. ABE and N. YANAIHARA, Immunocytochemical detection of the c-myc oncogene product in human fetuses, Biochem. Res., 7:161 (1986).

18. K.A. ZIMMERMAN, G.D. YANCOPOULOS, R.G. COLLUM, R.K. SMITH N.E., KOHL, K.A. DENIS, M.M. NAU, O.N. WITTE, D. TORAN-ALLERANOL, C.E. GEE, J.D. MINNA and F.W. ALT, Differential expression of myc family genes during murine development, Nature 319:780 (1986).

19. T. TANAKA, N. IDA, H. SHIMODA, C. WAKI, D.J.. SLAMON and M.J. CLINE, Organ specific expression of ras oncoproteins during growth and development of the rat, Mol. Cell. Biochem., 70:97 (1986).

20. N. FAUSTO and P.R. SHANK, Oncogene expression in liver regeneration and hepatocarcinogenesis, Hepatology, 3:1016 (1983).

21. N.L. THOMPSON, J.E. MEAD, L. BRAUN, M. GOYETTE, P.R. SHANK and N. FAUSTO, Sequential protooncogene expression during rat liver regeneration, Cancer Res., 46:3111 (1986).

22. R. MAKINO, K. HAYASHI and T. SUGIMURA, C-myc transcripts induced in rat liver at very early stage of regeneration or by cychloeximide treatment. Nature, 310:697 (1984).

23. J.C. SAEZ, M.V.L. BENNETT and D.C. SPRAY, Carbon tetrachloride at hepatotoxic levels blocks reversibly gap junctions between rat hepatocytes, Science, 236 : 967 (1987).

24. T. ENOMOTO and H. YAMASAKI, Lack of intercellular communication between chemically transformed and surrounding non transformed BALB/c 3T3 cells, Cancer Res., 44 : 5200 (1984).

25. R.A. WEINBERG, The action of oncogenes in the cytoplasm and nucleus, Science, 230:770 (1985).

26. D.A. SPANDIDOS, Mechanisms of carcinogenesis : the role of oncogenes, transcriptional enhancers and growth factors, Anticancer Res., 5:485 (1985).

27. R.F. DOOLITLE, M.W. HUNKAPILLER, L. HOOD et al. Simian sarcoma virus onc gene v-sis is derived from the gene (or genes) encoding a platelet-derived growth factor, Science, 221:275 (1983).

28. J. DOWNWARD, Y. YARDEN, E. MAYES, G. SCRACE, N. TOTTY, P. STOCKWELL, A. ULLRICH, J. SCHLESSINGER and M.D. WATERFIELD, Close similarity of epidermal growht factor receptor and v-erb-B oncogene protein sequences. Nature, 307:521 (1984).

29. C. WEINBERGER, C.C. THOMPSON, E.S. ONG, R. LEBO, D.J. GRUOL and R.M. EVANS. The c-erb-A gene encodes a thyroid hormone receptor, Nature, 324:641 (1986).

30. A. DEJEAN, L. BOUGUELERET, K.H. GRZESCHIK and P. TIOLLAIS, Hepatitis B virus DNA integration in a sequence homologousto v-erb-A and steroid receptor genes in a hepatocellular carcinoma, Nature, 322:70 (1986).

31. M. CORRAL, N. DEFER, B. PARIS, M. RAYMONDJEAN, D. CORCOS, L. TICHONICKY, J. KRUH, D. GLAISE, B. KNEIP and C. GUGUEN-GUILLOUZO, Isolation and characteriziton of complementary DNA clones for genes oververexpression in chemically induced rat hepatomas, Cancer Res., 46:5119 (1986).

The work was supported by FNLCC.

IN VITRO STUDIES IN LIVER CARCINOGENESIS

SEPARATION AND BIOCHEMICAL CHARACTERIZATION OF

RAT LIVER PARENCHYMAL CELL SUBPOPULATIONS

Pablo Steinberg, Beate Seibert and Franz Oesch

Institute of Toxicology, University of Mainz
Obere Zahlbacher Strasse 67
D-6500 Mainz, West Germany

INTRODUCTION

Parenchymal cells within the hepatic lobules of the rat are morphologically and biochemically heterogeneous (Shank et al., 1959; Novikoff, 1959; Loud, 1968; Jungermann and Katz, 1982). It has been previously shown that the concentration of cytochrome P-450 and the activities of most cytochrome P-450-dependent monooxygenases are relatively higher in the centrilobular regions than in the periportal regions of the rat liver (Baron et al., 1978; Gooding et al., 1978; Baron and Kawabata, 1983); further, these studies revealed that pretreatment of the animals with phenobarbital intensified this gradation across the liver lobule, whereas after administration of 3-methylcholanthrene the concentration of cytochrome P-450 and the monooxygenase activities were more uniformly distributed. Since very reactive and toxic metabolites are often formed during cytochrome P-450-catalyzed monooxygenations of hepatotoxins, the intralobular distribution of different cytochromes P-450 may be a crucial factor in determining the location of the damage within the hepatic lobules after exposure to several hepatotoxic compounds.

A method to isolate parenchymal cells originating in periportal or centrilobular regions of the liver would provide an extremely valuable tool for the study of the mechanism(s) underlying the toxic effects of many chemicals which only affect a particular cell subpopulation within the liver acinus. In an attempt to obtain fractions enriched in either periportal or centrilobular cells, liver parenchymal cells isolated from untreated and phenobarbital- or 3-methylcholanthrene-pretreated rats were separated into five subpopulations by centrifugal elutriation. The criterion used to assess the zonal origin of the separated subpopulations has been the measurement of cytochrome P-450 content as well as the activities of two cytochrome P-450-dependent monooxygenases, ethoxyresorufin O-deethylase and benzphetamine N-demethylase.

MATERIALS AND METHODS

Chemicals

Collagenase and DNAse I were purchased from Boehringer (Mannheim, FRG); phenobarbital from Merck (Darmstadt, FRG); 3-methylcholanthrene from Aldrich (Steinheim, FRG); ethoxyresorufin from Pierce (Rodgau, FRG); and benzphetamine from Upjohn Co. (Kalamazoo, USA). All other chemicals employed were of the highest purity available.

Animals and pretreatments

Male Sprague-Dawley rats (300-400 g body weight) from the Süddeutsche Versuchstierfarm (Tuttlingen, FRG) were housed in plastic cages on a fixed day and night cycle and fed a standard rat chow until used. The animals were pretreated i.p. with phenobarbital (100 mg/kg body weight/day) in 0.85 % saline or 3-methylcholanthrene (25 mg/kg body weight/day) for three consecutive days. Untreated rats received appropriate volumes of corn oil. Liver parenchymal cells were isolated 24 hours after the last injection.

Isolation of liver parenchymal cells

Total liver cell suspensions were obtained using a collagenase perfusion method described by Glatt et al. (1981). The buffer used for all steps of the cell isolation procedure was the complete Krebs-Henseleit buffer containing 25 mM 4-(2-hydroxymethyl)-1-piperazineethanesulfonic acid (HEPES, pH 7.4), 0.5 % D-glucose, insulin (8 mg/liter), and the mixture of amino acids recommended by Seglen (1976). Briefly, the liver was perfused for 5 min through the portal vein in a non-recirculatory manner with Ca^{2+}-free Krebs-Henseleit buffer. This was followed by a recirculatory perfusion of 10 min with 0.5 mM ethylene glycol bis(ß-aminoethyl ether) N,N,N',N'-tetraacetic acid (EGTA) in the above-mentioned buffer to disrupt the desmosomes. The buffer was then changed to a complete Krebs-Henseleit buffer without EGTA but containing 2.5 mM $CaCl_2$ and 0.05 % collagenase and the perfusion continued for 35-45 min. Glisson's capsule was removed from the liver and the cells filtered through gauze to remove clumps. The suspension was centrifuged and washed three times at 50 g for 3 min, and the supernatants discarded. The final pellet contained > 95 % parenchymal cells.

Fractionation of isolated liver parenchymal cells

The parenchymal cells in the pellet were resuspended and filtered through a 100 micron and then a 60 micron nylon mesh. Elutriation was performed as described by Bernaert et al. (1979). A JE-6B elutriator rotor with a standard separation chamber (Beckman Instruments, Palo Alto, California, USA) was used in a J-6M/E Beckman at a speed of 840 rpm. The rotor, the elutriation medium (Krebs-Henseleit buffer containing 0.5 % w/v bovine serum albumin and 0.01 % w/v DNAse I) and the samples collected during the separation were kept at 4 °C to preserve the integrity of the cells. The parenchymal cell suspension (5-10 x 10^7 cells) was loaded into the elutriation system with an initial flow rate of 15 ml/min. Parenchymal cell fractions I to V were obtained by using flow rates of 20, 25, 30, 35 and 45 ml/min, respectively; for each fraction 150 ml of eluate were collected. The viability of each preparation was assessed by determining the proportion of cells that excluded 0.4 % trypan blue. Morphometric data of the elutriated subpopulations were obtained by flow cytometry according to Willson et al. (1985); polystyrene beads (5, 10, 20 and 30 micron size) were used to calibrate the fluorescence activated cell sorter.

Assays

All determinations were performed on the 10,000 g supernatants of the sonicated cell subpopulations. In all assays reported, the amount of product formed was linear with both time and concentration. Cytochrome

P-450 content was measured as described by Omura and Sato (1964). Benz-phetamine N-demethylase activity was determined by colorimetrically following the formation of formaldehyde (Lu et al., 1972). Ethoxyresoru-fin O-deethylase activity was measured fluorimetrically according to the method of Burke and Mayer (1974). Proteins were measured by the method of Lowry et al. (1951) with bovine serum albumin as standard.

Statistics

Statistical analyses of the results were carried out using Dun-nett's test for multiple comparisons with a control (Dunnett, 1964).

RESULTS AND DISCUSSION

Liver parenchymal cells from untreated and phenobarbital- or 3-methylcholanthrene-pretreated rats were isolated by a collagenase per-fusion method and further separated into five subpopulations by centri-fugal elutriation. The cell recovery following elutriation was of about 90 % and the number of cells in the five fractions was similar for the three experimental groups. The viability of the cell suspensions before loading the elutriation chamber amounted to 88 $\pm$ 4 % (n = 18), whereas the percentage of cells excluding trypan blue in the elutriated subpo-pulations from untreated and induced animals averaged 95 %. Thus, a high number of non-viable cells was removed during the elutriation pro-cess.

The cell diameter distributions within the elutriated parenchymal cell subpopulations from untreated, phenobarbital-pretreated and 3-methylcholanthrene-pretreated rats are shown in Fig. 1. The peaks of fractions 1 to 5 from untreated animals correspond to cells with mean diameters of 19.6, 21.1, 21.8, 22.7 and 23.5 µm, respectively. The par-enchymal cell subpopulations from phenobarbital-pretreated rats had mean diameters of 20.3, 21.7, 23.1, 24.0 and 25.6 µm. Following 3-methylchol-anthrene administration, the mean diameters of the cells present in fractions 1 to 5 were 21.8, 22.7, 23.4, 23.9 and 24.4 µm, respectively. Our observations of differences in cell sizes between parenchymal cell populations separated by centrifugal elutriation are in accordance with previous reports (Bernaert et al., 1979; Wanson et al., 1980; Klinger et al., 1985; Wilson et al., 1985; Gumucio et al., 1986). Morphometric stu-dies from the intact liver (Schmucker et al., 1978) and isolated paren-chymal cell fractions (Drochmans et al., 1975; Tonda et al., 1983) show-ed that centrilobular cells were consistently larger than periportal cells. Furthermore, Wanson et al. (1975) reported that administration of phenobarbital to rats preferentially increased the size of centrilobular cells; interestingly, in the present study pretreatment of the animals with phenobarbital led to a significantly greater increase of cell size in fractions 3-5 (i.e. those containing the larger cells in the case of untreated rats) than in fractions 1 and 2.

In order to further characterize the elutriated subpopulations from untreated and induced animals the concentration of cytochrome P-450 and the activities of two cytochrome P-450-dependent monooxygenases, benz-phetamine N-demethylase and ethoxyresorufin O-dethylase, were measured.

Fig. 2 shows the cytochrome P-450 content in the five subpopula-tions from the three experimental groups. In untreated animals the cel-lular concentration of cytochrome P-450 increased from fractions 1 to 5, the amount of the hemeprotein being approximately 1.4-fold higher in fraction 5 than in fraction 1. The fact that the cytochrome P-450 con-tent was higher in the large than in the small cells is in agreement

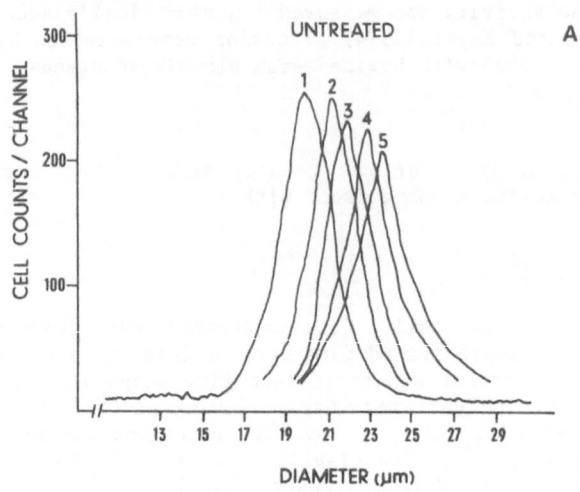

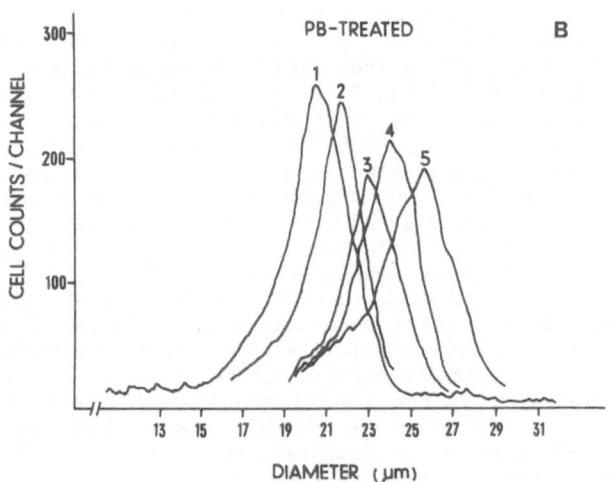

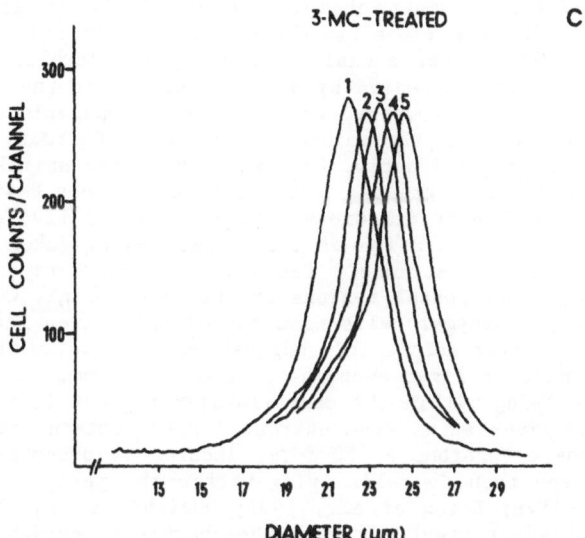

Figure 1: Cell diameter distribution within the five elutriated subpopulations from an untreated rat, a phenobarbital-treated rat and a 3-methylcholanthrene-treated rat; 1-5 = fractions.

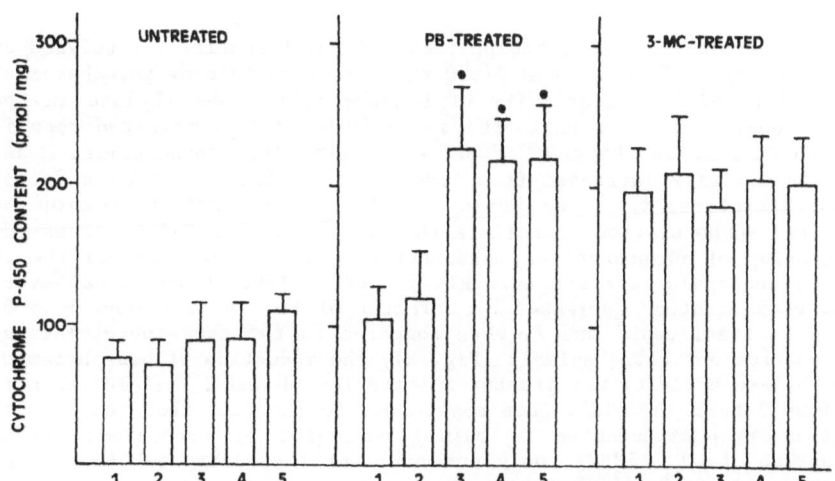

Figure 2: Cytochrome P-450 content in the elutriated parenchymal cell fractions from untreated and induced animals; 1-5 = fractions. Indicates significantly different from fraction 1 ($p < 0.05$, Dunnett's t-test).

with previous studies on parenchymal cell subpopulations isolated by centrifugal elutriation (Sumner et al., 1983; Willson et al., 1985), density gradient (Gooding et al., 1978) and sedimentation velocity (Sweeney et al., 1978). After administration of phenobarbital the content of cytochrome P-450 increased by a factor of two in the cells present in fractions 3-5 when compared to the same subpopulations isolated from untreated rats, whereas the amount of cytochrome P-450 in fractions 1 and 2 did not vary significantly. Pretreatment of the animals with 3-methylcholanthrene led to a greater increase of cytochrome P-450 content in fractions 1 and 2 than in fractions 3-5, so that all five subpopulations had a similar concentration of cytochrome P-450. Taken together, these data suggest that fractions 1 and 2 are enriched in parenchymal cells originating in periportal regions of the liver acini, while fractions 3-5 contain parenchymal cells from the distal halves (centrilobular regions) of the liver acini. This suggestion is based on the following observations made on liver sections by means of immunohistochemical methods: 1) cells lying within the centrilobular regions (i.e. the larger cells) of the liver acini from untreated rats contain greater concentrations of the cytochrome P-450 forms induced by phenobarbital and 3-methylcholanthrene than do cells lying within the periportal regions (Gooding et al., 1978; Baron et al., 1981; Ohnishi et al., 1982; Wolf et al., 1984); 2) after treatment with phenobarbital, cytochrome P-450 is primarily induced within centrilobular cells (Gooding et al., 1978; Smith and Wills, 1981; Ohnishi et al., 1982; Wolf et al., 1984); 3) the administration of 3-methylcholanthrene to rats results in similar degrees of induction of cytochrome P-450 within midzonal and periportal cells, but significantly less induction is detected within centrilobular cells, the concentrations of cytochrome P-450 within the three regions of the liver acini being therefore approximately equal (Baron et al., 1982).

The N-demethylation of benzphetamine is preferentially catalyzed by those isoenzymes of cytochrome P-450 that are inducible by phenobarbital (Lu et al., 1972). The activity of benzphetamine N-demethylase in the five subpopulations from untreated and phenobarbital-pretreated rats is shown in Fig. 3. In the case of untreated animals, benzphetamine N-demethylase activity increased from fraction 1 to fraction 5 by a factor of two. Therefore, the distribution of this enzyme activity within the elutriated subpopulations parallels that of cytochrome P-450. After administration of phenobarbital, benzphetamine N-demethylase activity in all five subpopulations was strongly induced. Although the total cytochrome P-450 content increased by a factor of two in fractions 3 to 5, but not in fractions 1 and 2, when compared to the same subpopulations isolated from untreated animals (Fig. 2), the induction of benzphetamine N-demethylase activity was greater in fractions 1 and 2 (4-fold) than in fractions 3 to 5 (3-fold). This may be due to the fact that the N-demethylation of benzphetamine is mainly catalyzed by cytochrome P-450b (Guengerich et al., 1982), only one of several cytochrome P-450 isoenzymes induced by phenobarbital.

The O-deethylation of ethoxyresorufin is catalyzed by the 3-methylcholanthrene-inducible isoenzymes of cytochrome P-450 (Burke and Mayer, 1974). Ethoxyresorufin-O-deethylase activity within the elutriated subpopulations from untreated and 3-methylcholanthrene-pretreated rats is shown in Fig. 4. In untreated animals the deethylating activity increased from fraction 1 to fraction 5 by a factor of 1.7. Pretreatment with 3-methylcholanthrene led to a 28- and a 20-fold induction of ethoxyresorufin O-deethylase activity in fractions 1 and 5, respectively. Thus, the enzyme activity was similar in large and small parenchymal cells from induced rats, an observation previously made by Tonda et al. (1983) in parenchymal cell subpopulations separated by density gradient centrifugation.

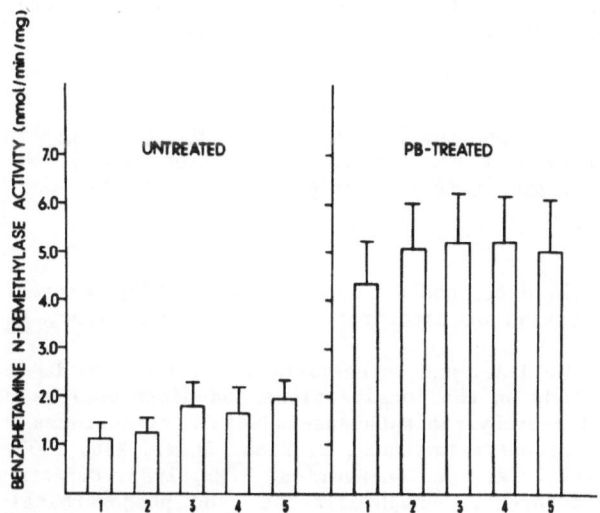

Figure 3. Benzphetamine N-demethylase activity in the elutriated parenchymal cell fractions from untreated and induced animals;
1-5 = fractions.

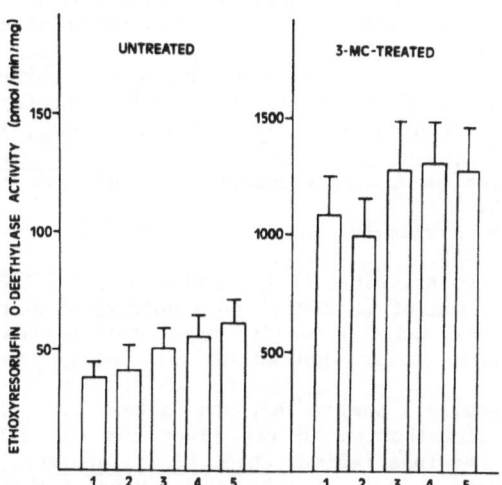

Figure 4: Ethoxyresorufin O-deethylase activity in the elutriated parenchymal cell fractions from untreated and induced animals;
1-5 = fractions.

In conclusion, isolated rat liver parenchymal cells could be separated by centrifugal elutriation into five subpopulations, which differed in: a) size; b) content of cytochrome P-450; c) activities of two cytochrome P-450-dependent monooxygenases; d) inducibility by 3-methylcholanthrene and phenobarbital. Thus, the elutriated liver parenchymal cells seem to preserve the heterogeneous distribution of drug metabolizing enzymes observed within the hepatic lobules.

Acknowledgements

This work was supported by the Deutsche Forschungsgemeinschaft (SFB 302) and the Alexander von Humboldt Foundation (P.S.). We also thank Ms. I. Böhm for typing this manuscript.

References

Baron, J., Redick, J.A., and Guengerich, F.P., 1978, Immunohistochemical localization of cytochromes P-450 in rat liver, Life Sci, 23: 2627.

Baron, J., Redick, J.A., and Guengerich, F.P., 1981, An immunohistochemical study on the localizations and distributions of phenobarbital- and 3-methylcholanthrene-inducible cytochromes P-450 within the livers of untreated rats, J. Biol. Chem., 256: 5931.

Baron, J., Redick, J.A., and Guengerich, F.P., 1982, Effects of 3-methylcholanthrene, ß-naphtoflavone, and phenobarbital on the 3-methylcholanthrene-inducible isozyme of cytochrome P-450 within centrilobular, midzonal, and periportal hepatocytes, J. Biol. Chem., 257: 953.

Baron, J., and Kawabata, T., 1983, Intratissue distribution of activating and detoxicating enzymes, in: "Biological Basis of Detoxication", J. Caldwell and W.B. Jakoby, eds., Academic Press, New York.

Bernaert, D., Wanson, J.-C., Mosselmans, R., De Parmentier, R., and Drochmans, P., 1979, Separation of adult rat hepatocytes into distinct subpopulations by centrifugal elutriation. Morphological, morphometrical and biochemical characterization of cell fractions, Biol. Cellulaire, 34: 159.

Burke, M.D., and Mayer, R.T., 1974, Ethoxyresorufin: direct fluorimetric assay of a microsomal O-dealkylation which is preferentially inducible by 3-methylcholanthrene, Drug Metab. Dispos., 2: 583.

Drochmans, P., Wanson, J.-C., and Mosselmans, R., 1975, Isolation and subfractionation on ficoll gradients of adult rat hepatocytes, J. Cell Biol., 66: 1.

Dunnett, C.W., 1964, New tables for multiple comparisons with a control, Biometrics, 6: 482.

Glatt, H.R., Billings, R., Platt, K.L., and Oesch, F., 1981, Improvement of the correlation of bacterial mutagenicity with carcinogenicity of benzo(a)pyrene and four of its major metabolites by activation with intact liver cells instead of cell homogenate, Cancer Res., 41: 270.

Gooding, P.E., Chayen, J., Sawyer, B., and Slater, T.F., 1978, Cytochrome P-450 distribution in rat liver and the effect of sodium phenobarbitone administration, Chem. Biol. Interact., 20: 299.

Guengerich, F.P., Dannan, G.A., Wright, S.T., Martin, M.V., and Kaminsky, L.S., 1982, Purification and characterization of microsomal cytochrome P-450s, Xenobiotica, 12: 701.

Gumucio, J.J., May, M., Dvorak, C., Chianale, J., and Massey, V., 1986, The isolation of functionally heterogeneous hepatocytes of the proximal and distal half of the liver acinus in the rat, Hepatology, 6: 932.

Jungermann, K., and Katz, N., 1982, Functional hepatocellular heterogeneity, Hepatology, 2: 385.

Klinger, W., Devereux, T., Fouts, J., Lohr, S., Crawford, D., Diliberto, J., and Sparks, R., 1985, Separation of immature and adult rat hepatocytes into distinct subpopulations by centrifugal elutriation, Arch. Toxicol., Suppl. 8: 469.

Loud, A.V., 1968, Quantitative stereological description of the ultrastructure of normal rat liver parenchymal cells, J. Cell Biol., 37: 27.

Lowry, O.H., Rosebrough, J., Farr, A.L., and Randall, R.J., 1951, Protein measurement with the Folin phenol reagent, J. Biol. Chem., 193: 265.

Lu, A.Y.H., Somogyi, A., West, S., Kuntzman, R., and Conney, H.H., 1972, Pregnenolone-16-alpha-carbonitrile: a new type of inducer of drug metabolizing enzymes, Arch. Biochem. Biophys., 152: 457.

Novikoff, A., 1959, Cell heterogeneity within the liver lobule of the rat (staining reaction), J. Histochem. Cytochem., 7: 240.

Omura, T., and Sato, R., 1964, The carbon monoxide binding pigment of liver microsomes, J. Biol. Chem., 239: 2370.

Ohnishi, K., Mishima, A., and Okuda, K., 1982, Immunofluorescence of phenobarbital inducible cytochrome P-450 in the hepatic lobule of normal and phenobarbital-treated rats, Hepatology, 2: 849.

Schmucker, D.L., Mooney, J.S., and Jones, A.L., 1978, Stereological analysis of hepatic fine structure in the Fischer 344 rat, J. Cell Biol., 78: 319.

Seglen, P.O., 1976, Incorporation of radioactive amino acids into protein in isolated rat hepatocytes, Biochim. Biophys. Acta, 442: 391.

Shank, R.E., Morrison, G., Cheng, C.H., Karl, I., and Schwartz, R., 1959, Cell heterogeneity within the hepatic lobule (quantitative histochemistry), J. Histochem. Cytochem., 7: 237.

Smith, M.T., and Wills, E.D., 1981, Effects of dietary lipid and phenobarbitone on the distribution and concentration of cytochrome P-450 in the liver studied by quantitative cytochrmistry, FEBS Lett., 127: 33.

Sumner, I.G., Freedman, R.B., and Lodola, A., 1983, Characterisation of hepatocyte sub-populations generated by centrifugal elutriation, Eur. J. Biochem., 134: 539.

Sweeney, G.D., Garfield, R.E., Jones, K.G., and Latham, A.N., 1978, Studies using sedimentation velocity on heterogeneity of size and function of hepatocytes from mature male rats, J. Lab. Clin. Med., 91: 432.

Tonda, K., Hasegawa, T., and Hirata, M., 1983, Effects of phenobarbital and 3-methylcholanthrene pretreatments on monooxygenase activities and proportions of isolated rat hepatocyte subpopulations, Molec. Pharmacol., 23: 235.

Wanson, J.-C., Drochmans, P., May, C., Penasse, W., and Popowski, A., 1975, Isolation of centrilobular and perilobular hepatocytes after phenobarbital treatment, J. Cell Biol., 66: 23.

Wanson, J.-C., Bernaert, D., Penasse, W., Mosselmans, R., and Bannasch, P., 1980, Separation in distinct subpopulations by elutriation of liver cells following exposure of rats to N-nitrosomorpholine, Cancer Res., 40: 459.

Willson, R.A., Liem, H.H., Miyai, K., and Muller-Eberhard, 1985, Heterogeneous distribution of drug metabolism in elutriated rat hepatocytes, Biochem. Pharmacol., 34: 1463.

Wolf, C.R., Moll, E., Friedberg, T., Oesch, F., Buchmann, A., Kuhlmann, W.D., and Kunz, H.W., 1984, Characterization, localization and regulation of a novel phenobarbital-inducible form of cytochrome P-450 reductase, glutathione transferases and microsomal epoxide hydrolase, Carcinogenesis, 5: 993.

GROWTH CONTROL OF HEPATOCYTES, THEIR IMMORTALIZATION AND TRANSFORMATION
BY TRANSFORMING GENES OF POLYOMA VIRUS AND OF SV40 VIRUS

Dieter Paul

Department of Cell Biology
Fraunhofer Institute of Toxicology
Nikolai-Fuchs-Str. 1
3000 Hannover 61, FRG

I. INDUCTION OF HCC IN RATS BY CARCINOGENIC CHEMICALS

Many experimental systems and protocols to induce cancer of the liver
in experimental animals, particularly in rats, have been described (1)
in attempts to understand the sequence of events that leads to Hepatocellular Carcinoma (HCC). The ultimate goal of this research is to identify tumor progenitor cells at the earliest point in their development (2).
It is undisputed that in the rat many morphological alterations take place
in the liver as result of toxic injury during the exposure to the carcinogen i.e. new populations of cells arise and populate the liver and morphologically abnormal hepatocytes appear. As a consequence, it has not been
possible to correlate such morphological abnormalities (e.g. degenerative,
regenerative, hyperplastic preneoplastic lesions or foci or nodules in
the liver 1-9) occurring in response to toxic injury with the appearance
of bona fide tumor precursor cells. An important conclusion that emerges
from the extensive work compiled in the literature is that beyond this
phenomenology little is known about the cellular basis of carcinogenesis
(3,4), because the fundamental question how to identify cell lineages,
i.e. precursor cells destined to become HCC at a later point in time, has
eluded experimentation. The central difficulties, in dealing with this
problem include (a) the observed large discrepancy between the frequency
of morphologically apparent "lesions" in the liver that occur in response
to treatment of experimental animals with hepatocarcinogens and the final
number of HCC; (b) the rare appearance of HCC in such "lesions", which
suggests fortuitous rather than predictable events; (c) the "lesions"
frequently regress; (d) spontaneously occurring "lesions" (indistinguishable
from those that appear in response to carcinogen treatment) are unrelated
to HCC (8,9).
In summary, the available data suggest that the evidence that cells present in liver "lesions" that develop in response to the exposure to a
carcinogen might be tumor cell precursors is to a large extent incon-
clusive. Postulated lineage relationships between the morphological abnormalities of cells in the liver and HCC are largely hypothetical and
available evidence is circumstantial.

To demonstrate direct lineage relationships between "initiated" cells
present in the liver of experimental animals that had been exposed to a
carcinogen can ultimately come from in vivo/in vitro systems, in which
the cultivation of abnormal liver cell populations has to take place to

select desired phenotypes thought to be characteristic for putative tumor precursor cells. Their properties could then theoretically be assayed for their supposed tumor progenitor characteristics by transplanting them into the liver of syngeneic normal hosts and by following the fate of grafted cells. Selection in vitro is mandatory because with the regimen of carcinogen application to the donor animals there is a constant flux and change in liver cell populations, manifested by the appearance of oval cells, proliferation of bile duct cells, tumors of parenchymal liver tissue etc., depending on the carcinogen used (1, 10).

II. CULTIVATION OF ADULT HEPATOCYTES AND OF LIVER NODULES

Although much progress has been made to culture adult liver cells and to induce them to proliferate in vitro, no succes has been reported in cultivating either cells derived from liver "lesions" or from apparently normal liver cells of carcinogen-treated adult animals (7, 11, 12) with the capacity to proliferate readily and to be maintained in long-term cultures, unless cells are manifestly malignant (13, 14). In contrast, fetal, newborn and baby rat or mouse hepatocytes can be readily grown in culture (15 - 18). The difficulties in culturing adult hepatocytes are due to their complex growth requirements, which are only partialy understood at this time. Also, local micro-environment in the liver (19), which are presumably affected by the carcinogen during long-term administration, may be essential for the growth of abnormal hepatocytes in vivo, but cannot be reconstructed as yet in culture systems. Transplantation of "nodular" cells without intermittent cultivation has been reported, however the efforts were not met by much success (20 - 23). Hepatocytes of rats treated with an initiation/selection/partial hepatectomy protocol (24) and subsequently transplanted into syngeneic hosts by injection into the portal system via the mesenteric vein, were shown to take in the livers of recipient animals (25 - 27). However, it seems to me that at the present time this approach is not amenable to detailed analysis because cells cannot be selected for the desired phenotypes. Thus, it would difficult to identify or to rescue grafted cells from recipient animals for further characterization (ref. 28).

III. ACTIVATION OF ras[H] BY CARCINOGENS

At the biochemical level, it is commonly thought that carcinogens induce mutations in target cells. One possibility is that oncogenes are direct targets of chemical carcinogens. It is known from recent work that a variety of different carcinogens activate normal ras genes into their activated counterparts in several tissues (ref. 29). Particularly interesting are animal systems involving just one single treatment with a carcinogen with minimal toxic side effects, which is sufficient to induce mutations and to induce tumors, such as in the mammary gland or in skin (1, 29). Unfortunately, similar protocols to induce liver cancer as a result of a single application of a carcinogen are not available, unless followed by partial hepatectomy and/or long-term treatments with a promoting agent (1). Oncogene activation cause transformation of normal cells in culture (cf. ref. 30 for review), and evidence that they are involved in the induction of tumors in vivo is beginning to emerge, e.g. in transgenic mice harboring an activated oncogene in their genome (ref. 31). For example, over-expression of c-myc driven by MMTV-LTR occurs in the mammary gland and causes mammary adenocarcinoma (32). When c-myc is driven by the Elastase I enhancer/promoter sequences adenocarcinomas of the pancreas develop (33). Thus, enhancer/promoter sequences coupled to an oncogene lead to tissue specific expression of the structural gene attached to them and direct tumorigenesis to the desired target organ (see ref. 34 - 37).

IV. HCC IN MAN

In human beings, liver cancer is one of the most frequent tumors, occurring mainly in Third World countries (42). It is closely associated with Hepatitis-B-Virus (HBV) (43), as shown by the presence of integrated HBV-DNA in the genome of virtually all HCC's (44), and by excellent epidemiological evidence indicating a high risk of chronic carriers of the virus to the occurrence of HCC later in life (45, 46). A similar association if not a causal relationship between distinct species specific Hepatitis-B-Viruses in woodchucks, ground squirrels and Peking ducks has recently been reported (47, 48). Moreover, clinical studies had shown that certain genetic factors pre-dispose to tumors of the liver in man, i.e. glycogenemia (Type I Gierke), an inborn error of metabolism (49). Also, there is evidence for unique chromosomal rearrangements in human hepatocarcinoma cells (50, 51). The region p 11 q 1 on human chromosome # 1 is trisomic through pentasomic. These are alterations common to all hepatoma cells that were studied. In addition, the presence of a re-arranged chromosome # 6 with a deletion of the majority of the long (q) arm as well as a translocation of unknown origin to the tip of the long arm of chromosome # 15, and also abnormalities on chromosome # 10 have been described in most, but not in all, the analyzed cells.

Together, these data suggest that specific genes might directly participate in the generation of HCC without necessarily involving the use of carcinogens. To investigate these questions in detail, we became interested a few years ago in utilizing cultured hepatocyte systems to study whether viral transforming genes could convert them into malignant hepatocytes.

V. TRANSFORMATION AND IMMORTALIZATION OF CULTURED HEPATOCYTES BY TRANSFORMING GENES OF POLYOMA VIRUS AND SV40 VIRUS

These studies were undertaken for several reasons: (a) to investigate the oncogenic potential of the Papova viruses Polyoma and SV40 in hepatocytes and (b) to obtain hepatocyte lines representative of the liver tissue from which they were derived.

This is of interest because in most previous studies aimed at culturing cells derived from HCC, which had been induced by chemical carcinogens in experimental animals, showed that they generally do not reflect the complete repertoire of liver-specific functions.

The results of our studies can be summarized as follows. Briefly, fetal and newborn hepatocytes of mice and rats can be cultured under conditions that permit their proliferation under the control of EGF, insulin and HC as hepatotrophic mitogens (18). Adult hepatocytes require additional serum (platelet) factor activities (38) which may be identical with the hepatocyte growth factor (HGF) that was recently purified (39). Such proliferating hepatocytes in primary culture with a limited lifespan can be utilized for transformation experiments aimed at inducing permanently growing hepatocyte lines. The results of the experiments, indicated that hepatocytes can indeed be converted into immortalized cells by using either the Polyoma virus early region (40) encoding LT-ag, MT-ag and sT-ag or SV40 virus early region encoding T-ag and t-ag. Resulting hepatocyte lines maintain stable expression of liver-specific functions. It thus appears, that immortalized hepatocyte lines can be produced which, when transformed by Polyoma virus genes, are tumorigenic (40). When, on the other hand, cells were infected with SV40 virus, cells were usually – at early time points after establishment - nonmalignant but nevertheless maintained permanent growth potential in culture (unpublished observations). The efficiency of transformation was low when transforming Polyoma virus genes were transfected (about 10^{-5}) (40) and was somewhat higher when transforming SV40 genes were introduced by infection of the cell with SV40 virus ($10^{-3} - 10^{-4}$).

Together, the results indicate that (a) hepatocytes at all developmental stages can be immortalized into permanently growing hepatocyte lines by viral transforming genes; (b) immortalization by SV40 virus rendered cells in a non-malignant state unless they were continuously subcultured, which resulted in the acquision of tumorigenic potential; (c) immortalization of growth properties occurred concomitantly with the stabilization of the expression of liver-specific genes. Unfortunately, the viruses used here do not induce liver tumors in rodents (41).

VI. INDUCTION OF HCC IN TRANSGENIC MICE

The usefulness of transgenic mice to study the effects of individual genes in vivo is well established (3). Brinster et al. had shown 1984 that introduction of SV40 genes into the germline of mice led to the development of chorioid plexus papilloma in transgenic mice (52). In more recent work, transgenic mice harbouring the SVAe-MGH construct 202 in which the SV40 virus transforming genes are driven by the metallothionin enhancer/promoter were constructed (35). The resulting transgenic animals expressed SV40 genes highly specifically in the liver because the metallothionine enhancer/promoter is particularly efficiently used in hepatocytes. The animals develop HCC after the 4th month of age, and die at about 7 months of age (53). The tumors grow to extreme sizes, as if most hepatocytes were involved in tumor formation. Histological analyses indicated (a) that the liver of tumor bearing animals showed morphological abnormalities indistinguishable from carcinogen-treated animals and (b) that hepatic tumors were bona fide HCC (Bannasch & Paul, unpublished observations).

VII. IMMORTALIZED HEPATOCYTE LINES DERIVED FROM FETAL TRANSGENIC MICE (STRAIN 202)

When hepatocytes of such transgenic animals were cultured at the fetal stage, hepatocyte lines grew out in primary culture, expressing SV40 genes and liver-specific markers including AFP and albumin (54). The emerging hepatocyte line no longer required EGF for growth as observed with normal fetal hepatocytes in primary cultures but responded to insulin plus HC in chemically defined MX-83 medium, which we had developed earlier to support proliferation of cultured hepatocytes (ref. 18). Up to passage 26, cells did not grow in agar and were not tumorigenic in nude mice. Thus, we confirmed our earlier observations that cultured hepatocytes can be transformed into immortalized cell lines by SV40 virus in vitro. It appears, that the acquisition of permanent growth potential by the cells in culture is not indicative of their tumorigenic potential: the hepatocyte lines are immortalized but are non-malignant. Additional evidence for their untransformed state was provided by the finding that cells arrest in the G_1 phase of the cell cycle in the absence of insulin. Upon re-addition of insulin to the culture, cells re-entered the cell cycle, entered S-phase partially synchronously and went on dividing (54).

With time in culture, the cells became increasingly autonomous of growth factors. Cells initially did not respond to hydrocortisone and did not multiply in the absence of growth factors but became arrested in G_1 as discussed above. After about 12 months of continuous culture, cells were clearly independent of exogenously supplied growth factors. Their growth rate was accelerated by HC in the absence of insulin. A more detailed analysis showed that the cells became responsive to extremely low levels of insulin or of hydrocortisone after about 2 years. It is not clear which mechanism underlies these changes in growth control of the cells. We have an indication for the production of growth-stimulating material by the cells in response of HC, suggesting that the steroid is not a bona fide growth factor. Together, it is possible that the increasing cell's autonomy of growth factors for cell multiplication may be one of the underlying reasons for the unrestricted growth of HCC in the animal between 4 and 7 months of age. The resulting growth factor independence observed in vitro could be the manifestation of tumor promotion taking place in the cultures. It remains to be seen whether hepatocyte lines derived from older animals and of tumor bearing animals display reduced growth factor requirements when placed into culture as predicted by our preliminary observations involving fetal hepatocyte lines (18,40,54).

VIII. CONCLUDING REMARKS

It appears, that the HCC induced by a viral transforming gene expressed in hepatocytes of transgenic mice is a powerful approach to answer some of the questions stated above. It offers most of the features that are necessary to dissect the cellular events within the liver during carcinogenesis: (a) hepatocyte lines of all developmental stages of the liver can be cultured, selected and purified for the desired phenotypes; (b) hepatocytes in the liver are destined to become HCC; (c) "immortalized" hepatocytes (i.e. cells expressing SV40-T-ag) can be identified in vivo by immunofluorescent staining using anti-T-ag antibodies. The results discussed here permit to approach a number questions regarding the development of cell lineages that lead to tumor formation in the liver. We are focussing our attention at the question concerning the time of T-ag induction during the development of the mouse embryo, which we consider the point at which cells become "initiated" and thus determined to become HCC.

It is clear that the mechanism by which carcinogens act, will not be elucidated by this approach. Rather, it will help providing answers to questions concerning causal relationships between the appearance of liver lesions including islands, foci, nodules and so on, and the development of HCC, i.e., cell lineage relationships between different hepatocyte phenotypes during the carcinogenic process in the liver.

IX. SUMMARY

Hepatocytes can be converted into permanently growing hepatocyte lines by the transforming genes of either Polyoma virus or SV40 virus. In transgenic mice (strain 202) most of the hepatocytes in the liver during late fetal development display an immortalized phenotype in culture, which is apparent immediately after placing liver cells into primary cultures. We conclude, that at the late fetal stage hepatocytes in the liver display similar properties which might be the "initiated" cell type discussed earlier which is untransformed but determined to become malignant at a later point in development.

Immortalized hepatocyte lines derived from the transgenic animals display reduced growth factor requirements in culture, i.e. increased autonomy. With time in culture, cells become increasingly autonomous by further reduction of their growth requirements until the final autonomous state has been attained, i.e. growth in the absence of any growth factor or hormone. It remains to be seen whether the development of the normal liver towards HCC is accompanied by a similar increased autonomy of growth factors as observed in cells in culture.

Acknowledgements

Transgenic mice (strain 202) were kindly provided by Dr. R. Brinster. The work described in this paper was supported by grants from the Deutsche Forschungsgemeinschaft, the Bundesminister für Forschung und Technologie (Bonn) and the Forschungsrat Rauchen und Gesundheit (Hamburg).

X. REFERENCES

1. Farber, E. & Cameron, R. Adv. Cancer Res. 31: 125 (1980)

2. Emmelot, P. & Scherer, E. Biophys. Biochim. Acta 105: 247 - 304 (1980)

3. Moore, M.A., Mayer, D. & P. Bannasch. Carcinogenesis 3: 1429 - 1436 (82)

4. Moore, M.A., Hacker, H.J. & P. Bannasch. Carcinogenesis 4: 595 - 603 (83)

5. Emmelot, P. & Scherer, P. Eur. J. Cancer 11: 689 - 696 (1975)

6. Pitot, H.C. et al. Nature 271: 456 - 458 (1976)

7. Sell, S. & Leffert, H.L. Hepatology 2: 77 - 86 (1982)

8. Schulte-Hermann, R. et al. Environmental Health Perspect. 50: 185 - 194 (1983)

9. Weinbren, K. in: Primary liver tumors (Remmer, H., Bolt, H.M., Bannasch, P. and Popper, H., editors). MTP Press, Lancaster, pp. 395 - 399 (1978)

10. Sell, S., Osborn, V. & Leffert, H.L. Carcinogenesis 2: 7 - 14 (1981)

11. Kitagawa, T., Michaelopolus, G. & Pitot, H.C. Cancer Research 35: 3682 - 3692 (1975)

12. Paul, D. & Piasecki, A. Unpublished observations

13. Novicki, D.L. et al. In Vitro 19: 191 - 202 (1983)

14. Morris, H.P. & Slaughter, L.J. in: Liver Carcinogenesis (Lapis, K. and Johannessen, J.V., editors), Hemisphere Publ., New York, N.Y. pp. 263 - 282 (1979)

15. Leffert, H.L. & Paul, D. J. Cell Biol. 52: 559 - 568 (1972)

16. Leffert, H.L. J. Cell. Biol. 62: 792 - 801 (1974)

17. Paul, D. & Walter, S. J. Cell Physiol. 85: 113 - 123 (1975)

18. Hoffmann, B., Piasecki, A. & Paul, D. Exptl. Cell Res. (submitted for publication)

19. Nicolson, G.L. & Rosenberg, N.L. BioEssays 6: 204-208 (1987)

20. Seller, M.I. Anat. Rec. 172: 149 - 156 (1972)

21. Le Duc, E.H. & Wilson, J.W. J. Nat. Cancer Inst. 30: 85 - 99 (1983)

22. Williams, G.M., Klaiber, M. & Farber, E. Am. J. Pathol. 89: 379 - 390 (1977)

23. Ohmori, T., Watanabe, K. & Williams, G.M. J. Nat. Cancer Inst. 65: 485 - 490 (1980)

24. Solt, D.B., Medline, A. & Farber, E. Am. J. Pathol. 88: 595 - 609 (1977)

25. Laishes, B.A., & Farber, E. J. Nat. Cancer Inst. Inst. <u>61</u>: 507 - 512 (1978)

26. Laishes, B.A. & Rolfe, P.B. <u>Cancer Research</u> <u>40</u>: 4132 - 4143 (1980)

27. Laishes, B.A. & Rolfe, P.B. <u>Cancer Research</u> <u>41</u>: 1731 - 1741 (1981)

28. Hunt, I.M. et al. <u>Cancer Research</u> <u>42</u>: 227 - 236 (1982)

29. Barbacid, M. <u>Trends in Genetics</u> <u>2</u>: 188 - 192 (1986)

30. Paul, D. <u>Drug Research</u> <u>35</u>: 772 - 779: 890 - 897 (1985)

31. Palmiter, R.D. & Brinster, R.L. <u>Ann. Rev. Genetics</u> <u>20</u>: 465 - 499 (1986)

32. Stewart, T.A. <u>et al.</u> <u>Cell</u> <u>38</u>: 627 - 637 (1984)

33. Quaife, C.J. <u>Cell</u> <u>48</u>: 1023 - 1034 (1987)

34. Hanahan, D. <u>Nature</u> 315: 115 - 122 (1985)

35. Palmiter, R.D. <u>et al.</u> <u>Nature</u> 316: 458 - 461 (1985)

36. Andres, A.C. <u>et al.</u> <u>Proc. Nat. Acad. Sci. U.S.A.</u> <u>84</u>: 1299 - 1303 (1987)

37. Adams, J.M. <u>et al.</u> <u>Nature</u> 318: 533 - 538 (1985)

38. Paul, D. & Piasecki, A. <u>Exptl. Cell Res.</u> <u>154</u>: 95 - 100 (1984)

39. Nakmura, T. <u>et al.</u> <u>Proc. Nat. Acad. Sci. USA</u> <u>83</u>: 6489 - 6493 (1986)

40. Höhne, M. <u>et al.</u> (submitted for publication)

41. Topp, W.C. <u>et al.</u> in: <u>DNA Tumor Viruses</u> (Tooze, J., editor) Cold Spring Harbor Laboratory, Cold Spring Harbor, N.Y. pp. 205 - 296 (1980)

42. Shafritz, D.A. <u>Hepatology</u> <u>2</u>: 35 S - 41 S (1982)

43. Tiollais, P. <u>et al.</u> <u>Nature</u> 317: 489 - 495 (1985)

44. Twist, E.M. <u>et al.</u> <u>J. Virol.</u> 37: 239 - 243 (1981)

45. Kew, M. In: Adv. Hepatitis Res. (ed. F.V. Chisari), Masson Publ. Co., New York, N.Y. pp. 203 - 215 (1984)

46. Beasley, R.P. <u>et al.</u> <u>The Lancet</u> <u>2</u>: 1129 - 1133 (1981)

47. Summers, J. <u>Hepatology</u> <u>1</u>: 179 - 183 (1981)

48. Omata, M. <u>et al.</u> <u>Gastroenterology</u> <u>85</u>: 260 - 267 (1983)

49. von Gierke, E. <u>Beitr. Pathol. Anat.</u> <u>82</u>: 497 (1929)

50. Knowles, B. <u>et al.</u> In: <u>Advances in Hepatitis Research</u> (F.V., editor). Masson Publications Inc. New York, N.Y. pp. 196 - 202 (1984)

51. Knowles, B. <u>et al.</u> <u>Int. J. Cancer</u> <u>30</u>: 27 - 33 (1982)

52. Brinster, R.L. et al. Cell 37: 367 - 379 (1984)

53. Messing, A. et al. Nature 316: 461 - 463 (1985)

54. Paul, D. et al. Exptl. Cell Res. (submitted for publication)

CHANGES IN HEPATOCYTE TGFβ RECEPTORS AND GENE EXPRESSION DURING NORMAL AND NEOPLASTIC LIVER GROWTH

Brian I. Carr*, Robert H. Whitson[+] and Keiichi Itakura[+]

Departments of Medical Oncology* and Molecular Genetics[+]
City of Hope National Medical Center
Duarte, CA 91010 USA

The Model

We have used the rat liver as a model system for studying the controls on normal and neoplastic growth in vivo and in vitro. Our working hypothesis has been that cell proliferation and the synthesis of specialized proteins are a consequence of gene action which in turn is strongly influenced by cellular environmental stimuli such as hormones and other growth regulatory molecules. The liver model permits the study of hepatocytes from resting normal liver, regenerating liver after a two-thirds partial hepatectomy (PH) and liver containing proliferating cells as a consequence of chronic carcinogen administration. We have studied these 3 aspects of growth using resting, regenerating, and carcinogen-altered liver as source material from which hepatocyte populations are prepared by the collagenase perfusion technique and after attachment to tissue culture dishes, the cells are then studied. Using this model system, we have been interested in determining how growth regulatory molecules (stimulants and inhibitors) influence hepatocyte growth and conversely, learning about growth controlling mechanisms through the study of how hepatocytes from resting, regenerating and carcinogen-altered liver differ in their interactions with model growth stimulants and growth inhibitors. We chose transforming growth factor type β (TGFβ) as a model growth inhibitor, based on our discovery of its potent, yet seemingly nontoxic growth inhibitory properties for adult rat hepatocytes stimulated by EGF, insulin and glucagon[1,2].

Background and Relevance

The ability of the mammalian liver to regenerate has been known since antiquity (the story of Prometheus). However, little is known about the factors that stimulate the regenerative growth or control it and limit over-growth. Similarly, although direct laboratory and clinical epidemiological evidence is available to suggest that chemicals are important in the causation of hepatocarcinogenesis, almost nothing is known about how the interaction of chemical carcinogens with hepatocytes actually results in cell proliferation. It is already known that after a two-thirds partial hepatectomy, there is a series of highly coordinated and controlled changes in the expression of several genes that are presumed to be involved in growth control. These include a sequential increase in the expression of the mRNA levels of c-fos, c-myc, c-ras, heat-shock gene transcripts for hsp83 and hsp70 and the β adrenergic receptor. There is a concomitant decrease in the EGF receptor and the alpha 1-adrenergic receptor, but no change in the insulin receptor. Several factors have been shown to be stimulatory for hepatocyte DNA synthesis in primary monolayer culture; these include EGF, norepinephrine, glucagon, and insulin. Whether these are actually relevant factors for hepatic proliferation in vivo however, is still speculative. We have made use of the known stimulatory properties of these factors in vitro, to study the consequences of their interaction with the hepatocyte membrane, and have compared this to hepatocytes from regenerating and neoplastic liver. We have used this approach to make inferences about growth-relevant membrane changes that may be important in hepatocytes from regenerating an carcinogen-altered liver. Similarly, we have begun to study the interaction of TGFβ, as a model growth inhibitor, with hepatocytes from resting, regenerating, neoplastic liver and hepatoma cell lines. Our experiments were designed to test the hypothesis that powerful, naturally occurring growth inhibitors limit normal growth and that changes in inhibitor activity or in sensitivity to inhibitor action may be important in permitting normal and neoplastic liver growth.

TGFβ Action, TGFβ Gene Expression and TGFβ Receptors

Effects on normal hepatocyte DNA synthesis: We originally noted that increasing doses of serum from a variety of species up to 50% concentration caused a dose-dependent inhibition of EGF-induced DNA synthesis in the primary cultures of adult rat hepatocytes[1]. Although at low doses such as 0.1 to 1%, stimulation by serum could be observed, inhibition was variable at > 10% serum concentration. Removal of the various cellular constituents from blood prior to the production of serum showed that the inhibitory factor was located in the platelets, since platelet-free plasma unmasked increased stimulatory activity in the serum that was produced from this plasma, and had less marked inhibitory action. As a consequence of this, we examined transforming growth factor type β (TGFβ) which is known to be produced in large amounts in platelets, as well as in placenta and kidney, and found that this was an exceedingly potent and seemingly non-toxic inhibitor of DNA synthesis with an ID_{50} of $4 \times 10^{-12}M$! Increasing the concentrations of insulin, EGF and glucagon or combining all three growth factors did not seem to be capable of overcoming the inhibitory action of TGFβ[1,2,3]. Our assay system for DNA synthesis was based upon the addition of ^{3}H-TdR into hepatocyte DNA at 72 to 96 hrs of culture. We examined the time course for the action of TGFβ, and found that it needed to be present in the first, second, or third 24-hour culture periods only, for DNA synthesis to be suppressed. However, if TGFβ was added at the same time as the ^{3}H-TdR, then no suppression of DNA synthesis was found. This was taken to indicate that either DNA synthesis could not be suppressed once it had actually begun, or that for TGFβ suppression of DNA synthesis to occur, something was required that took time. Presumably, this would reflect a requirement for the synthesis of a cellular protein under the influence of TGFβ that might be the actual intracellular inhibitor of DNA synthesis. If such an intermediary inhibitor is present, we did not find it secreted into the medium. If TGFβ is incubated with normal hepatocytes for the first 24 hrs of culture and then removed, subsequent DNA synthesis that would normally be induced by the presence of EGF at 72 to 96 hrs is completely suppressed. However, the medium conditioned by these hepatocytes that had been incubated with TGFβ for the first 24 hrs in culture was not inhibitory to fresh hepatocyte cultures when it was subsequently added to them. Other evidence that hepatocyte DNA synthesis is not inhibited once it has actually begun, is seen in the resistance of PH hepatocytes to the inhibitory actions of TGFβ (below).

We have found two conditions that can partially antagonize the inhibitory actions of TGFβ on adult rat hepatocytes. These are rat or rabbit serum and normal hepatocyte conditioned medium. When medium which has been conditioned by epidermal growth factor plus glucagon plus insulin for 72 hrs of normal hepatocyte culture is applied to fresh hepatocytes in the presence of TGFβ, then a marked shift to the right of the doses at which TGFβ will inhibit DNA synthesis was observed[1,3]. Similar results can be seen by incubating TGFβ for the first 24 hrs of culture in the presence of normal rat serum or rabbit serum. The reason for this partial antagonism of the inhibitory action of TGFβ by serum and conditioned medium is at present unclear.

Binding Studies of ^{125}I-TGFβ on Normal Hepatocytes

^{125}I-TGFβ was obtained by radiolabelling platelet-derived TGFβ with ^{125}I using chloramine T under very mild conditions, and was used for investigating the binding characteristics of TGFβ to rat hepatocytes. Equilibrium binding at 4°C was obtained by 4 hrs and then declined very slowly over the subsequent 24 hrs. At 37°C, however, binding peaked by 90 minutes then rapidly declined, probably due to degradation of bound TGFβ, as has been noted for many other ligands. We found that pre-incubation of rat hepatocytes at 37°C with normal rat or rabbit serum increased the subsequent binding of ^{125}I-TGFβ at 4°C, but that serum from cow, chicken, goat and horse had no effect on the binding of ^{125}I-TGFβ. This increase in binding was rapidly reversible, since removal of the serum after an overnight incubation resulted in a 50% loss of the increase in binding in the subsequent 3 hrs when serum was removed[4]. Serum factors may be important for control of the TGFβ receptor, since 24 hrs after plating adult rat hepatocytes in the presence of EGF, most of the ^{125}I-TGFβ binding capacity is lost. Therefore, we routinely perform ^{125}I-TGFβ binding on freshly prepared adult rat hepatocytes on the day that the rat is perfused. Insulin at 200 ng/ml also increases the binding of TGFβ to its hepatocyte receptor, but the effect is less marked than that observed with serum. We have found some evidence for internalization of ^{125}I-TGFβ. After 4 hrs of incubation of hepatocytes with ^{125}I-TGFβ at 4°C, we found that 90% of the radioactivity could be removed from the hepatocytes by a wash with pH 2.5 buffer. The reason for the residual 10% cell associated activity is not yet clear. However, when this acid wash technique is applied to hepatocytes that have been incubated for 90 min with ^{125}I-TGFβ at 37°C, approximately 50% of the cell-associated radioactivity is resistant to acid washing. This is taken as indirect evidence for some form of internalization. We also investigated whether TGFβ could induce a down-regulation of its receptor. We found that preincubation of hepatocytes with TGFβ 10 ng/ml at 37°C for 3 hrs did not cause any statistically significant change in subsequent total binding of ^{125}I-TGFβ at 4°C. We initially took this as evidence for a lack of down-regulation; however, subsequent studies with affinity labelling (see below) revealed that there was a marked decrease in the high molecular weight receptor, but this was not reflected in the overall binding. We interpret these results to indicate that there is a selective down-regulation of TGFβ receptors. Because of the complex kinetics of the interaction of

^{125}I-TGFβ with hepatocytes as well as the complicated kinetics when TGFβ binding studies was subjected to Scatchard analysis, we investigated the TGFβ hepatocyte receptors in more detail by binding ^{125}I-TGFβ with its hepatocyte receptors using the cross-linking agent, disuccinimidyl suberate. The cross-linked cells were then solubilized and subjected to PAGE electrophoresis using 9% acrylamide slab gels. The resulting autoradiogram revealed at least 3 major classes of TGFβ receptor molecular weight forms in normal hepatocytes, the main bands having molecular weights of 85 and 65 kD, a lesser proportion of molecular weight forms at 135 kD and a very low affinity form at 280 kD. These molecular weight forms correspond to the molecular weights described for TGFβ receptors in other cell types[4].

Hepatocytes from regenerating liver

(A) ^{125}I-TGFβ Binding Studies: Hepatocytes were obtained at various times after a two-thirds partial hepatectomy (PH) and placed in primary monolayer culture. By 5 hrs after PH, hepatocytes were found to have lost most of their high affinity binding for TGFβ but had no change in their binding characteristics for ^{125}I-insulin[5]. By contrast, sham hepatectomized rat hepatocytes had no change in their ^{125}I-TGFβ binding characteristics. In order to examine the significance of this observation, we measured the levels of DNA synthesis in normal and PH hepatocytes in the presence of EGF ± TGFβ. At 72-96 hrs of culture, we found no differences, since both cell types were equally inhibited by TGFβ. Daily measurements of ^{125}I-TGFβ binding however, revealed that after 2 days in culture, TGFβ receptors in normal and PH hepatocytes had become similar. We therefore changed the DNA synthesis measurement protocol, and measured incorporation of ^{3}H-TdR from 0 to 48 hrs in the presence of EGF and insulin ± TGFβ, and continuous ^{3}H-TdR. Under these conditions, we found that whereas normal hepatocytes were inhibited as expected, PH 5 hour hepatocytes were remarkably resistant to the inhibitory action of TGFβ. Thus, in the early stages of hepatic regeneration, hepatocytes become less sensitive to inhibition by TGFβ, possibly through a decrease in the binding sites for TGFβ. Hepatocytes were also removed from rats at 20 hrs after a two-thirds partial hepatectomy and placed in primary monolayer culture. Two peaks of DNA synthesis were found. The first peak was seen when ^{3}H-TdR was added at 0 to 24 hrs of culture, and was independent of the presence or absence of any growth factors. This was presumed to reflect the DNA synthesis that was actually occurring in vivo at the time that the hepatocytes were prepared, and this peak of DNA synthesis was not inhibitable by TGFβ up to 10 ng/ml. However, a second peak of DNA synthesis was found at 72 to 96 hrs, which was dependent upon the presence of EGF in the cultures. As with normal hepatocytes, this peak was inhibited by the presence of TGFβ in the cultures.

(B) TGFβ gene expression: We wished to observe whether there was a concomitant alteration in the synthesis of TGFβ in rat liver during hepatic regeneration. We had expected that if rat liver in vivo reflected what we have observed with the primary cultures of rat hepatocytes in vitro, then during hepatic regeneration there would be a decline in the ambient TGFβ levels, which we supposed would permit the hepatocytes to respond to circulating mitogens or hormones. Using a full length cDNA probe for the human TGFβ gene, we measured the TGFβ mRNA levels on Northern gels under stringent conditions, using total hepatic RNA. We found, to our surprise, that resting liver had exceedingly low but detectable levels of TGFβ mRNA. However, after a PH, the levels of TGFβ mRNA started to increase from about 6 hrs, reached a peak at 36 hrs and did not start to decline until at least 96 hrs after the PH, finally reaching baseline levels by 10 days. In order to investigate whether these increased levels of TGFβ mRNA reflected an increase in TGFβ protein levels, 2 experiments were devised. In the first, cells from liver perfusates were stained with a TGFβ antibody, using a double antibody technique in order to visualize the cells. There was an almost complete absence of staining in the normal hepatocytes but a strong appearance of stain for TGFβ protein in cells from PH liver. In a second approach, acid/ethanol extracts have been prepared from normal and PH livers, and the amount of functional TGFβ is currently being assessed using a radio-immunoassay technique, as well as by inhibition of DNA synthesis on adult rat hepatocytes. Thus, TGFβ mRNA levels start to increase in the early prereplicative phase of DNA synthesis and reach a peak well after the first round of DNA synthesis and mitosis. It is thus conceivable that TGFβ could represent a physiological stop signal preventing liver overgrowth. Curiously, when we purified hepatocytes from rat liver 36 hours post PH (peak signal for TGFβ mRNA levels) using Percoll gradients, we found little increase in TGFβ mRNA levels on Northern gels. However, when the non-hepatocyte cell RNAs were probed, we found the increased TGFβ mRNA. This raises the distinct possibility that liver cell growth may be regulated in part by TGFβ in a paracrine fashion, i.e., non-hepatocyte liver cells producing growth-regulatory molecules which control hepatocyte proliferation.

Carcinogen-altered hepatocytes and hepatomas

(A) Carcinogen Action on Rat Liver: From a cell biologist's point of view, the uncontrolled growth of neoplasia could result from an increase of cell stimulants, an increased sensitivity to the action of cell stimulants, a decrease in cell inhibitors or a loss of sensitivity to the action of cellular inhibitors. We investigated whether there might be a decreased response to the inhibitory action of TGFβ, our model growth inhibitor, using carcinogen altered rat hepatocytes and established hepatoma lines. Rats were fed dietary 2-acetylaminofluorene 0.02% (w/w) (AAF) continuously for 12 weeks, which produced macroscopic liver nodules. The livers were perfused with collagenase and the largest nodules were scooped out, dissociated and placed in primary monolayer culture. EGF 10 ng/ml was found to induce DNA synthesis in AAF cells as in normal hepatocytes, and the DNA synthesis in AAF cells could also be inhibited by TGFβ. However, the inhibition of DNA synthesis by TGFβ showed a marked shift to the right, with increasing doses of TGFβ needed to suppress the EGF-induced DNA synthesis. Despite this, complete suppression of DNA synthesis could be induced although much larger doses (5 ng/ml instead of 0.3 ng/ml) were required to completely suppress it. Thus, AAF-altered hepatocytes lost sensitivity to the inhibitory actions of TGFβ although suppression could still be obtained. Interestingly, the carcinogen-induced liver nodules contained high levels of TGFβ mRNA. Primary hepatocellular carcinomas were obtained using three different regimens and were examined one year after a three month-feeding of dietary 2-acetylaminofluorene, one year after the start of the regimen of Solt and Farber, and one year after administration of dietary phenobarbital 0.5% (w/w) given after a single initiating dose of diethyl-nitrosamine 200 mg/kg. The tumors produced by all 3 regimens had increased levels of TGFβ mRNA compared to age-matched controls. The significance of this interesting and unexpected result is not clear at the present. Whether this represents a mutated form of TGFβ, an altered receptor in which the TGFβ has stimulatory rather than inhibitory actions, an invasion of TGFβ-producing cells, or a loss of response of the cells to the normal actions of TGFβ with subsequent overproduction of TGFβ, are all explanations which are currently being investigated.

(B) <u>Rat and Human Hepatoma Cell Lines</u>: Growth curves were performed in the presence of 0.3, 1, 3, and 10 ng/ml TGFβ with the human hepatoma cell lines PLC/PRF/5, Hep-G2, Hep-3B, HuH 7, and SK/Hep-1, and the rat hepatoma cell lines MH_1C_1, MH7777, HTC and H-4-II-E. All the cell lines were resistant to the inhibitory actions of TGFβ compared to normal hepatocytes, as noted by others[7]. Hep-3B and HuH 7 showed > 50% inhibition of growth after TGFβ 10 ng/ml (0.3 ng/ml causes 80% inhibition of DNA synthesis in normal adult rat hepatocytes) but still continued growing. All the other cell lines showed super-imposable growth curves for TGFβ 10 ng/ml and 0 ng/ml, indicating neither a growth-inhibitory nor a growth-stimulatory effect. Cross-linking studies were also done using ^{125}I-TGFβ with the hepatoma cell lines, in order to determine whether there was a change in distribution for the various molecular weight forms of TGFβ receptor. The affinity cross-linking gels for Hep-3B and SK/Hep-1 appeared similar to the gels obtained from normal rat hepatocytes. However, PLC/PRF/5, Hep-G2 and HUH 7 all showed a preponderance of the high molecular weight (280 kD) receptor, which was present as only a minor component in normal rat hepatocytes. By contrast, the rat hepatoma cell lines were similar to normal rat hepatocytes in the molecular weight distribution of their TGFβ receptors, except that the 65 and 85 kD receptors had a much higher affinity for TGFβ, since maximum binding occurred at the lowest input amounts of ^{125}I-TGFβ and no increase in binding occurred when larger amounts were added, in contrast to our results in normal rat hepatocytes. These results would seem to indicate, that for some hepatomas at least, resistance to the inhibitory action of TGFβ might reside at a post-receptor level; while in others, an alteration in receptor activity is a candidate mechanism for resistance to the inhibitory actions of TGFβ. Those cellular sites which could be important in resistance to the inhibitory action of TGFβ might include TGFβ processing, second messenger action or degradation. The human hepatoma cell lines also differed from the rat hepatoma cell lines in respect of their expression of TGFβ gene. The human hepatoma lines all expressed high levels of TGFβ mRNA on Northern gels compared to normal human or rat liver or rat hepatocytes. Increases in TGFβ were not found in mRNA transcripts of the rat hepatomas.

In summary, hepatocytes for normal rat liver have high-affinity, saturable receptors for TGFβ, and their mitogen-induced DNA synthesis is inhibited by TGFβ in a dose-dependent manner. Hepatocytes from early regenerating rat liver lose high affinity binding for TGFβ at early time points and concomitantly lose sensitivity to the inhibitory effects of TGFβ. However, TGFβ does not appear to inhibit DNA synthesis once it has started, since it does not inhibit the DNA synthesis <u>in vitro</u> of hepatocytes obtained 20 hrs after partial hepatectomy or in normal hepatocytes at the time of DNA synthesis. TGFβ mRNA levels are increased during hepatic regeneration, with the peak occurring at approximately 36 hrs with a plateau until 96 hrs before starting to decline. The liver cell which produces this strong TGFβ mRNA signal has not yet been identified but may not be the hepatocyte. Whether this is reflected in TGFβ protein production and at sufficient levels to cause inhibition of growth <u>in vivo</u>, has yet to be determined. Human and rat hepatomas have <u>decreased</u> sensitivity to the inhibitory actions of TGFβ, yet retain normal over-all levels of TGFβ binding, although the receptor characteristics are quite different from normal. Primary rat hepatomas appeared to produce TGFß although this was not seen in the rat hepatoma cell lines. This would appear to indicate that some cells other than the carcinogen-altered hepato-cyte are producing the TGFß in primary rat hepatomas. In contrast, five human hepatoma cell lines over-produced TGFß mRNA and TGFß pro-tein compared to normal human or rat liver.

References

1. I. Hayashi and B. I. Carr, DNA synthesis in rat hepatocytes: Inhibition by a platelet factor and stimulation by an endogenous factor, J. Cell. Physiol. 125:82-90 (1985).
2. B. I. Carr and I. Hayashi, DNA synthesis in cultured rat hepatocytes is inhibited by platelet-derived transforming growth factor ß in a non-toxic, dose-dependent manner, Proc. Amer. Assoc. Cancer Res. 26:791 (1985).
3. B. I. Carr, I. Hayashi, E. L. Branum, and H. L. Moses, Inhibition of DNA synthesis in rat hepatocytes by platelet-derived type ß transforming growth factor, Cancer Res. 46:2330-2334 (1986).
4. B. I. Carr, Control of hepatocyte TGFß receptors during growth stimulation, J. Cell. Biochem. 11A:A212 (1987).
5. B. I. Carr, A. Thall, R. H. Whitson, and K. Itakura, Transforming growth factor type ß receptors decrease early in hepatic regeneration, J. Cell. Biol. 103(5):1650 (1986).
6. J. Massague, Subunit structure of a high-affinity receptor for type ß transforming growth factor, J. Biol. Chem. 260: 7059-7066 (1985).
   J. Massague and B. Like, Cellular receptors for type ß trans-forming growth factor, J. Biol. Chem. 260: 2636-2645 (1985).
   S. Cheifetz, B. Like, and J. Massague, Cellular distribution of type I and type II receptors for transforming growth factor type ß, J. Biol. Chem. 261:9972-9978 (1986).
7. J. B. McMahon, W. L. Richards, A. A. del Campo, M. K. H. Song, and S. S. Thorgeirsson, Differential effects of transforming growth factor-ß on proliferation of normal and malignant rat liver epithelial cells in culture, Cancer Res. 46: 4665-4671 (1986).

REGULATION OF CARBOHYDRATE METABOLISM IN A GLYCOGEN-STORING

LIVER CELL LINE

Doris Mayer

Institut für Experimentelle Pathologie,
Deutsches Krebsforschungszentrum
6900 Heidelberg, FRG

INTRODUCTION

Synthesis and breakdown of glycogen is a very complex and tightly controlled process involving substrates, intermediates, cofactors, activators, inhibitors, enzymatic interconversions and hormonal balances. Glycogen metabolism occurs in many different tissues. The various metabolic controls are different in each tissue and are adapted to the particular environment and metabolic requirements. In normal rat liver glycogen is stored physiologically as an osmotically inactive polysaccharide from which glucose molecules can be rapidly provided for metabolic processes. The hormonal, dietary and circadian control of its metabolism has been investigated in great detail[1-4].

Different pathologic conditions either occurring spontaneously or induced experimentally have been described where glycogen is accumulated in excessive amounts[5-9]. Thus, an abnormally high storage of glycogen has been observed in hepatic tumors and especially in preneoplastic lesions of animals treated with chemical carcinogens[8,10]. In the case of rats glycogen storage foci consisting of large glycogen-storing hepatocytes represent the earliest lesions which are microscopically visible after carcinogen application.

Biochemical and cytochemical investigations of glycogen metabolism in livers of carcinogen-treated rats were performed in order to understand the metabolic alterations leading to excessive glycogen storage during early stages of hepatocarcinogenesis. However, since the glycogen storage foci represent only a few percent of total liver parenchyma[11] total liver homogenates turned out to be not appropriate for biochemical studies designed to measure metabolite and enzyme alterations of the lesions[12]. Biochemical studies on microdissected material are very difficult and time-consuming[13]. Due to the very limited amount of material obtained it is almost impossible to perform experiments on enzyme kinetics or on metabolic regulation of enzymes in microdissected tissue.

Enzyme histochemical studies have provided very useful insights into the alterations of the enzymatic pattern in these lesions[14]. Thus, it has been shown that especially the activity of the key enzymes of carbohydrate metabolism is either increased or decreased which indicates that intermediates of carbohydrate metabolism are channeled in a different way in glycogen storage cells compared with normal hepatocytes. Enzyme histochemical studies are usually of qualitative nature, quantitative data are difficult to obtain. The method does not allow detailed quantitative studies on metabolic regulation.

A third methodological approach, namely the isolation of glycogen storage cells by density gradient centrifugation or by elutriation from single cell suspensions obtained by perfusion of carcinogen-treated livers with collagenase, was hampered by various facts:
1) Part of the glycogen was degraded during the perfusion procedure.
2) The glycogen storage cells were not changed in density, only in size.
3) "Twin-cells" and triplets which were either not completely dissociated or which had reaggregated after isolation, were elutriated together with large glycogen-storing cells.
A pure population of glycogen-storing hepatocytes has never been obtained by both centrifugation techniques.

For that reason we have tried to obtain an _in vitro_-system consisting of a pure population of glycogen-storing cells. We succeeded in establishing a glycogen-storing liver cell line _in vitro_ which shared a number of properties with preneoplastic glycogen storage cells occurring _in vivo_. This cell line was used as a model to study some aspects of the regulation of glycogen metabolism in a glycogen-storing liver cell. For comparison, a glycogen-poor liver cell line, as well as a transplantable Morris hepatoma and normal adult hepatocytes were investigated.

ESTABLISHMENT AND CHARACTERIZATION OF THE CELL LINES

The two liver cell lines studied in this paper have been established from a primary culture of normal adult rat hepatocytes by single cell cloning[15]. C_1I was a cell line storing large amounts of glycogen, and C_2I was poor in glycogen. The glycogen-free, well characterized Morris hepatoma 3924A[16] was adapted to tissue culture from the ascitic form of the tumor[17].

Light and electron microscopic characterization of C_1I and C_2I

C_1I and C_2I are epithelial liver cells of polygonal shape growing as contact-inhibited monolayers. Under phase contrast C_1I cells show large clear areas localized around the nuclei (Fig. 1a) which proved to be strongly positive with the PAS-reaction. Electron microscopically these areas were shown to be composed of monoparticulate glycogen, they were lacking any other organelles (Fig. 2a). In the remaining cytoplasm mitochondria of both normal and atypical structure were observed. Rough endoplasmic reticulum was reduced compared with freshly dissociated hepatocytes, smooth endoplasmic reticulum was well developed and was intermingled with small glycogen particles[15].

In C_2I cells no glycogen deposits were visible by phase contrast microscopy (Fig. 1b), after PAS-staining only small spots of PAS-positive material were detected. Under the electron microscope these spots turned out to be small clusters of α-particulate glycogen (Fig. 2b).

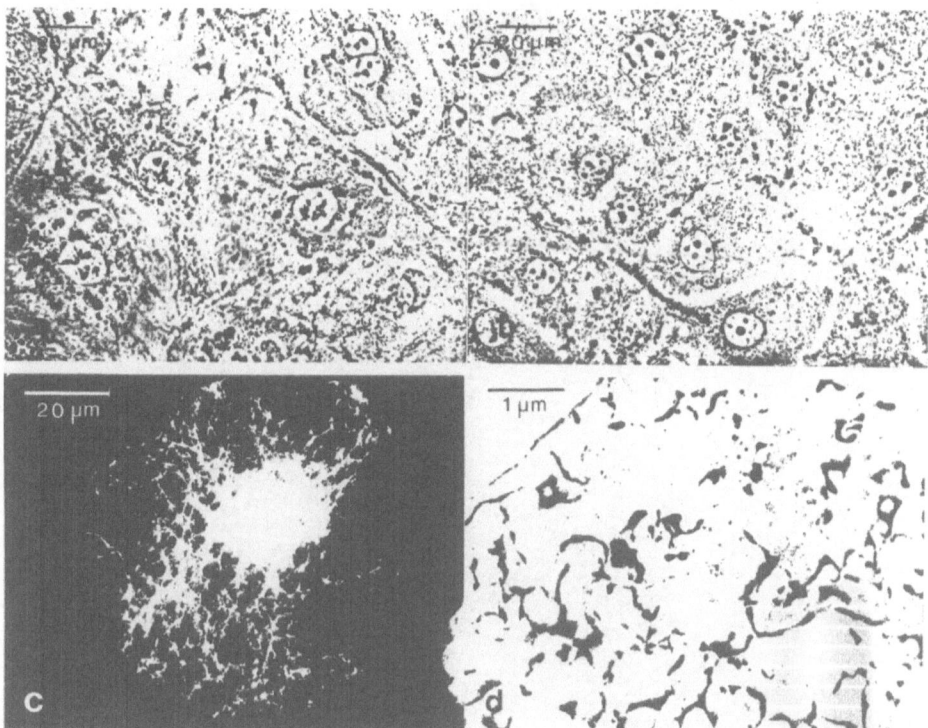

Figure 1. Phase micrographs of C_1I (a) and C_2I (b). Note large clear
areas in C_1I around the nuclei. These areas represent glycogen,
they are lacking in C_2I. Both cell lines are stainable by anti-
prekeratin (c, C_2I) proving that they are of epithelial
origin. The distribution of glucose-6-phosphatase activity is
demonstrated ultrahistochemically (d, C_2I). The pattern is typical as observed for hepatocytes.

Table 1. Markers for the Selection of Epithelial and Hepatocyte-derived
Cells

Epithelial Cells	Hepatocyte-derived Cells
Prekeratin	Prekeratin polypeptide pattern[19]
Desmosomes	Glucose-6-phosphatase pattern[15]
Glucose-6-phosphatase	SER-glycogen-pattern[15]
activity	Glucokinase activity
	β_2-Adrenoceptors[18]

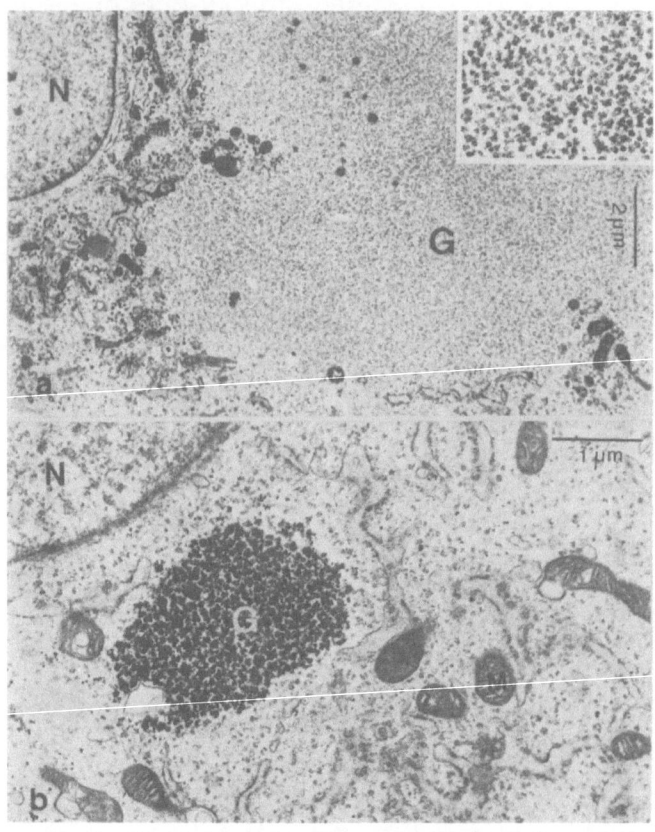

Figure 2. Survey electron micrograph of a glycogen-
storing cell of C_1I (a). N, nucleus, G,
glycogen, M, mitochondrium. The glycogen
zone is free of any organelles. Inset:
Higher magnification of the glycogen zone
reveals β-particles. (b) shows a detail
of a cell of C_2I with hepatocyte-like
morphology and α-particles of glycogen.

Criteria for the selection of epithelial liver cells

It was of importance to know what type of cells had been selected
by cloning. Both cell lines contained prekeratin filaments as demonstrated immunocytochemically (Fig. 1c) proving that they were of epithelial
origin. Some other properties observed which prove the epithelial origin
of the liver cells are summarized in the left part of Table 1. Additional
markers which point to a hepatocellular origin of the cells are presented
in the right part of Table 1, such as the distribution of glucose-6-
phosphatase activity (Fig. 1d) which is typical for hepatocytes, the presence of glucokinase activity which is the hepatocyte-specific isoenzyme
of the hexokinases, the presence of the hepatocyte-specific subtype $β_2$ of
adrenoceptors[18] and the polypeptide pattern of prekeratins[19]. However,

the cells did not produce albumin or α-fetoprotein. Thus, although the cells revealed a number of properties indicating their hepatocellular origin, they cannot be definitely designated as hepatocytes.

Criteria for the selection of "preneoplastic" cells

C_1I and C_2I were rapidly growing cells with a doubling time of about 28 hours compared to 16 hours observed for MH 3924A. They were growing to confluence on plastic dishes (Table 2), final cell density was only 27% of that obtained by MH 3924A. C_1I cells showed a very low potency for anchorage independent growth (colony forming efficiency in soft agar < 1%), C_2I cells did not grow in soft agar. So far, C_1I and C_2I did not produce tumors after transplantation into nude mice.

Table 2. Growth Characteristics of Epithelial Liver Cells

	C_1I	C_2I	MH 3924A
Lag phase	36 h	36 h	24 h
Log phase	48 h	48 h	48 h
Doubling time	28 h	28 h	16 h
Final cell density (25 cm² growth area)	1.3×10^6	1.2×10^6	4.5×10^6
Colony forming efficiency (% of plated cells)	86	65	81
Growth on dishes	confluent	confluent	criss-cross
Growth in soft-agar	(+)	–	+++
Growth in nude mice	–	–	+

ACTIVITY OF KEY ENZYMES OF CARBOHYDRATE METABOLISM

Preneoplastic hepatocytes induced chemically in vivo reveal typical alterations in the pattern of enzyme activities of carbohydrate metabolism. Thus, a strong reduction of glucose-6-phosphatase activity, a key enzyme of gluconeogenesis and a reduction of glycogen phosphorylase activity were observed. By contrast, the activities of glucose-6-phosphate dehydrogenase, the key enzyme of pentose phosphate pathway and of the glycolytic enzyme glyceraldehyde-3-phosphate dehydrogenase were increased[14]. This prompted us to characterize our cell lines according to their pattern of key enzymes of carbohydrate metabolism. The enzymes investigated are summarized in Table 3. It is evident that the activity of the glycolytic enzyme pyruvate kinase was increased, while that of the gluconeogenetic enzymes fructose-1,6-bisphosphatase and glucose-6-phosphatase were decreased compared with normal hepatocytes. Glucose-6-phosphate dehydrogenase activity was very high, and glycogen phosphorylase activity was low. It was of interest that C_1I and C_2I both revealed high hexokinase activity and that glucokinase was reduced, but still present (Fig. 3). Glucokinase activity is usually reduced or absent in hepatocellular tumors while hexokinase which has an extremely low activity in normal hepatocytes is strongly expressed in hepatocellular tumors.

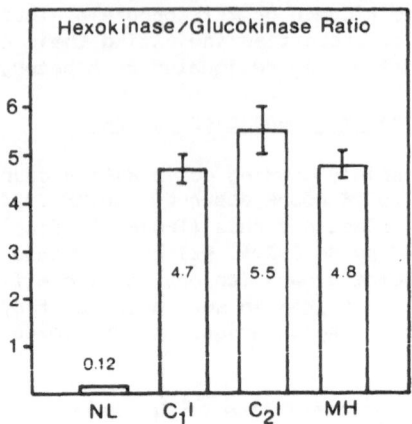

Figure 3. Activity ratios of hexokinase and glucokinase
in normal rat liver (NL),
C_1I, C_2I and MH 3924A.

From the data given in Table 3 it can be concluded that C_1I and C_2I
cells have spontaneously transformed in vitro, although they are not or
not yet tumorigenic after transplantation into nude mice. In that respect
they might be considered as "preneoplastic-like" cells.

INVESTIGATION OF GLYCOGEN PHOSPHORYLASE AND GLYCOGEN SYNTHETASE

Glycogen synthetase and glycogen phosphorylase are the two enzymes
directly involved in the synthesis and degradation of glycogen. Both enzymes exist in two ore more interconvertible forms. Glycogen metabolism is
known to be mediated through the covalent modification of glycogen synthetase and phosphorylase by phosphorylation and dephosphorylation
processes[1,3,20,21].

The activation of glycogen synthesis involves the conversion of the
phosphorylated inactive synthetase b into dephosphorylated active synthetase a. Phosphorylation is performed by various synthetase kinases, dephosphorylation by synthetase phosphatase. Recently, Tan has shown[22] that
in vivo glycogen is not synthesized by synthetase a which is present only
in trace amounts in liver of fed rats, but by an intermediate form R which
has also a high affinity for UDPG but is activated by glucose-6-phosphate.

Glycogen phosphorylase activation and inactivation are mediated
through phosphorylase kinase and phosphorylase phosphatase which themselves
are regulated by cAMP and Ca^{2+}-ions in the case of phosphorylase kinase, and
by glucose and the ratio of phosphorylase a/a+b in the case of
phosphatase[1,23]. It has been generally agreed that only the a-form of
phosphorylase is able to catalyze phosphorolysis of glycogen in vivo while
phosphorylase b is completely inactive[1,2].

Table 3. Activity of enzymes of carbohydrate metabolism in C_1I, C_2I, MH 3924A and normal rat liver

	Normal liver	C_1I	C_2I	MH 3924A
Glycogen phosphorylase (a+b)	213.5 ± 2.5	29.3 ± 0.9*	25.7 ± 0.7*	22.7 ± 0.7
Glycogen synthetase (a+b)	2.8 ± 0.1	5.2 ± 0.1*	1.6 ± 0.1*	1.9 ± 0.1*
Hexokinase + Glucokinase	4.0 ± 0.4	9.2 ± 0.9**	10.8 ± 1.0**	20.7 ± 0.8**
Pyruvate Kinase	88.5 ± 13.7	2561.0 ± 95.1**	1544.3 ± 16.7*	1437.0 ± 90.1**
Lactate dehydrogenase	1077.0 ± 99.2	1515.3 ± 43.9	951.0 ± 99.9	507.7 ± 13.6
Glucose-6-phosphatase	17.1 ± 1.9	4.9 ± 0.3*	3.2 ± 0.4**	2.3 ± 0.3**
Fructose-1,6-bisphosphatase	23.4 ± 2.4	0	0	0
Glucose-6-P-dehydrogenase	5.3 ± 1.9	76.8 ± 1.5**	812.1 ± 3.2**	69.1 ± 4.8**

Activity is expressed as $nmol \times mg\ protein^{-1} \times min^{-1}$
Values are means ± SEM of 5 determinations
Significantly different from normal liver: *$p \leqslant 0.01$; **$p \leqslant 0.001$

Influence of glucose on synthetase and phosphorylase in intact cells

Addition of glucose to hepatocytes isolated from normal starved rat liver first leads to inactivation of phosphorylase and subsequently to activation of synthetase [24],[25]. The mechanism underlying these processes is supposed to be the following[2],[25]: Glucose binds to phosphorylase a, the resulting complex is a superior substrate for phosphorylase phosphatase. Phosphorylase is inactivated and glycogenolysis is stopped. Removal of phosphorylase a, which is a strong inhibitor for glycogen synthetase phosphatase, allows the latter enzyme to convert synthetase b to a, resulting in the activation of glycogen synthesis.

We have investigated whether this mechanism is impaired in any way in C_1I cells and thus might give some indication on the mechanism leading to excessive glycogen accumulation. Figure 4 shows the changes of enzyme activities obtained when cells kept in glucose-poor medium for 24 hours are refed with low (5 mM) and high (50 mM) glucose concentrations. In both cases phosphorylase was rapidly inactivated with a subsequent activation of synthetase. Although the effect was less marked than in normal isolated hepatocytes[25], it is obvious that this regulation mechanism is intact in C_1I cells.

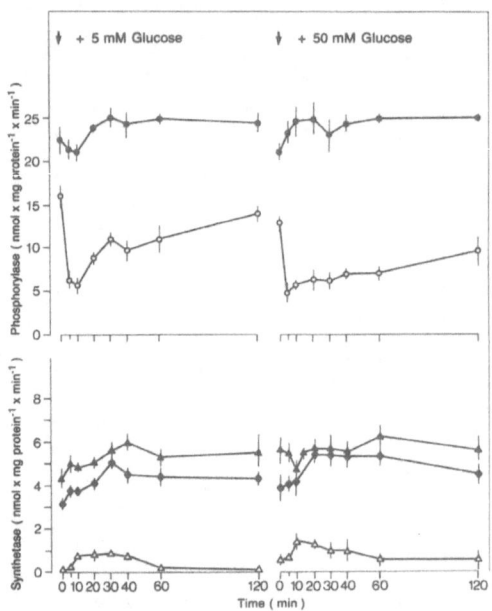

Figure 4. Effects of two glucose concentrations on the inactivation of phosphorylase and the activation of synthetase in C_1I cells. Cells were preincubated for 24 h in 2 mM glucose before addition of 5 or 50 mM glucose. o, phosphorylase a; ●, total phosphorylase; △, synthetase a; ◆, synthetase R; ▲, total synthetase.

Table 4.

Kinetic data of glycogen phosphorylase

Cells	phosphorylase a				phosphorylase a+b			intracellular G6P mM
	Spec. act. mU/min (% of normal liver)	$K_m(G1P)$ mM	K_m^{**}(glycogen) mM	K_i(app) mMG6P	spec. act. mU/min (% of normal liver)	% $\frac{a}{a+b}$	$K_m(G1P)$ mM	
C_1I^* (glycogen-storing)	17.3 ± 0.7 (8.3)	2.4 ± 0.4	0.28	0.45	29.3 ± 0.9 (13.7)	59	2.4 ± 0.3	3.0 ± 0.7
C_2I^* (glycogen-poor)	11.7 ± 0.1 (5.6)	3.4 ± 0.1	n.d.	0.19	25.7 ± 0.7 (12.0)	46	2.8 ± 0.1	0.16 ± 0.05
MH3924A	19.5 ± 0.7 (9.3)	1.9 ± 0.3	0.28	0.55	22.7 ± 0.7 (10.6)	86	2.3 ± 0.3	0.58 ± 0.12
normal rat liver	208.3 ± 3.8 (100)	2.8 ± 0.2	0.44	>25	213.5 ± 2.5 (100)	98	3.1 ± 0.2	0.25 ± 0.05

* confluent cells
** calculated as glucose equivalents
n.d. = not determined

Kinetic properties of phosphorylase and synthetase

We have studied the activities of the various forms of phosphorylase and synthetase and some of their kinetic properties in order to get more insight into differences in the regulation of glycogen metabolism of normal rat liver, the glycogen-free tumor MH 3924A, the glycogen-storing cell line C_1I and the glycogen-poor cell line C_2I. Cells from the 5th day of culture were used when C_1I and C_2I cells were confluent and MH 3924A was in stationary phase.

Glycogen phosphorylase: The kinetic properties of phosphorylase are summarized in Table 4. The specific activities of phosphorylase a and total phosphorylase (a+b) were markedly reduced in the cell lines compared to normal liver. The ratio of active form a to total phosphorylase (a+b) was also reduced. Whereas in normal liver phosphorylase was almost completely in its phosphorylated state (98%), the a-form represented only 59% and 46% in C_1I and C_2I cells and 85% in MH 3924A cells.

K_m-values for glucose-1-phosphate were about the same for all cells and tissues described. K_m-values for glycogen were determined taking into consideration the endogenous glycogen content of the samples and were calculated in terms of glucose equivalents. There was no significant difference in K_m for glycogen between the cell lines and normal liver.

In contrast to phosphorylase a from liver, the enzyme of the cell lines C_1I, C_2I and MH 3924A was inhibited by physiological concentrations of G6P. The apparent K_i-values for G6P were 0.45, 0.19 and 0.55 mM G6P for C_1I, C_2I and MH 3924A, respectively. From the type of kinetics observed (Fig. 5), it can be concluded that G6P acts competitively to G1P. In the presence of AMP the enzyme was not inhibited by G6P-concentrations up to 25 mM. It is supposed that in the cell lines the liver type phosphorylase is replaced by an isoenzyme which might be characteristic for tumor cells[26].

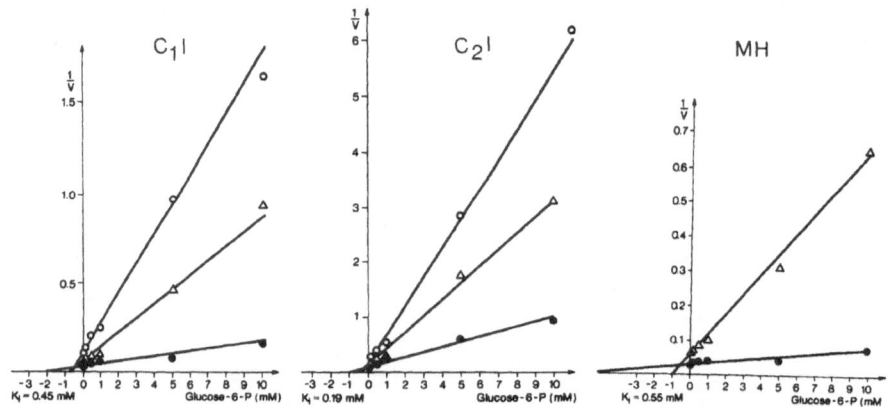

Figure 5. Dixon plots illustrating the inhibitory effect of glucose-6-phosphate on phosphorylase a from C_1I, C_2I and MH 3924A. Phosphorylase was measured in the presence of 25 mM (●), 5 mM (Δ) and 2.5 mM glucose-1-phosphate (o).

Glycogen synthetase: The kinetic data obtained for synthetase are summarized in Table 5. The specific activities of synthetase a were very low

Table 5.

Kinetic data of glycogen synthetase

Cells	Synthetase a Spec. act. mU/min (% of normal liver)	Synthetase R Spec. act. mU/min (% of normal liver)	Synthetase a+b Spec. act. mU/min (% of normal liver)	K_m(app) mM UDPG	% $\frac{a}{a+b}$	Synthetase a+b $A_{0.5}$ mM G6P	intracellular G6P (mM)
C_1I* (glycogen-storing)	0.25 ± 0.11 (100)	0.92 ± 0.04 (65)	5.2 ± 0.1 (189)	0.18 ± 0.01	2.4	0.79 ± 0.08	3.0 ± 0.7
C_2I* (glycogen-poor)	0.06 ± 0.03 (24)	0.77 ± 0.05 (54)	1.6 ± 0.1 (56)	0.15 ± 0.01	1.9	1.05 ± 0.25	0.16 ± 0.05
MH 3924 A	0.08 ± 0.05 (32)	n.d.	1.9 ± 0.1 (67)	0.14 ± 0.01	2.1	0.79 ± 0.11	0.58 ± 0.12
normal rat liver	0.25 ± 0.10 (100)	1.42 ± 0.16 (100)	2.8 ± 0.1 (100)	0.37 ± 0.04	4.5	0.17 ± 0.06	0.25 ± 0.05

* confluent cells
n.d. = not determined

in all tissues investigated. It may be concluded that this enzyme form is only of minor importance for glycogen accumulation in C_1I cells. The two G6P-dependent forms R and b had higher specific activities in the glycogen-storing cell line C_1I than in glycogen-poor C_2I cells. The apparent K_m-values of total synthetase for UDPG were lower in the cell lines than in normal liver. The G6P-concentration needed for half maximum activation ($A_{0.5}$) of synthetase was much higher in the cell lines than in normal liver.

INTRACELLULAR GLUCOSE-6-PHOSPHATE CONTENT

Since glucose-6-phosphate seemed to play a predominant role for the regulation of synthetase and phosphorylase activity, we have measured the intracellular G6P-content of the cells and related it to the $A_{0.5}$ of synthetase and the K_i of phosphorylase in the different cell lines and to their glycogen content. As shown in Tables 4 and 5 the G6P-concentration in C_1I cells was much higher than in all other cell types investigated. The reason for that extremely high G6P-concentration is not known so far. It is about seven times higher than the K_i of phosphorylase a for G6P and four times higher than $A_{0.5}$ for synthetase. It may be concluded that in C_1I cells phosphorylase a can be inhibited and synthetases b and R can be activated by the intracellular G6P-concentration. In C_2I cells and MH 3924A the intracellular G6P-concentration corresponds to the respective K_i-values of the enzyme, thus phosphorylase may be partly inhibited. However, the G6P-concentrations are too low to activate synthetases b and R. Since no or only trace amounts of glycogen is present in MH 3924A and C_2I cells, it is obvious that glycogen accumulation is rather the consequence of activation of glycogen synthesis and only to a minor extent of phosphorylase inhibition. This is also supported by the fact that in normal liver a net glycogen synthesis is observed although phosphorylase is present in its active form. The intracellular G6P-concentration in normal liver is high enough to activate synthetase b.

CONCLUSIONS

The excessive accumulation of glycogen in C_1I cells may be due to the following mechanism:

1.) G6P is kept on a very high intracellular concentration, the reason for the G6P-accumulation is not known so far.

2.) The specific activity of the active form of glycogen phosphorylase is low. In addition, phosphorylase a activity can be inhibited by the high intracellular G6P-concentration.

3.) Synthetase R and b reveal high specific activity, both enzyme forms can be activated in the presence of the high intracellular G6P-concentration.

REFERENCES

1. H. G. Hers, The control of glycogen metabolism in the liver, Annu. Rev. Biochem. 45:167 (1976).
2. W. Stalmans, The role of liver in the homeostasis of blood glucose, Curr. Top. Cell. Regul. 11:51 (1976)

3. P. Cohen, Well established systems of enzyme regulation by reversible phosphorylation, in: "Molecular Aspects of Cellular Regulation", P. Cohen, ed., Elsevier North-Holland Biochemical Press, New York (1980).

4. A. Gutman, Regulation of glycogen metabolism, in: "Regulation of Carbohydrate Metabolism", R. Beitner, ed., CRC Press Inc., Boca Raton, Florida (1985).

5. P. Bannasch, H. J. Hacker, F. Klimek, and D. Mayer, Hepatocellular glycogenosis and related pattern of enzymatic changes during hepatocarcinogenesis, Adv. Enzyme Regul. 22:97 (1984).

6. J. Bienvenu, H. Carrier, F. Freycon, and M. Mathieu, Hétérogénéité de la glycogénose par déficit en alpha-1,4-glucosidase: Etude enzymatique dans trois familles, Clin. Chim. Acta 84:277 (1978).

7. B. Lederer, F. van Hoof, G. van den Berghe, and H. G. Hers, Glycogen phosphorylase and its converter enzymes in haemolysates of normal human subjects and of patients with type VI glycogen-storage disease, Biochem. J. 147:23 (1975).

8. S. W. Moses, N. Bashan, and A. E. Slonim, Effects of the abnormal carbohydrate metabolism present in glycogen storage disease on intermediary amino acid and lipid metabolism, in: "Regulation of Carbohydrate Metabolism", R. Beitner, ed., CRC Press Inc., Boca Raton, Florida (1985).

9. R. Malthus, D. G. Clark, C. Watts and J. G. T. Sneyd, Glycogen-storage disease in rats, a genetically determined deficiency of liver phosphorylase kinase, Biochem. J. 188:99 (1980).

10. P. Bannasch, D. Mayer, and H. J. Hacker, Hepatocellular glycogenosis and hepatocarcinogenesis, Biochim. Biophys. Acta 605:217 (1980).

11. M. A. Moore, D. Mayer, and P. Bannasch, The dose dependence and sequential appearance of putative preneoplastic populations induced in the rat liver by stop experiments with N-nitrosomorpholine, Carcinogenesis 3:1429 (1982).

12. D. Mayer, M. Moore, and P. Bannasch, Biochemical correlation of glycogen content and activity of some enzymes of carbohydrate metabolism in rat liver during early stages of carcinogenesis, J. Cancer Res. Clin. Oncol. 104:99 (1982).

13. F. Klimek, D. Mayer, and P. Bannasch, Biochemical microanalysis of glycogen content and glucose-6-phosphate dehydrogenase activity in focal lesions of the rat liver induced by N-nitrosomorpholine, Carcinogenesis 5:265 (1984)

14. H. J. Hacker, M. A. Moore, D. Mayer, and P. Bannasch, Correlative histochemistry of some enzymes of carbohydrate metabolism in preneoplastic and neoplastic lesions in the rat liver, Carcinogenesis 3:1265 (1982).

15. D. Mayer, and B. Schäfer, Biochemical and morphological characterization of glycogen-storing epithelial liver cell lines, Exp. Cell Res. 138:1 (1982).

16. H. P. Morris, and P. B. Wagner, Induction and transplantation of rat hepatomas with different growth rate (including "minimal deviation" hepatomas). Methods Cancer Res. 4:125 (1968).

17. C. Denis, D. Mayer, V. Trocheris, V. Viallard, H. Paris, and J. C. Murat, Study of carbohydrate metabolism in glycogen storing cell lines derived from cultured rat hepatocytes, Int. J. Biochem. 17:247 (1985).

18. C. Cortinovis, D. Mayer, B. Bouscarel, H. Paris, and J. C. Murat, Study of β-adrenoceptors and β-adrenergic responsiveness in cultured "preneoplastic-like" and neoplastic rat hepatocytes, Gen. Pharmacol. 16:259 (1985).

19. W. W. Franke, D. Mayer, E. Schmid, H. Denk, and E. Borenfreund, Differences of expression of cytoskeletal proteins in cultured rat hepatocytes and hepatoma cells, Exp. Cell Res. 134:345 (1981).

20. J. Larner, and C. Villar-Palasi, Glycogen synthetase and its control, Curr. Top. Cell. Regul. 3:195 (1971).

21. E. G. Krebs, Protein kinases. Curr. Top. Cell. Regul. 5:99 (1972).

22. A. W. H. Tan, Glycogen synthase R in livers of starved rats and starved rats given glucose, J. Biol. Chem. 257:5004 (1982).

23. W. Stalmans, M. Laloux, and H. G. Hers, The interaction of liver phosphorylase a with glucose and AMP, Europ. J. Biochem. 49:415 (1974).

24. L. Hue, F. Bontemps, and H. G. Hers, The effect of glucose and of potassium ions on the interconversion of the two forms of glycogen phosphorylase and of glycogen synthetase in isolated rat liver preparations, Biochem. J. 152:105 (1975).

25. M. Bollen, L. Hue, and W. Stalmans, Effects of glucose on phosphorylase and glycogen synthase in hepatocytes from diabetic rats, Biochem. J. 210:783 (1983).

26. K. Sato, K. Satoh, T. Sato, F. Imai, and H. P. Morris, Isoenzyme patterns of glycogen phosphorylase in rat tissues and transplantable hepatomas, Cancer Res. 36:487 (1976).

TECHNIQUES IN MEASURING DNA SYNTHESIS AND MITOSIS INDUCED BY TUMOR

PROMOTERS IN HEPATOCYTE PRIMARY CULTURES

Wolfram Parzefall and Franziska A. Pühringer

Institut für Tumorbiologie-Krebsforschung,
Borschkegasse 8a, A-1090 Vienna, Austria

SUMMARY

Repeated regenerative liver growth and adaptive liver growth stimuli (of hormonal or xenobiotic nature) applied in vivo have been closely connected with liver tumor promotion. Therefore, from a practical point in toxicology it is of interest to elucidate whether or not a given chemical is a liver growth stimulator. Identification of a test compound as liver growth stimulator justifies the suspicion that on long term administration tumor development may be a corollary event. Such a conclusion may be often confirmed by detection of the induction of drug metabolizing enzymes. Short term tests in vivo for the induction of liver growth and drug metabolizing enzymes have been described for different classes of compounds. Short term tests in vitro are currently under development. They would provide the possibility to check for hormonal and xenobiotic actions on liver cell replication not only in animal cells but more importantly on human material as well.
During the last 5 years it has become obvious that onset of DNA synthesis in primary hepatocyte cultures is inversely related to cell density. More importantly progression of these cells through G2 into mitosis seems to take place only in cultures of sufficiently low cell density in cultures. Nevertheless it appears that control of this step in the hepatocyte cell cycle is not yet fully understood. Two main techniques have been used to monitor DNA synthetic activity which are discussed: biochemical measurement of incorporated tritium-labelled nucleotide precursors into DNA by liquid scintillation counting and autoradiograpy. The first technique has been widely used because results are on hand rapidly. Their drawbacks, however, were noticed soon, as there were unspecifically incorporated label due to nucleotide metabolism, inadequate relation of data to cell protein or per culture dish instead on purified hot acid soluble DNA leading to unreliable results, and finally lacking information on the number of non-parenchymal cells incorporating label and on cells undergoing mitosis.
Autoradiographic techniques, although more laborious for the collection of data, had to be used in order to look for hepatocytes in mitotis. And this finally has helped to identify cell density as one of the regulators of hepatocyte replication in culture. Induction of hepatocyte DNA replication by hormones and tumor promoters under various conditions are discussed as examples and the use of both techniques will be demonstrated.

INTRODUCTION

A large number of nongenotoxic compounds may produce liver cancer in rodents after long-term treatment. Administration to animals previously treated with a subcarcinogenic dose of an initiating carcinogen in most cases leads to a drastic shortening of the latency period until to the eventual appearance of liver tumors. The compounds in question include drugs, hormones and environmental pollutants. As a common property most of them reversibly induce characteristic sets of enzymatic activities and liver growth. From a practical point in toxicology it is of interest to elucidate whether or not a given chemical is an inducer of such adaptive changes because they semm to be closely connected with liver tumor promotion (1,2).

The role played by these agents in human hepatocarcinogenesis is even more difficult to estimate. However, human hepatocytes from biopsies could be a valuable system for testing the potency of such compounds to induce liver DNA synthesis and mitosis in vitro. In a similar way, first rat liver cells (3) and then human hepatocytes have been used in the DNA repair test to check for DNA damaging properties of chemicals (4,5) short-term tests in vivo for the induction of liver growth and drug metabolizing enzymes have been described for different classes of compounds (6). Screening in vitro for cellular reactions connected to liver growth by validated methods would be mandatory. Such methods are currently under development (7,8). Studies on liver growth regulation in vitro, mainly conducted with rat hepatocytes, have been performed during the last 10 years (9-12). It has become obvious that regulation of DNA synthesis induction is highly dependent on the culture system used (8,10,11,13,14). Findings in culture should therefore be compared with what is known from in vivo in order to be relevant.

METHODS - RESULTS - DISCUSSION

Measurement of growth reactions in cultured hepatocytes from adult rat liver cannot rely on increases in cell numbers, because these cells rarely undergo cellular division and if so, cell attrition often obscures a growth response. Moreover, counting cell numbers from cultured hepatocytes is highly impeded because these cells hardly can be harvested as single cell suspensions. They rather come off the cultures as patchy sheets from the monolayer no matter whether they were havested by trypsin/EDTA or by collagenase or by sequential treatment with calcium-free, EGTA containing buffer and subsequent collagenase treatment.

However, semiconservative DNA synthesis can be observed in hepatocyte primary cultures. The techniques used are
1. incorporation of radioactive precursors and determination of label
    a)   by liquid scintillation counting,
    b)   or by autoradiography,
2. assays of DNA content by colorimetric or fluorimetric techniques or by flow-cytometry.
3. counting of mitoses.

Application of tritiated thymidine as a specific precursor of DNA is the method mostly used. With this tracer experimental designs have to take into account several points, which will influence the results. First, the specific activity of thymidine must be carefully selected. Specific activities of 10 to 60 Ci/mmole are in use. They are added to the cultures at activities of 0.1 to 10 µCi/ml. This results in thymidine concentrations in the nanomolar range unless no further cold thymidine is added for dilution. These concentrations stay well below the concentrations causing feedback inhibition of ribonucleotide reductase (>10 µM). This is the key enzyme for the production of deoxycitidine and pyrimidine nucleotides for DNA synthesis. Its inhibition will stop largely overall DNA synthesis.

Secondly, unspecific binding of thymidine to macromolecules as well as thymidine metabolism and reutilization of tritium label into other macromolecules have been uncoverd as causes for overestimations in DNA synthesis (15). Figure 1 illustrates this fact. Considerable portions of acid precipitable label are associated with the protein fractions (10, 50 and 30 % in the three examples) and a smaller proportion with RNA (3 to 10%). The hot acid soluble fraction contained between 40 and 66% of the lable. Therefore either of the following steps or combinations thereof may be applied. Avoiding long labelling periods rather short exposure of cells to tritium-labelled thymidine of high specific activity would be preferred. Extensive washing of the samples, facultativly isolation of nuclei, digestion of RNA and protein prior to measurement of radioactivity in the acid precipitable hot acid soluble fraction can be employed. Additional steps like purification of DNA on cesiumchloride-gradients may be taken.

Treatment of adult rat hepatocytes in culture with drugs of genotoxic activity might also induce DNA repair synthesis. Tomita et al. (10) have used a reasonable approach to eliminate the accouts of DNA repair synthesis and of unspecificly incorporated label. For every treatment group cultures with 10 mM hydroxyurea (HU) and without are provided. Total incorporation of label is determined in cultures without HU. Semiconservative DNA synthesis is largely inhibited in cultures including HU. In this case only unspecific labelling and DNA repair will be measured. By subtracting the latter from the total counts an estimate for replicative DNA synthesis is obtained.

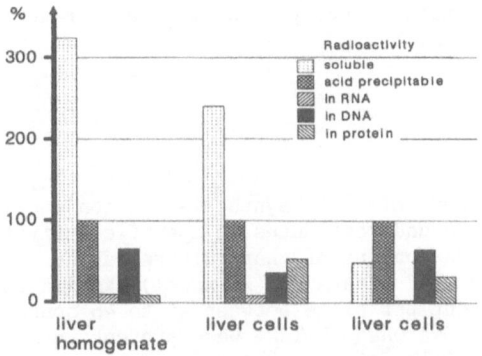

Fig. 1. Radioactivity from ^{3}H-thymidine (^{3}H-TdR) associatied with macromolecular fractions. Labelling times and specific activity used were as follows, left panel, 2 hours, 6.7 Ci/mmole; middle, 6 hours, 20 Ci/mmole; right, 24 hours, 47 Ci/mmole. Data were taken from references (16-18).

Finally it must be pointed out that reliability of results taken from radioactivity data is highly dependent on the basis to which counts are normalized. Every cytotoxic dose of a drug a culture is treated with will decrease the cell number in relation to controls. Therefore, the amount of radioactivity incorporated per culture as well as that per cellular protein must be used with caution. The only reliable basis seems to be the DNA content of a culture. Although, as shown by the example in figure 2 prolonged

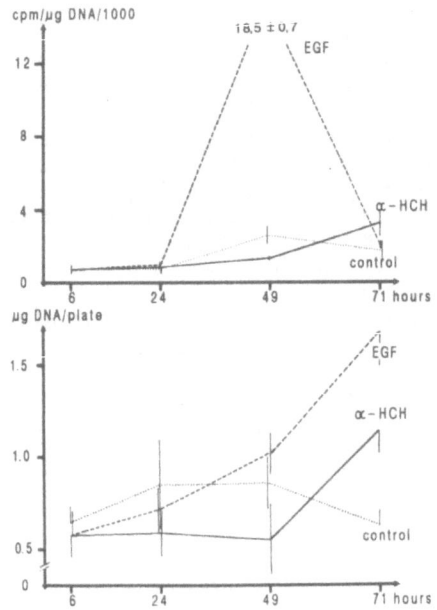

Fig. 2   Time course of stimulation of hepatocyte DNA synthesis by EGF (20 ng/ml) and α-HCH (10 μM). Treatment commenced at 2 hs after plating. Upper panel, specific activity following a 2 hour labelling period with 1 μCi/ml of ³H-TdR. Lower panel, DNA content of the cultures. Every point is the average of 5 to 6 replicate cultures. Bars, S.D.

exposure to an inducer of DNA synthesis in conjunction with short-term labelling will lead to underestimates in specific activity. This may be due to increases in DNA content of that culture during the course of mitogen treatment (figure 2). EGF treatment (20 ng/ml) has led to an almost twofold increase of DNA content per plate between 24 to 48 hours. The increase in specific activity of DNA when ³H-TdR was present for a 2 hour period only is approximately 20-fold. After continued exposure for further 24 hours to the growth factor the DNA content of the cultures increased by 50%.

Therefore, DNA synthesis, as estimated by the measurement of the specific activity of the DNA is presumably by a factor of 3 lower than it should be in comparison with controls. DNA content in control cultures did not change. In this particular case the drastic reduction in specific activity in the EGF-treated cultures cannot be explained alone by increases in DNA multiplication. Rather down regulation of EGF receptors or traverse of cells from S into another GO or Gl (19). In such cases of short-term labelling cell protein may be an alternative basis to relate counting data to.

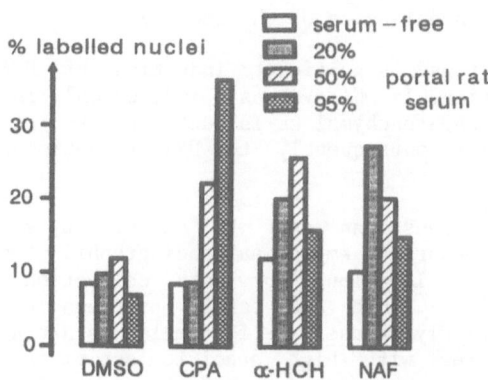

Fig. 3   Hepatocytes from young adult rats seeded on collagen gels in primary culture for 0.5 hours in serum-free medium. At that time they were turned to the different serum concentrations. Treatment with drugs lasted from 17 hs to 65 hours. CPA, α-HCH and NAF were added at a final concentration of 10 μM. ^{3}H-TdR was present during the same interval. (CPA = cyproterone acetate, NAF = nafenopin)

An example for the induction of DNA synthesis by a known liver growth stimulator and liver tumor promoter namely alpha-hexachlorocyclohexane (α-HCH, 10 μm) is given in the same graph (fig. 2). After a rather long-lasting lag period (60 to 70 hours) of treatment a significant increase in DNA content per plate and in the specific activity was observed. It is of importance to note that the hepatocytes were cultured under serum-free conditions. DNA contents shown in figure 2 were measured by use of the fluorescence dye HOECHST 33258. The method of Labarca and Paigen (20) was optimized for cultured hepatocytes to give homogenous and linear fluorescence. The advantage of the method is that it can be used with small numbers of cells (50 000 cells / ml) and that it is rapid.

A response to α-HCH has been seen previously only in the presence of rat serum containing media (figure 3) (21).

Among the assays that use radioactive label a particularly rapid procedure has been proposed by Althaus (22) for detection of DNA repair. This procedure circumvents all needs for purification of DNA. In a kind of double labelling assay cultures treated with the test compound are exposed to ^{3}H-TdR and parallel cultures remaining untreated are exposed to ^{14}C-TdR. Both types of cultures should contain identical numbers of cells. After termination of incubation cells of both cultures are homogenized, mixed and counts of ^{3}H over ^{14}C measured. As a control two additional cultures must be set up. Both will remain untreated but again the first will be labelled with ^{3}H-TdR and the other with ^{14}C-TdR. The resulting ratio of counts from ^{3}H over ^{14}C in this homogenate is taken to compare the ratio of treated cultures to. It is obvious that treatments which will alter cell numbers in the cultures (e.g. cytotoxic events) will in an uncontrolled manner lead to incorrect findings. In addition the high amount of radioactivity needed and the fact that for every treated culture an untreated counterpart must be set up are some inconveniencies of this method.

After one has found significant induction of DNA synthesis several other questions arise. Is DNA synthesis induced only in parenchymal cells? To what extent do nonparenchymal cells contribute to the increase in label per DNA? Do the cells subsequently to DNA synthesis enter mitosis and to what extent?

All these questions can only be answered by morphologic criteria. Therefore it is necessary to employ autoradiographic techniques. Although this method is more laborious for data collection the advantages are obvious. Technically, there are rarely problems encountered with high background if relatively insensitive fotoemulsions are used. After treatment of the cultures with high specific activities of the precursor thymidine exposure times as short as 24 hours may be sufficient. By this means interference due to the detection of labeled repair patches or even mitochandrial DNA synthesis are avoided, which only can be detected with sensitive emulsions and long exposure times.

Distinction of parenchymal from non parenchymal cells in hepatocyte cultures is easily accomplished in hematoxylin stained specimens. The cytoplasm of nonparenchymal cells stains only very weakly whereas parenchymal cells absorb the dye readily. An additional indication for nonparenchymal cells after prolonged stimulation in culture is that they form colonies with many labelled nuclei. By these criteria the portion of nonparenchymal cells can be excluded from labelling indices.

Some further valuable information may be won by observation of the culture morphology in autoradiographs. By this means it has been found that in cultures with lower cell density labelling indices were higher (8,11,14, 23). Systematic examination has brought about a negative correlation between cell density and DNA synthetic activity in hepatocyte cultures (8,14). As a consequence one has to consider that every treatment affecting the cell number of cultures will possibly influence the number of cells entering S phase. Besides the fact that lowering of cell density by itself enhances the rate of entry of hepatocytes into the S phase it has been found that treatment with growth factors and hormones is a further stimulus for DNA synthesis (9-11). In most instances EGF plus insulin is the mixture of choice for induction of DNA synthesis. At sufficiently low cell densities hepatocytes continue their cell cycle progression through mitosis as has been shown by Michalopoulos (14).

We have induced DNA synthesis and mitosis by EGF and cyproterone acetate. The results are shown in figure 4.

In contrast to cultures of other cell types mitoses in hepatocyte cultures do not round up or tend to detach. They remain attached to the substratum and are well spread. Autoradiographic technique can also be combined with different stains for phenotypic markers. Thereby the state of differentiation of replicating and non replicating cells has been monitored (14,24).

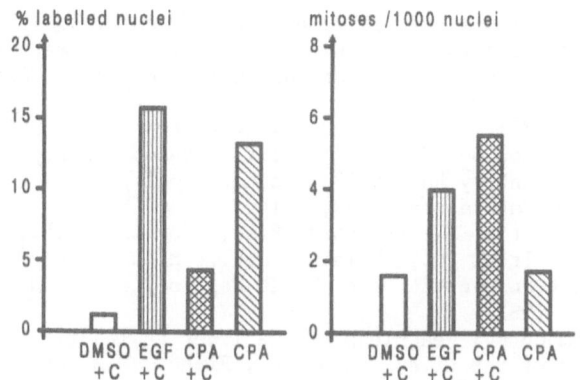

Fig. 4 Hepatocytes after seeding on collagen gel were treated with EGF (20 ng/ml) from 20 to 44 hs, or with 10 μM CPA or the solvent DMSO (0.2%). Prior to harvesting cells received 0.5 μCi/ml ^{3}H-TdR and during the last 14 hs of culture colcemide (+C, 0.25 μg/ml) or not. All cultures were extensively washed and then fixed for autoradiography at 68 hs.

Finally in autoradiographies topologic and general morphologic features can be recorded simultaneously. It has been found for example that labelling at the edges of patches of the monolayer was more intense (11), that cell density of one part of a culture seems to influence labelling in another part of the same culture (23). On collagen gels we have observed a more localized influence of cell density on hepatocyte labelling (8). Furthermore we have repeatedly found that in most cultures irrespective of the substrate used the cells at the periphery of the dish were generally heavier labelled than cells in the center of the culture. The reason for this behaviour is not clear yet.

In conclusion, autoradiography appears to be the method which provides the most complete information on hepatocyte replication in culture. Liquid scintillation counting of incorporated label, however, will be the method of choice for screening for growth inducing activities, and for the establishment of dose response curves. For particular questions and for confirmation of results both methods will have to be used simultaneously.

REFERENCES

1. Schulte-Hermann R.: Tumor promotion in the liver. Arch. Toxicology, 57: 147-158, 1985.
2. Schulte-Hermann R., Parzefall W. and Wilfried Bursch Role of stimulation of liver growth by chemicals in hepatocarcinogenesis. Banbury Report 25: Nongenotoxic Mechanisms in Carcinogenesis, Cold Spring Harbor Laboratory, 1987, B.E. Butterworth, T.J. Slaga eds.
3. Williams G.M.: Carcinogen induced DNA repair in primary rat liver cell cultures; a possible screen for chemical carcinogens. Cancer Letters 1, 231-236, 1976.
4. Butterworth B.E., Doolittle D.J., Working P.K., Strom S.C., Jirtle R.L., Michalopoulos G.: Chemically induced DNA repair in rodent and human cells, Banbury Report 13: Indicators of genotoxic exposure: Cold Spring Harbor Laboratory, 1982, 1-14.
5. Strom S.C., Jirtle R.L., Jones R.S., Novicki D.L., Rosenberg M.R., Novotny A., Irons G., Mclainn J.R., Michalopoulos G.: Isolation, culture and transplantation of human hepatocytes. J. Natl. Cancer Inst. 68, 771-777, 1982.
6. Schulte-Hermann R.: Reactions of the liver to Injury: Adaptation. In: Toxic Injury of the Liver. Farber E., Fisher, M.M. eds., Marcel Dekker, New York, 1979, 385-444.
7. Edwards A.M., Lucas C.M.: Phenobarbital and some other liver tumor promoters stimulate DNA synthesis in cultured rat hepatocytes. Biochem. Biophys. Res. Commun. 131, 103-108, 1985
8. Parzefall W., Galle P.R., Schulte-Hermann R.: Effect of calf and rat serum on the induction of DNA synthesis and mitosis in primary cultures of adult rat hepatocytes by cyproterone acetate and epidermal growth factor. In Vitro Cellular & Developmental Biology 21: 665-673, 1985.
9. Richman R.A., Claus T.H., Pilkis S.J., Friedman, D.L.: Hormonal stimulation of DNA synthesis in primary cultures of adult rat hepatocytes. Proc. Natl. Acad. Sci. USA 73: 3589-3593; 1976.
10. Tomita Y., Nakamura T., Ichihara, A.: Control of DNA synthesis and ornithine decarboxylase activity by hormones and amino acids in primary cultures of adult rat hepatocytes. Exp. Cell Res. 135, 363-371, 1981.
11. McGowan J.A., Strain A.J., Bucher N.L.R.: DNA synthesis in primary cultures of adult rat hepatocytes in a defined medium: effects of epidermal growth factor, insulin, glucagon, and cyclic-AMP. J. Cell. Physiol. 108: 353-363; 1981.
12. Hasegawa K., Namai K., Koga, M.: Induction of DNA-synthesis in adult rat hepatocytes cultured in a serum-free medium. Biochem. Biophys. Res. Commun. 95: 243-249; 1980.
13. Andreis P.A., Armato U.: Effects of Epidermal Growth Factor/ Urogastrone and associated pancreatic hormones on mitotic cycle phases and proliferation kinetics of neonatal rat hepatocytes in primary culture. Endocrinology, 108, 1954-1964,1981.
14. Michalopoulos G., Cianciulli H.D., Novotny A.R., Kligerman A.D., Strom S.C., Jirtle R.L.: Liver regeneration studies with hepatocytes in primary culture. Cancer Res. 42: 4673-4682; 1982.
15. Morley C.G.D., Kingdon H.S., Use of H-Thymidine for measurement of DNA synthesis in rat liver - a warning. Analytical Biochem. 45, 298-305, 1972.

16. Goldspink D.F. Goldberg A.L., Problems in the use of Me- H thymidine for the measurement of DNA synthesis. Biochim. Biophys. Acta, 299, 521–532, 1973.
17. Yager J.D., Miller J.A.: DNA repair in primary cultures of rat hepatocytes.
18. Galle P.R.: Thesis, Marburg 1987.
19. Tomomura A., Sawada N., Sattler, G.L. Kleinman, H.K., Pitot H.C.: the control of DNA synthesis in primary cultures from adult and young rats: Interactions of extracellular matrix components, epidermal growth factor, and the cell cycle. J. Cell. Physiol. 130, 221–227, 1987.
20. Labarca C., Paigen K.: A simple, rapid, and sensitive DNA assay procedure. Analytical Biochem. 102, 344–352, 1980.
21. Parzefall W., Galle P.R., Schulte-Hermann R.:Induction of DNA synthesis in hepatocyte primary cultures. Europ. J. Cell Biol. 33, Suppl 5, 27, 1984.
22. Althaus F.R., Lawrence S.D., Sattler G.L., Longfellow D.G., Pitot H.C.: Chemical quantification of unscheduled DNA synthesis in cultured hepatocytes as an assay for the rapid screening of potential chemical carcinogens. Cancer Res. 42, 3010–1015, 1982.
23. Nakamura T., Tomita Y., Ichihara, A.: Density-dependent growth control of adult rat hepatocytes in primary culture.
J. Biochem. 94, 1029–1035, 1983.
24. Sirica A.E., Richards W., Tsukada Y., Sattler C.A., Pitot H.C.: Fetal phenotypic expression by adult rat hepatocytes on collagen gel/nylon meshes.
Proc. Natl. Acad. Sci. USA 76, 283–287, 1979.

CONCLUSIONS

WHAT HAVE WE LEARNED IN THE LAST THREE YEARS ABOUT HEPATOCARCINOGENESIS AND WHERE SHOULD WE BE GOING?

Rolf Schulte-Hermann

Institut für Tumorbiologie-Krebsforschung
der Universität Wien
A-1090 Wien, Borschkegasse 8a

We are at the end of a meeting that many of us consider as of very high quality. I will briefly summarize some of the crucial issues considered and some trends emerging during the meeting.

If we are critical, we must admit that, <u>with certainty</u>, we still know very little about hepatocarcinogenesis. We feel certain that some chemical compounds are, or were, involved in the genesis of human liver cancer under specific conditions, e.g. vinylchloride, thorotrast, ethanol, probably aflatoxin B_1, and also viruses. To detect further risk factors as yet unknown, and for design of a more rational therapy we need to understand which properties of these agents and which responses of the biological system are crucial for the development of cancer.

In the laboratory most of us have been working with one or the other model agent, such as nitrosamines, aflatoxines, thioacetamide, methapyrilene, peroxisome stimulators, phenobarbital, certain estrogens or hepatitis B virus. All these agents have in common the ability to induce liver cancer under appropriate experimental conditions even though they are widely different in terms of their (other) biological activities. We therefore believe that the agents interfere with different steps of the process of carcinogenesis, and use them in our attempts to elucidate the biological nature of these steps. However, as expressed during this meeting almost all of us experienced inconsistencies in our models. We have to accept that biology (of cancer) is not as simple as our models, and although models are indispensable for the design of rational experiments, we must keep alert about the discrepancies between models and reality.

Probably all of us accept that cancer formation in the liver and elsewhere is a multi-step phenomenon. The discovery of altered cell foci which are putative intermediates between normal and malignant cells strongly supports this concept, and the enormous expansion, in the past few years, of papers on this subject indicates how many scientists have detected the

potential merits of the "foci" as a tool in cancer research.
Nevertheless, the existence of prestages appears not proven in
all models. Thus, we learned that for certain virally induced
cancers prestages so far could not be identified.

For most of our experimental models of carcinogenesis we
feel fairly sure about the existence of a first step or
initiation; however, with respect to the biological and molecular nature of initiation crucial questions remain unsettled:
    (1) In biological terms the classical two-stage-model of
carcinogenesis predicts that an initiated cell will not develop
into a growing tumor unless promotion is effected by additional
(exogenous or endogenous) factors. Alternatively, some of us
consider initiation as an early event that triggers a process
autonomously leading to cancer.
    (2) Is DNA always and necessarily the crucial target for
the initiating action of chemical carcinogens? How do the so
called non-genotoxic agents lead to cancer and vice versa: is
every agent with genotoxic activity a potential carcinogen?
    (3) Which parts of DNA are the target crucial for initi-
ation? Specifically: are known (proto)oncogens the target? We
heard that several of the oncogens now known can be overexpressed in liver tumors. However, none of these oncogens seems
to be overexpressed consistently in all tumors. Thus, are there
multiple pathways to cancer also in terms of oncogens involved?
Furthermore: most oncogens studied so far appear to be related
to growth control. Tumor formation in the liver and elsewhere,
however, is probably not simply a defect in growth control but
involves additional changes in cell function. Thus the next per-
tinent question is: are we looking at the "right" (onco)gens, or
are the crucial genes involved in initiation and later steps of
carcinogenesis still to be discovered? In any event, successful
transfection of hepatocytes in vitro by oncogenes as reported
during the meeting should open a new approach to study the role
of specific genes in hepatic carcinogenesis.
    (4) What role do cell proliferation and cell death play in
formation and maintenance of initiated cells? Results presented
suggest that at least not all means to induce cell proliferation
are equally effective in supporting initiation by genotoxic
agents; alternatively, specific mechanisms may exist to eliminate initiated cells. In favour of this latter possibility it
was reported that cell death by apoptosis preferentially occurs
in putative preneoplastic foci.

Cancer is a "disease of differentiation" and not merely a
disease of genes. Therefore, results presented on the biochemical programs expressed in (pre)neoplastic lesions were very
useful. Hopefully, the many different pieces of information soon
can be put together into the mosaic that makes up the
"biochemical phenotype" of these lesions.

Differentiation control during carcinogenesis is intimately
related to tumor promotion. As promotion is currently defined it
describes a process through which initiated cells have a selective growth advantage resulting in the formation of a focus or,
possibly, a benign tumor. Historically a promoter is defined as
a compound incapable of initiation. However, it is not clear -
and impossible to prove - whether "pure promoters" really exist.
I suggest that we abandon to use the term "promoter" as meaning
"pure promoter". Rather we should understand a promoter

310

as a factor capable of tumor promotion and which, under specified conditions, may exert its main effect on carcinogenesis
through promotion.

On the molecular level even less is known about tumor promotion than about initiation. The key will probably be the elucidation of the interaction of promoting compounds with regulatory networks that control cell growth and function, and
intriguing new findings on growth factors and growth inhibitors
and on receptors on the cell membrane or inside the cell have
been presented during this meeting. Furthermore, do promoters
switch on expression of oncogens? Is the normal function of such
"oncogens" to control expression of specific phenotypes in the
liver cell? Studies on the effects of promoters on the phenotype
of (pre)neoplastic lesions will be helpful to answer such
questions, and vice versa will help the toxicologist to assess
health risks of non-genotoxic compounds such as peroxisome
proliferators which so far resisted any broadly acceptable
classification.

What will we learn until the next meeting on experimental
hepatocarcinogenesis will open in hopefully three years' time
from now? We will probably not answer definitely all those
crucial questions. However, if we combine the powerful modern
techniques provided by molecular biology with the more tradi-
tional ones provided by cell biology, pathology, toxicology,
biochemistry etc. we will get new insights, improve our models
and eventually ameliorate preventive and therapeutic strategies.

I should like to conclude by expressing the gratitude of
all of us to Drs. Marcel Roberfroid, Veronique Preat, and their
colleagues from Brussels for having organized this excellent and
highly stimulating meeting.

CONTRIBUTORS

Alexandre M., Free University of Brussels, Brussels,
    Belgium
Andersson G., Huddinge Hospital, Huddinge, Sweden
Andersson N., Huddinge Hospital, Huddinge, Sweden
Atermann K., University of Brunswick, Fredericton, Canada
Baffet G., INSERM U 49, Rennes, France
Bannasch P., German Cancer Research Center, Heidelberg, FR
    Germany
Barbason H., University of Liège, Liège, Belgium
Becker K., Institute for Veterinär physiology, Giessen, FR
    Germany
Betetta B., University of Cagliari, Cagliari, Italy
Bouzahzah B., University of Liège, Liège, Belgium
Brumioul D., University of Liège, Liège, Belgium
Bursch W., Institute for Tumor Biology and Cancer
    Research, Vienna, Austria
Carr B., City Hope National Medical Center, Duarte, USA
Castelain Ph., Free University of Brussels, Brussels,
    Belgium
Columbano A., University of Cagliari, Cagliari, Canada
Coni P., University of Cagliari, Cagliari, Canada
Corcos D., Institute of molecular Pathology, Paris, France
Corral M., Institute of molecular Pathology, Paris, France
Daino L., University of Sassari, Sassari, Italy
Defer N., Institute of molecular Pathology, Paris, France
Deleener A., Free University of Brussels, Brussels,
    Belgium
Delzenne N., Catholic University of Louvain, Brussels,
    Belgium
Dessi S., University of Cagliari, Cagliari, Italy
Eigenbrodt E., Institute for Biochemistry and
    Endocrinology, Giessen, FR Germany
Enzmann H., German Cancer Research Center, Heidelberg, FR
    Germany
Eriksson L., Huddinge Hospital, Huddinge, Sweden
Etienne P.L., INSERM U 49, Rennes, France
Feo F., University of Sassari, Sassari, Italy
Garcea R., University of Sassari, Sassari, Italy
Gerbracht H., Institute for Biochemistry and
    Endocrinology, Giessen, FR Germany
Glaise D., INSERM U 49, Rennes, France
Guguen Guillouzo Ch., INSERM U 49, Rennes, France
Hacker H.J., German Cancer Research Center, Heidelberg, FR
    Germany
Haesen S., Free University of Brussels, Brussels, Belgium
Herens Ch., University of Liège, Liège, Belgium

Itakura K., City Hope National Medical Center, Duarte, USA
Jungermann K., Georg-August University, Göttingen, FR
    Germany
Kirsch-Volders M., Free University of Brussels, Brussels,
    Belgium
Klietzen R., German Cancer Research Center, Heidelberg, FR
    Germany
Klimek F., German Cancer Research Center, Heidelberg, FR
    Germany
Kruh J., Institute of molecular Pathology, Paris, France
Lapis K., Semmelweis Medical University, Budapest, Hungary
Ledda-Columbano G.M., University of Cagliari, Cagliari,
    Canada
Massart S., University of Liège, Liège, Belgium
Mayer D., German Cancer Research Center, Heidelberg, FR
    Germany
Mihailovich N., University of Chicago, USA
Möller Ch., Huddinge Hospital, Huddinge, Sweden
Negri S., University of Chicago, USA
Neumann H.G., University of Würzburg, Würzburg, F.R.
    Germany
Norstedt G., Huddinge Hospital, Huddinge, Sweden
Oesh F., University of Mainz, Mainz, FR Germany
Pani P., University of Cagliari, Cagliari, Canada
Pani P., University of Cagliari, Cagliari, Italy
Parzefall W., Institute for Tumor Biology and cancer
    Research, Vienna, Austria
Pascale R., University of Sassari, Sassari, Italy
Paul D., Fraunhofer Institute of Toxicology, Hannover, FR
    Germany
Peschke P., German Cancer Research Center, Heidelberg, FR
    Germany
Préat V., Catholic University of Louvain, Brussels,
    Belgium
Puhringer F., Institute for Tumor Biology and cancer
    Research, Vienna, Austria
Rabes H., University of Munich, Munich, FR Germany
Reinacher M., Institute for Veterinär Pathology, Giessen,
    FR Germany
Rissler P., Huddinge Hospital, Huddinge, Sweden
Robaye B., University of Liège, Liège, Belgium
Roberfroid M., Catholic University of Louvain, Brussels,
    Belgium
Roth E., Surgical University Hopital, Vienna, Austria
Ruan Y., German Cancer Research Center, Heidelberg, FR
    Germany
Saeter G., Institute for Cancer Research, Oslo, Norway
Sarma D.S.R., University of Toronto, Toronto, Canada
Schaff Z., Semmelweis Medical University, Budapest,
    Hungary
Schulte-Hermann R., Institute for Tumor Biology and Cancer
    Research, Vienna, Austria
Schwarze P., Institute for Cancer Research, Oslo, Norway
Seelman-Eggebert G., German Cancer Research Center,
    Heidelberg, FR Germany
Seglen P., Institute for Cancer Research, Oslo, Norway
Seibert B., University of Mainz, Mainz, FR Germany
Steinberg P., University of Mainz, Mainz, FR Germany
Vesselinovitch S., University of Chicago, USA
Weber E., German Cancer Research Center, Heidelberg, FR
    Germany

Whitson R., City Hope National Medical Center, Duarte, USA
Zerban H., German Cancer Research Center, Heidelberg, FR
    Germany

INDEX

14 C Acetate, 189–190
2–Acetylaminofluorene, 6–11, 32–
    34, 42–45, 177–183,196–
    204, 222–229, 232
  As promoter, 222–229
2–Acetylaminophenanthrene, 6–11
Acid mucopolysaccharides, 98
Acyl–CoA : cholesterol
    aycltransferase, 187, 188
Adaptive program, 143
Adenoid structures, 96
Adenomas, 51–60
Adenosine–5'–triphosphatase, 66,
    80–81
Adenylate cyclase, 95
Adrenaline, 81–88
Alfa–hexachlorocyclohexane, 143,
    151–156, 300–301
Alpha–fetoprotein, 65–67
Alpha–naphthylisothiocyanate, 16–
    24
Amino acids, 163, 166, 171, 172
Androgen, 58–59
Angiomas, 97
Angiosarcomas, 97
Anthracene, 16–23
Antipromotion, 204
Apoptosis, 134, 139, 143–156, 199
  In normal liver, 143–151
  Preneoplastic lesions, 151–156
Apoptotic bodies, 145–156, 201
Aromatic amines, 6–11
Aromatic hydrocarbon, 10
Asialo–glycoprotein receptor, 175–
    183
Asialo–glycoprotein, 177–179
Autoradiography, 297–298, 302–304

6–Bisphosphatase, 80
Benzphetamine N–demethylase, 259–
    263
Bile ductular epithelia, 90
Bile formation, 80–81
Binding sites, 175–179
Binucleated hepatocytes, 222–226,
    232, 235, 238–242

Butylated hydroxytoluene, 43, 47

C–abl, 245–251
C–erb–A, 247
C–erb–B, 247
C–fos, 246–251
C–Ha–ras, 126, 232, 238–242, 246–
    251
C–Ki–ras, 246–251
C–mos, 245–251
C–myc, 26, 126–127, 245–251
C–sis, 245–251
C–src, 245–251
Carbohydrate metabolism, 80, 83–
    84, 86, 94–95, 109, 283–
    294
Carbohydrate metabolites, 163,
    165–166, 170
Carbohydrate metabolizing enzymes,
    163–171
  In hepatocellular carcinomas,
  In normal liver, 166–170
    166–170
Carbon tetrachloride, 84, 133–138
Carcinogen–altered liver, 275,
    279–280
Carcinogenesis, 29–37
  Multistep process 29, 30
  Two stage theory, 29–37
Carcinomas, 51, 56
Cell cycle, 121–127
Cell death, 143–156, 310
Cell diameter, 259–266
Cell kinetics, 125–126
Cell loss, 199
Cell proliferation, 93, 121–127,
    133–139, 185–192, 250–251,
    310
  Cholesterol metabolism 185–192
  Hepatocarcinogenesis, 121–127
  Initiation, 133
  Oncogenes, 250–251
Cell–cell interaction, 249–251
Centrifugal elutriation, 257–264
Centrilobular, 257, 262
Cholangiocarcinomas, 96–97

Cholangiofibrosis, 96
Cholesterol, 16-23, 44, 185-192
   DNA synthesis, 185-192
   Esterification, 185-187, 188
   Metabolism, 185-192
   Synthesis, 185, 189-191
Choline methionine deficient diet,
     44
Chromosomal aberrations, 211, 218,
     235, 240
Chromosome karyotype, 232, 238
Cirrhosis, 65-66, 89-90
Clofibrate, 43, 163-169
Clonal growth, 124-127
Clonal origin, 94
Collagenase perfusion, 223, 226,
     232, 236-237, 258-275
Compensatory cell growth, 133,186
Complete hepatocarcinogens, 6-8
Concentration gradients, 80-81
Connective tissue, 15, 19, 22
Compensatory cell proliferation,
     133-139, 186
   Versus Hyperplasia, 133-139
Culture of liver cells, 268-271,
     276-281, 294-299, 297-300
Cyproterone acetate, 134-138, 143-
     151, 301-303
Cystic cholangiomas, 96
Cytochrome P-450, 80, 257-264
Cytodensitometry, 233
Cytogenetic, 231-242
Cytogenetic Alterations, 231-242
   During hepatocarcinogenesis,
     231-242
Cytoskeleton, 90-91
Cytotoxic, 8

4-Dimethylaminoazobenzene, 15-23
DDT, 6-7, 43-47
Deoxycholic acid, 44
Diazepam, 43
Dietary factors, 42, 44, 48
Diethylhexylphtalate, 43
Diethylnitrosamine, 42-45, 51-60,
     135-136, 196-204, 214-217,
     222-228, 232, 245
Differentiation, 89-98, 250
   During Neoplasic development,
     89-98
   Oncogenes, 250
Dihydroepiandrosterone, 94
Dimethylnitrosamine, 212-214
Diploid, 125, 221-229, 233-242
Dissociation constants, 179-180
DNA adducts, 6
DNA breaks, 211-214
DNA content, 144-145, 232, 300-301
DNA damage, 6-8
  Hepatocarcinogenesis, 6
DNA repair, 299, 302

DNA synthesis, 185-189, 199, 201,
     275-276, 297-304
Dose, 31, 33, 36, 42, 47, 51
Dose-response relationship, 57
Dose-response, 92
Ductular cells, 96

Endogenous compounds, 42, 44, 48
Enolase, 163-165, 169
Enzymehistochemistry, 108-114
Epidermal growth factor receptor,
     175
Epidermal growth factor, 177, 179,
     275-278
Epithelial liver cells, 284-286
Epoxide hydrolase, 80
Estradiolphenylpropionate, 44
Estrogen, 59
Ethinylestradiol, 44
Ethoxyresorufin O-deethylase,
     259-263
Ethylene dibromide, 134-138

Fasted rats, 186-191
Fetal liver, 180, 249
Fibroblastic cell, 19, 20
Fibrosarcomas, 15, 19
Flow-cytometry, 221-222, 226
Focal proliferations, 30, 47
Foci, 33-38, 46, 92-96, 106, 309
   Adicophilic, 92-96
   Amphophilic, 94
   Basophilic, 92-96
   Clear, 92-96
   Intermediate, 92-96
   Localization, 92-96
   Mixed cell, 92-96
   Tigroid, 92-96
Fructose 1,6-bisphosphatase, 163-
     165, 167
Fructose 1,6-bisphosphate, 163,
     171

Gamma-glutamyl transferase, 66,
     115, 134-138, 163, 165-
     169, 196, 223
Gene expression, 275-281
Genetic alterations, 231-242
   During hepatocarcinogenesis,
     231-242
Genotoxic, 5-11
GGT-positive foci, 7, 154, 155,
     197-201
Glucagon, 81-86
Glucokinase, 109, 163, 287-289
Gluconeogenesis, 80-81, 83, 86,
     109
Glucose release, 81, 83, 85
Glucose uptake, 81, 83, 85
Glucose-6-phosphatase, 80, 96,
     108-109, 113, 163, 170,
     285-287, 289

Glucose-6-phosphate dehydrogenase, 80–81, 95–96, 109–111, 115, 163–165, 168, 186, 190–192, 287–292
Glucose-6-phosphate, 292, 294
Glucostat, 79–83
Glutathione peroxidase, 80–81, 84
Glutathione S-transferase, 80, 136
Glutathione, 84
Glyceralde hyde-3-phosphate dehydrogenase, 95
Glyceraldehyde-3-phosphate, 109
Glycine, 163, 171
Glycogen phosphorylase, 95, 108–113, 287–292
Glycogen storage foci, 283
Glycogen synthetase, 290–294
Glycogen, 81, 83–84, 86, 93–96, 106–108, 283–298
  Demonstration, 106–108
  Metabolism, 108
  Storage, 93–96
Glycogen-storing liver cell line, 283–294
Glycogenosis, 94–95
Glycolysis, 81, 82, 86, 109
Gonadectomies, 52–60
Growth control 267–271, 275–281
Growth factors, 270–271
Growth fraction, 214–216
Growth inhibitors, 275–281
Growth regulation, 275–281, 298

HBV antigens, 64–67
Hepadna virus, 63, 67–68
Hepatitis B virus, 63
Hepatitis B, 89–90
Hepatocarcinogens, 15–24
  Implantation, 15–24
Hepatocarcinogens, 5–13
Hepatocarcinoma, 89, 222–224
Hepatocellular carcinomas, 15, 19, 21, 22, 32, 92–96, 163–172, 197–205
Hexokinase, 287
Hexose monophosphate, 185–190
High fat diet, 33–34, 44–45
Histochemistry 105–116
Hormones, 79–86
Human hepatocarcinomas, 247–248, 269
Human hepatocellular carcinoma, 63–67, 69–71
  Etiologic factors, 63–70
Hydroxy-methyl-glutaryl coenzyme A reductase, 185–186, 190
Hyperplasia, 133–139, 143–149, 156

Immortalization by viral trans- forming genes, 267–271

Initiation, 121–122
Immunohistochemistry, 108–115
In vitro hepatocyte growth, 202
In vitro models, 247–250, 284–288
In vivo/in vitro systems, 267
Incidence of cancer, 41–48
Inhibition of promotion, 195
Initiation, 5–11, 29–30, 44–48, 133
Insulin 81–86
Insulin-like growth factors, 175–177, 180, 182
Intermediate filaments, 90–91
Iron, 177–179
Isoprenoid units, 185–187

Labeling index, 125, 199–203, 216–217
Lactate dehydrogenase, 163, 165–167
Latency period, 36–37, 41
Lead nitrate, 133–139, 186, 188–191
Lecithin : cholesterol acyltransferase, 187, 188
Ligand, 175–183
Lipoprotein, 185–188
Lipotropes, 195–205
  Content, 195–199
Liver growth, 143–144
Liver regeneration, 249

2-Methyl-4-dimethylaminoazobenzene 8
3-Methylcholanthrene, 15–23, 257–264
5'-Methylthioadenosine, 195–205
Malic enzyme, 162–165, 168
Markers, 66, 94, 115
Mestranol, 44
Metabolic zonation, 79–86, 92, 105
Metabolism of xenobiotics, 83
Metaphase chromosomes, 232–242
Micronuclei, 211–217
  Effect of diethylnitrosamine, 211–217
  Index, 214–216
  Precancerous rat liver, 211–217
Mitogens, 133–139, 186
Mitosis, 297–304
Mitotic activity, 212
Models, 196, 215, 309
Modulating Factors of Hepatocarcinogenesis, 41–48, 51, 60
  Nature, 42–46
Modulation, 35–37, 41–42, 56
Mononucleated hepatocytes, 221, 232, 235
Multi-stage process, 5

Mutations, 231

N-Hydroxy derivatives, 7
N-methyl-N-nitrosourea, 122–123,
    136, 138
N-myc, 246–251
N-nitrosomorpholine, 42, 94–97,
    105–106, 163–173
N-ras, 247
NADPH, 188–198
Nafenopin, 33–34, 43, 47, 135–136,
    138, 152–156, 301
Necrosis, 15, 133
Negative modulation, 37, 41–42
Neonatal liver, 180
Neoplastic Liver, 89–96, 175–183,
    275–281
Nitrogen detoxification, 80–81
Nitrosamines, 211
Nodules, 22–23, 32–34, 46–48, 51–
    56, 91–95, 177–189, 197–
    205, 222, 224, 246–247
Non genotoxic xenobiotics, 42–48
Non-A, Non-B hepatitis, 69–70
Non-parenchymal cells, 79
Noradrenaline, 81
Nuclear alterations, 221–229
    During hepatocarcinogenesis,
        221–229

O6-alkylguanine, 211
Octaploid, 234–242
Oncofetal, 66–67
Oncogenes, 126, 231, 238–240, 245–
    251, 310
    Activation, 245–251
    Expression, 245–251
    Role in hepatocarcinogenesis,
        245–251
Orchidectomy, 53–60
Ornithine decarboxylase, 10–11,
    196, 199–203
Orotic acid, 44
Ovariectomy, 44, 54–55
Oxazepam, 43, 47
Oxidative energy metabolism, 80–81
Oxygen tensions, 81, 82
O6-methylguanine, 123

6-Phosphogluconate dehydrogenase,
    163, 170, 186, 190–192
Parenchymal cells, 79
Partial hepatectomy, 212–216, 221
Partial hepatectomy, 8, 45, 133–
    138, 177–180, 186, 196–
    204, 212–216, 221–226,
    232, 234–235, 278–279
Peliosis hepatis, 47–98
Pellets, 16
Pericytoma, 97–98

Periportal hepatocyte, 80–86, 257–
    262
Perisinusoidal cells, 90
Perivenous hepatocyte, 80
Persistent lesions, 92
Phases, 29–37, 82
Phenobarbital, 8, 32–34, 43–47,
    143, 151–156, 163–172,
    215–217, 232–243, 257–264
Phosphoenolpyruvate carboxykinase,
    80–82, 85
Phosphofructokinase, 163, 170
Ploidy, 221–229, 232–242
Polyamines, 195–199, 201–204
Polyploidization, 221–229
Portocaval anastomosis, 83–84
Portocaval shunt, 33–34, 45
Portocaval transposition, 45
Positive modulation, 36–37, 41–48
Precancerous liver, 211–218
Preclastogenic lesion, 212, 214
Preneoplastic lesions, 33, 34, 46,
    143–156
Primary liver tumors, 90
Process, 35–36
Progression, 30
Proliferative stimulus, 8
Promoters, 43, 151–156, 297–304
Promotion, 5–11, 30–37, 195–205,
    221–229, 232–242, 310
Protocols, 29–36, 41–48
Pure initiators 5, 6–11, 32, 34
Pure promoters, 6
Pyruvate kinase, 80, 83, 113–114,
    63–166, 171
Pyruvate, 81

Ras genes, 268
Rat and Human Hepatoma Cell Lines,
    280–281
Rat liver parenchymal cell
    subpopulation, 257–264
Reactive oxygen species, 9
Receptors, 31, 10, 175–183
    In neoplastic liver, 175–183
    In regenerating liver, 175–183
Regenerating liver, 177–179, 275–
    279
Regeneration, 186, 199
Remodeling, 152, 155, 199, 204
Resistance, 42
Resistant hepatocyte, 8, 196–205,
    224
Reversion, 92

S-adenosyl-L-methionine, 115–205
S-adenosylhomocysteine, 195–196
Selection, 42–44, 232–235
Semipermeable membrane technique,
    110

Serine dehydratase, 163, 170–171
Sex hormones, 51–60
   As modulators, 51–60
Short treatment, 42–48
Single dose, 31, 33, 36, 42, 47,
      51
Sinusoidal, 90–97
Skin carcinogenesis, 30–32, 48
Spongiosis hepatis, 97–98
Stages, 5, 29–37
Starvation, 83, 84
Steps, 29–37, 47
Stimulants, 275–281
Subfractions, 177–181
Succinate dehydrogenase, 80–82
Surgery, 42, 45, 48
Synergistic effects, 10–11

Target cells, 90
Tetraploid, 221–229, 234–242
TGGB Receptors, 275–281
   During normal, 275–281
   Neoplastic liver growth, 275–281
H3 Thymidine labelling, 146, 148
H3 Thymidine, 93, 124–125, 136–
      137, 189, 214, 216–217,
      276, 298–303

Trans–4–acetylamino–stilbene, 6–11
Transferrin 175, 177–180
Transferrin receptor, 175
Transformation by viral transform
      ing genes, 267–271
Transforming growth factor type B,
      275
Transgenic mouse, 95–96, 270–271
Transplantation of hepatocytes,
      222
Tritium–labelled nucleotide
      precursors, 297
Tumor cell precursors, 267
Tumor classification, 89

UDP–glucuronosyl transferase, 80

Viruses, 63–70
   Hepatocellular carcinoma, 63–70

X–irradiation, 211–213

Yield, 41

Zonal heterogeneity, 79–86, 80